DOING
CRITICAL
SOCIAL
WORK

DOING CRITICAL SOCIAL WORK

Transformative Practices for Social Justice

Edited by Bob Pease • Sophie Goldingay •
Norah Hosken • Sharlene Nipperess

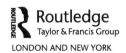
Routledge
Taylor & Francis Group
LONDON AND NEW YORK

First published 2016 by Allen & Unwin

Published 2020 by Routledge
2 Park Square, Milton Park, Abingdon, Oxon OX14 4RN
605 Third Avenue, New York, NY 10017

Routledge is an imprint of the Taylor & Francis Group, an informa business

Cataloguing-in-Publication details are available
from the National Library of Australia
www.trove.nla.gov.au

Typeset in 11/14 pt Minion by Post Prepress Group, Brisbane
Index by Puddingburn

ISBN-13: 9781760110840 (pbk)

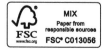

MIX
Paper from
responsible sources
FSC   FSC® C013056
www.fsc.org

Printed and bound in Great Britain by
TJ Books Ltd, Padstow, Cornwall

Contents

Tables and figures

Acknowledgement of traditional land owners

As non-Aboriginal editors with settler backgrounds, we acknowledge that the university sites where we work are located on the lands of Australia's traditional custodians. We pay our respects to their elders past and present, and also to all Aboriginal and Torres Strait Islander peoples involved with this book as contributors or readers.

Professor Mick Dodson explains that in Aboriginal culture, the meaning of country is more than ownership or connection to land, as:

> When we talk about traditional 'country' . . . we mean something beyond the dictionary definition of the word. For Aboriginal Australians . . . we might mean homeland, or tribal or clan area and we might mean more than just a place on the map . . . For us, country is a word for all the values, places, resources, stories and cultural obligations associated with that area and its features. It describes the entirety of our ancestral domains . . . So when we acknowledge traditional country, as increasingly people do in Australia, it is no empty ritual: it is to acknowledge who we, the Aboriginal people, are and our place in this nation. It is to take special note of a place and the people who belong to it (2009: 1–2).

Aboriginal and Torres Strait Islander peoples belong to these lands; they have walked on them for thousands of years, and continue to care for and nurture them. We, who are from settler backgrounds, continue to benefit from Aboriginal lands including living and working rent-free on them.

We are concerned about our impact on this earth, particularly the consumption practices of those with the greatest privileges and sense of entitlement. We are grateful for the care and examples provided by the rich Aboriginal traditions to live lightly and harmoniously with all creatures on earth.

Australia has never had a cohesive 'whiteness'; since colonial invasion, the social construction of whiteness has always been part of the racialised context of Australian political culture. At various times in Australia's history, different groups or nationalities of people have been considered or accepted as 'white' or 'not white', depending on how immigration served the workforce needs of the settler economy. Hence there is a particular responsibility for academics, practitioners and students of social work in Australia who are not Aboriginal and Torres Strait Islander Australians (who are from Eurocentric settler backgrounds) to better understand, and challenge how these racially privileged positions affect how social work is understood, positioned and problematised in a colonised country. This involves recognising social work's complicity in its cumulative legacies of discriminatory practices.

We commence this exploration of critical social work from the primarily Australian authors living on Aboriginal and Torres Strait Islander lands, by considering colonialism and imperialism as continuing oppressive processes that have shaped critical social work practices. We hope for a future when this colonial context will be transformed and continue to work towards decolonising practice in our research, writing and everyday practices.

Reference

Dodson, M. 2009, Speech at the Australian of the Year at the National Press Club, 17 February 2009, Canberra

Foreword

Doing Critical Social Work explores pivotal social work practice issues in these times of government austerity measures, and the deepening of neoliberalism in everyday life. This book explores how to foster hope, resilience and dissent in everyday social work practice in the face of consumerist, risk-adverse, marketised, individualising, depoliticising, ideology, policy and social practice. These chapters are timely and important for the lively critical social work debates by academics and practitioners that are occurring across the globe. Social workers everywhere are dealing with the growth of managerialism, decreased government funding, ongoing restructuring, and the decline of social care and justice. Commenting on this context, Gray and Webb call for a new politics for social work, in the belief that it bears a public responsibility to confront injustice while seeking justice for all (2013: 3).

As noted in this collection, part of this new politics needs to be a renewed analysis of the state in its leading role to sustain and legitimise racially stratified, patriarchal capitalism, even when the current form of capitalism clearly created the global financial crisis of 2007 and the subsequent years of suffering, recession and unemployment around the globe. An energetic, multidisciplinary debate existed about the state in the 1960s to 1980s, including a debate about whether social workers were the 'soft cops of capitalism' (Poulantzas 1987), angels of mercy, catalysts for change or all three (Galper 1975; 1980; Corrigan & Leonard 1978; Bailey & Brake 1980; London-Edinburgh Weekend Return Group 1980). Galper argued that while the state represented the interests of the capitalist class, most social service workers work with oppressed populations and are well-positioned to foster resistance and help build a new socialist society (1980). Feminists also noted that social welfare legitimised capitalism and accumulation while maintaining and extending patriarchal relations for those providing and receiving services, as well as for the larger society (Showstack 1987; Ng 1988; Fraser 1993; Orloff 2009). Asserting the interests of subordinate groups, feminists, anti-racists and others, also argued that though the state reproduces conditions that favour exploitation and oppression, it simultaneously reflects the successes and failures of struggles for equity, and hence, may also contain progressive policies and practices (Ng 1988; Walker 1990; Warskett 1993; Evans & Werkle 1997).

Much of this debate was supplanted by post-structural and governmentality analyses which explained to social workers why they increasingly felt ruled by decentralised and often remote governments through the standardised forms, assessment tools, outcome metrics and practices that the social workers were increasingly required to use in their everyday work (Rose 1996, 1990; Cruikshank 1999; MacDonald & Marston 2002; Marston & MacDonald 2006).

In the last few years, managerialised conditions in the social work profession suggest the need to return to debates concerning the state. In particular, the debates need to tackle whether the profession's links to the austerity-embracing state makes social work a practice of care, control, coercion, resistance or all four combined. Rather than exclusively caring or controlling, Taylor-Gooby has argued that the social care professionals, who grew in numbers and influence under the welfare state, reflect the multiple ambiguities of that state in which social justice, equity and care motives intertwined unevenly with motives of control, and at times, coercion (2000; see also, Bailey & Brake 1980; London-Edinburgh Weekend Return Group 1980; Lavalette 2011). It could be argued that, currently, social workers reflect the multiple agendas of the neoliberal state with its emphasis on market solutions to all social problems and denial that the social even exists, much less that it merits policy responses that promote equity and collective care.

My recent research confirms these complex dynamics and suggests that, under managerialism, control of social workers by employers and those funding programs has increased dramatically in recent decades (largely through the standardised tools and outcome metrics). In the name of efficiency and cost saving, these managerial practices increase the pace of work and size of caseloads (Baines 2011; Baines et al. 2014). Social workers, who are rushed to complete documentation on time and address the increasingly complex needs of service users in increasingly difficult circumstances, often feel they have little choice but to exert downward control on service users to provide any level of service and to avoid disciplinary actions from management. Coercion has also grown in these workplaces, saturated by austerity measures, often in unexpected forms such as violence and abuse from service users, and bullying from management or co-workers. Further research is required to understand these often highly gendered dynamics, their intermingling with state legitimation and capital accumulation agendas, and to further develop the critical analysis and practices shaped by the state, as discussed in the following chapters.

Fortunately, as Galper noted in 1980, social workers do not just robotically oppress service users in the name of the employer or funding providers or both (usually the government). Rather, social workers work at the dynamic interface of social solidarity, social care and the potential for oppressive force of the state. This means that even though they are placed by employers and funding providers to be increasingly controlling, they are also very well-positioned to initiate unique forms of dissent, foster resilience and resistance and nurture hope as a critical social work practice, and create opportunities for others to do likewise. Many of the following chapters focus on this critical nexus in the social work workplace, where committed social workers create space for themselves, each other, service users and community members to develop alternative narratives, shared dissident identities and build practices that step outside management and government control to critically reflect and act on situations that are harmful and socially unjust.

As has been characteristic of critical social work debates, this book expands beyond national boundaries to engage with challenges encountered in other countries particularly those with liberal welfare states (Esping-Andersen 2013). As such, this collection will be useful to academics, students and practitioners in Canada, the US, the UK, Australia, New Zealand and beyond. It is very interesting that this book engages closely with the critical debates that I identified as requiring further analysis in the second edition of a collection I edited on doing anti-oppressive, social justice social work (Baines 2011). These debates included critical management and supervision in social work; connecting with indigenous knowledge, practice and theory and exploring its relationship to critical/social justice theory and practice; and transforming radical critique into practice. *Doing Critical Social Work* discusses skills, practice vignettes, limitations, strengths and issues for further development in all these areas, providing the reader with fresh new insights into critical practices and analysis. It is ironic to note that critical and other social-justice social work approaches are rarely, if ever, critiqued for not being able to analyse and theorise social struggle and injustice, though we are endlessly accused of not adequately translating theory into practice. As this book confirms, we actually translate theory into practice quite well, though dominant groups have an interest in discrediting and minimising critical approaches regardless of the clarity of our explanations and examples.

This book also explores social work practice in areas that are emerging as increasingly important in the context of constrained resources such as critical social work practice in government programs providing income support such as Centrelink; new and old forms of community work and mobilisation in the context of globalisation and the wordwide growth of poverty; work with LGBTI people and struggles, an increasingly recognised but still marginalised population; and the larger question of critical social workers as everyday activists in their workplaces, communities and on the streets. There are important chapters on populations that have been medicalised, marginalised and depoliticised (such as people with disabilities and aged people), whereby these issues are reframed as social issues and these populations are encouraged to resist and express their rights. Also important are the chapters on critical social work education, and how to make critical practice and theory come alive in the classroom and the field. Though some would ask what social work and environmental issues have in common; at their core, environmental struggles are all about collectivity and relationships between individuals, communities, ecosystems, economies, capitalism and all life on earth. Ecological notions of mutual dependence and shared interests are anathema to the neoliberalist position, and one of the main sources of this movement's connection to social work, resistance and the building of equitable and sustainable relations across the planet, as well as in local communities. Chapter 18 'Environmental social work as critical decolonising practice' deals with the complexity of this pressing social problem and provides thoughtful analysis and possibilities for new practices.

There are a number of strong, common themes that thread through these chapters that will be useful to practitioners, students and academics alike. These include challenges to taken-for-granted, Western, patriarchal, privileged voices; the notion of hope as critical practice and one of many ways to nurture and build resilience and resistance; strategies and observations on how to develop ways to build oppositional narratives, shared dissident identities; dissent, resistance, activism and social justice. By exploring the 'doing' of critical social work, this collection extends our capacity to speak back to power and build an alternate future where inter-dependency and equity are the central planks of an agenda for social justice and care.

Donna Baines
University of Sydney

References

Bailey, R. & Brake, M., 'Contributions to a radical practice in social work' in R. Bailey and M. Brake (eds), 2008, *Radical Social Work*, London: Edward Arnold, pp. 7–25

Baines, D. (ed.) 2011, *Doing Anti-Oppressive Practice. Building transformative, politicized social work*, 2nd edn, Halifax: Fernwood Books

Baines, D., Charlesworth, S., Turner, D. and O'Neill, L. 2014, 'Lean social care and worker identity: The role of outcomes, supervision and mission', *Critical Social Policy*, vol. 34, no. 4, pp. 433–53

Corrigan, P. & Leonard, P. 1978, *Social Work Practice under Capitalism: A Marxist approach*, London: Macmillan

Cruikshank, B. 1999, *The Will to Empower: Democratic citizens and other subjects*, Ithaca: Cornell University Press

Esping-Andersen, G. 2013, *The Three Worlds of Welfare Capitalism*, London: John Wiley & Sons

Evans, P.M., and Wekerle, G.R. (eds) 1997, *Women and the Canadian Welfare State: Challenges and change*, University of Toronto Press, Toronto

Fraser, N. 1993, 'Clintonism, welfare, and the antisocial wage: The emergence of a neoliberal political imaginary', *Rethinking Marxism*, vol. 6, no. 1, pp. 9–23

Galper, J. 1980, *Social Work Practice: A radical perspective*, Englewood Cliffs: Prentice-Hall

Galper, J. 1975, *The Politics of Social Services*, Englewood Cliffs: Prentice-Hall

Gray, M. & Webb, S. (eds) 2013, *The New Politics of Social Work,* London: Palgrave MacMillan

Lavalette, M. (ed.) 2011, *Radical Social Work Today: Social work at the crossroads*, London: The Policy Press

London Edinburgh Weekend Return Group. 1980, *In and Against the State,* London: Pluto Press

Marston, G. & McDonald, C. (eds) 2006, *Analysing Social Policy: A governmental approach*, Cheltenham: Edward Elgar Publishing

McDonald, C. and Marston, G. 2002, 'Fixing the niche? Rhetorics of the community sector in the neoliberal welfare regime', *Just Policy*, vol. 27, pp. 3–10

Ng, R. 1988, *The Politics of Community Services: Immigrant women, class and state*, Toronto: Garamond Press

Poulantzas, N. 1969, 'The problem of the capitalist state', *New Left Review*, vol. 58, no. 1, pp. 67–8

Orloff, A. 2009, 'Gendering the comparative analysis of welfare states: An unfinished agenda', *Sociological Theory*, vol. 27, no. 3, pp. 317–43

Rose, N. 1990, *Governing the Soul: The shaping of the private self,* London: Taylor & Frances/Routledge

Rose, N. 1996, 'Governing "advanced" liberal democracies' in A. Sharma and A. Gupta (eds), *The Anthropology of the State: A reader,* Malden: Wiley-Blackwell, pp. 144–62

Showstack Sassoon, A. 1987, *Women and the State,* London: Hutchinson

Taylor-Gooby, P., 2000, 'Risk and welfare' in *Risk, Trust and Welfare,* in P. Taylor-Gooby (ed.), Houndmills, Macmillan, pp. 1–18

Walker, G. 1990, *Family Violence and the Women's Movement*, Toronto: University of Toronto Press

Warskett, R. 1993, 'Democratizing the state: Challenges from public sector unions', *Studies in Political Economy*, vol. 42, pp. 129–40

List of contributors

Ann Carrington, PhD, BSW (Hons), is a lecturer in Social Work at James Cook University, North Queensland. Her practice has been predominantly with those who have experienced domestic violence or sexual assault or both. She developed the 'Vortex of Violence' practice model for working with women who have experienced domestic violence as published in the *British Journal of Social Work*. Her other area of research and practice is the integration of spiritual theory and practice in social work. Areas of interest within this field include: the integration of spirituality in social work theory, practice, research, ethics and pedagogy; the exploration of how spiritual theory and practice may add to social work's understanding of issues of power, control, privilege, vicarious trauma/burnout and reflective practice; the exploration of the potential for spiritual practice to be critical practice; and the examination of the tensions that may present in attempts to integrate spiritual theory and practice within social work.

John Coates, PhD, is a founding member of the Canadian Society for Spirituality and Social Work. He has been a longstanding advocate of ecological social work. He has published widely on issues related to the environment and social work, the indigenisation of social work, and spirituality and social work. His most recent work explores the relationship between these aspects of social work. John has now retired from academic life, but he continues to work actively to advance global and ecological concerns within the professional and academic social work communities. His most recent books include *Decolonizing Social Work* (with Gray, Hetherington & Yellow Bird, Routledge 2013) and *Environmental Social Work* (with Gray & Hetherington, Routledge 2013).

Sherrine Clark is a social worker and founding member of the Asylum Seeker Resource Centre (ASRC) based in Melbourne. She is currently Director of Humanitarian Services (which includes Foodbank, Community Meals, Material Aid, Health, Casework, Counselling, General Access programs and Housing). Sherrine has over ten years' experience developing a holistic, human rights-based model of practice working with asylum seekers in the Australian non-government organisation (NGO) context and is committed to upholding the rights and entitlements of asylum seekers. As a social work practitioner, she has also had experience working in the community mental health and family services areas.

Lesley Ervin coordinates the social work student field placements for both the Bachelor of Social Work and Master of Social Work, qualifying, degrees at Deakin University. Prior to this, Lesley was a practicing social worker in the health sector, working for a number of years in the acute hospital setting as well as the sub-acute community rehabilitation setting. As a component of her Master of Public Health, she was involved in a joint project between La Trobe University and the Public Health Agency of Canada. This project attempted to map the public health competencies of both countries with learning objectives from online learning modules developed by the two organisations. (L. Ervin, B. Carter and P. Robinson, 2013, 'Curriculum mapping: Not as straightforward as it sounds', *Journal of Vocational Education & Training,* vol. 65, no. 3, pp. 309–18).

Stephanie Gilbert, PhD, is Associate Professor for Teaching Quality and Development at The Wollotuka Institute, The University of Newcastle. Having trained in welfare and social work at James Cook University, North Queensland, Stephanie has had a long involvement in social work with Aboriginal people and communities, child protection and out-of-home care. Stephanie has contributed significantly to the published material available on Aboriginal people and social work. She was one of four co-editors on the first book based in the Australian context that examined Aboriginal social work practice and social work with Aboriginal people in 2012. Completing a Master of Arts and PhD in History, Stephanie's research has predominantly centred on the identity and experience of people who were removed from their families on the basis of Aboriginal heritage. Stephanie has served the profession of social work through the Australian Association of Social Workers and has now worked in Aboriginal education for over twenty years.

Sophie Goldingay is a senior lecturer in the School of Health and Social Development at Deakin University, and is currently Bachelor of Social Work

Course Leader and School of Health and Social Development Teaching and Learning Coordinator. Her research interests include qualitative research with institutionalised populations such as prisoners and people with psychiatric disabilities, people with learning disabilities, and equity and access in higher education. She led a Strategic Teaching and Learning Grant (STALG) team to create a Multidimensional Framework for Embedded Academic Skill Development which won the Vice Chancellor's award for Outstanding Contributions to Equity and Access. The project has led to significant developments across the Faculty of Health, including a Pathways project with the local Technical and Further Education (TAFE) provider in Geelong and a number of projects that embed academic skills into the Bachelor of Social Work.

Mel Gray, PhD, is Professor of Social Work in the School of Humanities and Social Science at the University of Newcastle. Mel has published widely on international social work and has a critical interest in social work's transferability across cultures and contexts, and professional and disciplinary borders. Recent books interrogating these issues include *Environmental Social Work* (Coates, Gray & Hetherington, Routledge 2013), *Decolonizing Social Work* (Coates, Gray, Hetherington & Yellow Bird, Ashgate 2013), *The New Politics of Social Work* (Gray and Webb, Palgrave 2013) *Sage Handbook of Social Work* (Gray, Midgely & Webb, Sage, 2012) and *Social Work Theories and Methods* (Gray & Webb, 2nd edn, Sage, 2013). Mel is also the book review editor for the *Asia-Pacific Journal of Social Work and Social Development.*

Norah Hosken is a senior lecturer in social work in the School of Health and Social Development at Deakin University, and a PhD candidate, with 30 years' experience as a practitioner and educator in social work, community work, welfare and women's sectors. Norah has worked alongside, and learned with individuals, groups and communities who have been highly discriminated against, and who are in urban, regional, rural and remote locations. This has included work with: the Women's Refuge Group of WA; the Coalition of Welfare Workers against Poverty; Women Protesting Social Security Prosecutions; The Geelong South Sudan (Agouk) Community Coming Together Group and TAFE4ALL. Her current PhD research is an institutional ethnography exploring how experiences of social justice and social injustice in Australian social work higher education are structured by inflections of race, class and gender, and how they are shaped within the practices and dominant narratives of neoliberalism. Norah has published in cross-cultural research, education and social work supervision.

Peter Humphries has practised in the areas of education, rehabilitation, mental health and more recently as the Deputy National Manager (occasionally Acting National Manager) in Centrelink's social work services. During his time in Centrelink, Peter was instrumental in developing the social work service in Centrelink's call centres, Centrelink's response to homelessness and the social work practice frameworks that helped explain and promote the work of the organisation's social workers. Peter is currently a Lecturer in the School of Social Work at the Australian Catholic University in Canberra where he teaches in the areas of mental health, group work, community work and working with families. Peter has presented and published in the areas of mental health, working with men, homelessness, social policy development and social work as an organisational practice.

Jude Irwin is Professor Emerita of Social Work and Social Justice at the University of Sydney. Jude has worked at the University of Sydney for over 30 years and her teaching, research, practice and policy interests span a number of areas including violence against women, children and young people, discrimination against gay men and lesbians, professional practice supervision, community development and learning in practice settings. She has been successful in attracting a number of research grants. In her most recent research projects, she has used action research and focused on improving collaboration between domestic violence and mental health services, and working with residents in social housing areas. Jude has been on a number of committees including the NSW Ombudsman's Child Death Advisory Committee, the New South Wales (NSW) Child Death Review Team, the NSW Council on Violence Against Women (Deputy Chair) and the Advisory Group, Australian Child Protection Research Centre. She was a founding member and past Director of the Australian Centre for Lesbian and Gay Research and the Council of the Heads of Schools of Social Work.

Tina Kostecki is a Lecturer in Social Work at Deakin University. She has been a social work practitioner, primarily in the women's services sector, and also an advocate, educator and researcher for the past 30 years. Her interests include the application of critical theoretical perspectives such as feminism and critical gerontology to inform social work practice. Working towards the redress of oppression, marginalisation and inequality have always been at the core of her commitment to social work practice. She has recently completed her PhD at Deakin University.

Jody Laughton has worked as a social worker for over twenty years in the child, youth and family fields, and in services for separated families, in both government and community-based organisations, alongside work for over ten years in social work field education programs at Melbourne University, and more recently at Deakin University. Jody's coursework Master of Social Work focused on program planning and evaluation, and organisational and human-resource management subjects. Jody has been a member of the Victorian Combined Schools of Social Work field education group for a number of years, and co-contributor to a presentation and article on the development of a common assessment tool (H. Cleak, L. Hawkins, J, Laughton & J. Williams, 2015, 'Creating a standardised teaching and learning framework for social work field placements', *Australian Social Work,* vol. 68, no. 1, pp. 49–64).

Selma Macfarlane, PhD, is a lecturer in social work in the School of Health and Social Development, Deakin University. Over the past fifteen years she has taught and developed course materials across many social work units, as well as being involved in field education, honours and higher-degree research supervision. Her publications include book chapters and journal articles on diverse topics such as women and ageing, critical reflection, social work education, and mental health. Her most recent publication is a co-authored book for students, practitioners and educators on critical social work.

Robyn Miller, PhD, is a social worker and family therapist with over thirty years' experience in the community sector, local government and child protection. She was a senior clinician and teacher for fourteen years at the Bouverie Family Therapy Centre, La Trobe University, and part of an innovative team working with families who had experienced trauma and sexual abuse. Robyn has practised in the public and private sectors as a therapist, clinical supervisor, consultant and lecturer and was a member of the Victorian Child Death Review Committee for ten years. She was the recipient of the inaugural Robin Clark memorial PhD scholarship in 2004 and the statewide award for Inspirational Leadership in 2010. From 2006–15 she provided professional leadership as the Chief Practitioner within the Department of Human Services in Victoria, which has embraced many positive reforms. She is currently working as a consultant with the Royal Commission into Institutional Responses to Child Sexual Abuse.

Christine Morley is Associate Professor of Social Work at the Queensland University of Technology, Australia. Formally foundation Head of Social Work at the University of the Sunshine Coast, her intellectual passions include exploring the possibilities for critical social work and critical reflection to make a contribution to social work as an emancipatory project. Previously at Deakin University, Christine has published more than 40 papers in national and international refereed journals, conference proceedings and in edited books as invited chapters. She is author of *Practising Critical Reflection to Develop Emancipatory Change* (Ashgate, 2014), and co-author (with Selma Macfarlane and Phillip Ablett) of *Engaging with Social Work: A Critical Introduction* (Cambridge, 2014).

Jessica Morrison is the Executive Officer of both the Australia Palestine Advocacy Network (APAN), a lobbying and advocacy organisation, and the Palestine Israel Ecumenical Network. She is engaged in community and social change activities, with a focus on peace and nonviolence, including being part of Christian peacemaker teams. Jessica has had a range of roles in teaching social work and has worked in a variety of community-based organisations. Her publications include: J. Morrison & E. Branigan, 2009, 'Working collectively in competitive times: Case studies from New Zealand and Australia', *Community Development Journal,* vol. 44, no. 1, pp. 68–79; J. Morrison & J. Goldsworthy, 2002, 'Resurrecting a model of integrating individual work with community development and social action', *Community Development Journal,* vol. 37, no. 4, pp. 327–37; J. Morrison, 2015, 'Emancipatory social work education: Why it is so difficult to practise instead of preach', *Advances in Social Work and Welfare Education,* vol. 17, no. 1, pp. 98–111.

Sharlene Nipperess is a lecturer in social work at RMIT University. Her practice, teaching and research interests are diverse and include: human rights and critical social work; social work ethics, in particular the ethical challenges relating to technology; and the fields of practice of social work with refugees and asylum seekers, and people experiencing mental distress. She also has a strong interest in sustainability and environmental social work and its place in the social work curriculum. Sharlene completed her PhD on human rights and its relationship with critical social work practice and education at the Centre for Human Rights Education at Curtin University. She is President of Australia and New Zealand Social Work and Welfare Education and Research (ANZSWWER) association and is a member of the newly formed Social Work Without Borders.

Carolyn Noble is the inaugural Professor of Social Work at Australian College of Applied Psychology, Sydney, and Professor Emerita at Victoria University, Melbourne. Her research is in the area of professional education, supervision, and community engagement, theory development in social work and equal employment opportunities for women in higher education and the human services. She is the executive editor of the social dialogue magazine, a production linked to the International Association for Schools of Social Work (IASSW), www.social-dialogue.com.

Bob Pease is Professor of Social Work at the University of Tasmania. He has published extensively on masculinity politics and critical social work practice, including four books as single author and ten books as co-editor, as well as numerous book chapters and journal articles. His most recent books include: *Critical Social Work: Theories and practices for a socially just world* (J, Allan, L. Briskman & B. Pease, eds, 2nd edn, Allen & Unwin 2009), *Migrant Men: Critical studies of masculinities and the migration experience* (M. Donaldson, R. Hibbins, R. Howson & B. Pease (eds), Routledge, 2009), *Undoing Privilege: Unearned advantage in a divided world* (Zed 2010), *Men and Masculinities Around the World: Transforming men's practices* (E. Ruspini et al., eds, Palgrave 2011), *Men, Masculinities and Methodologies* (B. Pini & B. Pease, eds, Palgrave 2013) and *The Politics of Recognition and Social Justice: Transforming subjectivities and new forms of resistance* (M. Pallotta-Chiarolli & B. Pease, eds, Routledge 2014).

José Ramos is a social change researcher, trans-disciplinary collaborator, and advocate for commons-oriented social alternatives. Originally from California, from Mexican-American heritage, he currently resides in West Footscray, Melbourne, Australia with his family, and works on both local and international social change projects. He is founder of the consulting network Action Foresight (www.action-foresight.net), a group which helps organisations respond creatively to the landscape of changes that they face. He has held academic teaching and research roles at the National University of Singapore, Swinburne University of Technology (Melbourne), Queensland University of Technology (Brisbane), Victoria University (Melbourne) and Leuphana University (Germany). He is senior consulting editor for the *Journal of Futures Studies*.

Noel Renouf has worked for well over thirty years as a mental-health social worker and educator. He is an Honorary Research Senior Fellow at the University of Queensland and a volunteer caseworker at the Asylum Seeker Resource Centre (ASRC) in Melbourne. He is co-author (with Robert Bland and Ann Tullgren) of *Social Work Practice in Mental Health: An introduction* (Allen & Unwin, 2015).

Russell Shuttleworth is a Senior Lecturer in the School of Health and Social Development, Deakin University. He has both a Master of Social Work and a PhD in medical anthropology. His practice has been with elderly and physically disabled people, providing casework and counselling services. He was also a long-time support worker for men with a range of different physical impairments. Russell has conducted disability and chronic illness-related research on issues such as sexuality, gender, leadership, access to health care contexts and speech impairment, as well as an evaluation of several disability organisations. He has also conducted research on both psychogeriatric and sexuality issues in aged care. Russell is currently part of an Australian Research Council (ARC) discovery project researching the transition to adulthood for young people with physical impairments. For many years, he has been a supporter of the Disability Movement and is currently working alongside a group of young disabled adults in the state of Victoria formulating policy guidelines around facilitated sex.

Acknowledgements of contributors

Chapter 2: Christine Morley kindly acknowledges Kaila White, University of the Sunshine Coast, for her research assistance in the preparation of this chapter.

Chapter 7: Norah Hosken would like to acknowledge Bob Pease, Chagai Gum Malong, and the many students and service users who have taught her so much about the relations of class, gender and race, and of the class-based structural violence of poverty.

Chapter 12: Parts of this chapter are based on Norah Hosken's current PhD study and draw from the principles as they were first developed in Chapter 7 this volume.

Chapter 15: Ann Carrington acknowledges Amanda Lee-Ross, Manager at Cairns Regional Domestic Violence Service, for her contribution to this chapter. As a colleague over the years, Amanda has helped Ann to consolidate her understanding and practice of feminism. More directly, their shared discussion and relating to this chapter acted as a foundation for the reflections presented here. The opinions expressed within this chapter are solely those of the author and are not necessarily reflective of her colleague.

Chapter 20: Russel Shuttleworth acknowledges Helen Meekosha's contribution to some of the ideas discussed in parts of this chapter, especially the introduction.

PART I

Addressing the tensions in critical social work

1

Doing critical social work in the neoliberal context: working on the contradictions

Bob Pease and Sharlene Nipperess

Introduction

The premise of the book is that significant opportunities exist for critical social work practice within spaces provided by contradictions within the state organisation of social work as well as within the wider terrain of the state, which includes the non-profit sector. Critical social work only exists within specific sites, where the agency, the larger context and its impact, the client's subjectivity and the background and structural position of the worker give it a distinct form. That is, critical social work can only be found where social work is actually practised. For example, in state-based social work such as child protection, mental health, Centrelink or correctional services, with particular client groups such as asylum seekers, Aboriginal and Torres Strait Islander people, people with disabilities, aged people or women escaping men's violence or in community-based campaigns and social movements. All of these sites of practice and more are addressed in this book. Unlike many other books on radical and critical social work, this book provides specific guidance for forms and practices of critical social work and outlines the knowledge and skill base necessary for critical practice (see the definition below 'Exploring the history of critical social work').

While all of the contributors are committed to the critical tradition in social work, they do not all articulate the same model of critical social work practice. For example, contributors may position themselves differently in relation to post-structural and discursive frameworks and structural and materialist frameworks of practice. While particular contributors may adopt one of these positions exclusively, we, as editors, do not see these approaches as mutually exclusive.

Most of the contributors hold academic positions within universities. However, all are involved in critical practice both within and outside the university sector. Also, we have worked very closely with practitioners in the field, in some cases as authors and co-authors, to ensure the book reflects everyday social work practice.

Exploring the history of critical social work

'Critical social work' is an umbrella term that describes a group of approaches in social work that are diverse but share a common commitment to both personal and structural change (Allan, Briskman & Pease 2009; Dominelli 2009; Payne 2014). The term has been widely used in Australia since the late 1990s but other terms such as emancipatory social work, progressive social work and transformative social work are also used to describe critical approaches to social work practice.

The critical tradition has a long history in social work. Certainly a tension between so-called mainstream and emancipatory views of social work can be identified from its earliest history (Mendes 2009). This history is illustrated by the contrast between the Charity Organisation Society movement with the Settlement House movement. The Charity Organisation Society started in the US in 1877 and was primarily concerned with distributing charity to reduce poverty. It differentiated between 'deserving' and 'non-deserving' poor and explained poverty according to personal character deficits. Mary Richmond (1861–1928) was particularly significant in the Charity Organisation Society and shaped the development of social work through the casework method. In contrast, the Settlement House movement, which commenced in England in 1884, rather than viewing poverty as an individual deficit explained poverty as the consequence of an unjust social order. The 'self-help' method, which emphasised community development and social action, was developed as a key approach (Mullaly 2007). Jane Addams (1860–1935), who in 1931 was awarded the Nobel Peace Prize, was particularly significant in the US Settlement House movement.

The approach represented by Jane Addams and the Settlement House movement fits within the critical tradition and indicates the long history of such an approach in social work. However, notwithstanding this long history, critical approaches were peripheral in social work until the 1960s and 1970s. It was during this period that a radical critique of mainstream social work re-emerged, particularly in the Marxist critiques of Corrigan and Leonard (1978), Gough (1979) and others, primarily in the UK, but in the US and Australia as well. Also, in many non-Western countries, the work of Paulo Freire (1993), the Brazilian educator, became influential. Critical social work approaches have continued to develop since (Hick, Fook & Pozzuto 2005; Allan, Briskman & Pease 2009; Gray & Webb 2013a). These approaches include: radical casework (Fook 1993); critical practice (Ife 1997); critical postmodernism (Pease & Fook 1999; 2005; Fook 2012); feminist social work (Dominelli 2002); structural social work (Mullaly 2007); anti-racist social work (Dominelli 2008); radical social work (Ferguson 2008; Ferguson & Woodward 2009; Lavalette 2011a; Turbett 2014); anti-oppressive social work (Mullaly 2010; Baines 2011); human rights-based social work (Lundy 2011; Ife 2012); and anti-discriminatory social work (Thompson 2012).

Allan (2009:40–1) suggests five principles that are shared by contemporary critical approaches to social work:

- A commitment to work towards greater social justice and equality for those who are oppressed and marginalised within society.
- A commitment to work alongside the oppressed and marginalised populations.
- A commitment to question taken-for-granted and dominant assumptions and beliefs.
- An analysis of power relations which serve to marginalise and oppress particular populations in society.
- An orientation towards emancipatory personal and social change.

These principles take into account the diversity of approaches in critical social work and emphasise the commitment to social justice and social change as well as personal emancipatory change. They will be drawn upon in a number of chapters throughout this volume.

Critical theory and critical social work practice

While there are many definitions of critical social work, as noted earlier, we use it as an umbrella term for designating approaches to social work practice that are informed by an eclectic range of critical social theories. We argue that critical theory is fundamentally important in shedding light on the issues facing social workers. We also believe that it enables social workers to understand the relationship between their localised practice settings, and the wider social and political forces that are shaping social work practice.

There is a wide range of theoretical influences on critical social work. We are excited by issues arising from the dialogue between Fraser and Honneth (2003) in relation to the politics of redistribution and recognition (for example, Garrett 2010; Houston 2013; Pallotta-Chiarolli & Pease 2014). One of the key points of disagreement between Fraser and Honneth relates to whether or not the injustices associated with misrecognition and prejudice that subject people to discriminatory practices (based on their gender, sexuality, race or ability)are primarily psychological or not. Fraser prefers to talk about the wounds of this misrecognition as a form of status inequality (Fraser & Honneth 2003). This dialogue has made a significant contribution to social workers' understanding of subjectivity and agency in the context of power relations (Pallotta-Chiarolli & Pease 2014).

Discourse analysis provides an insight into the broad-ranging dimensions of critical social work (Garrity 2010). In particular, it focuses on language and how language practices construct our understandings of 'reality' and subsequently how we act on this reality (Healy 2005). Marston (2013), for example, argues that discourse analysis assists practitioners to become more aware of their own discourse and how it shapes their practice. He draws attention to how social workers can reframe dominant discourses in their practice with service users and power holders.

The work of Foucault helps investigate risk discourses, governmentality and surveillance in encouraging self-disciplining of populations (Kemshall 2010; Powell 2012). While Foucault's work is sometimes seen as deterministic, because it emphasises how people become complicit in the process of internalising dominant ideologies, we believe that people can develop awareness of these processes and have the capacity of individual and collective agency to resist them (Pallotta-Chiarolli & Pease 2014).

Garrett (2007; 2013) has argued that Bourdieu's theory has continued relevance for social work. Bourdieu (1999) draws attention to the psychic injuries caused by injustice. He uses the language of social suffering to convey the ways in which people's experience of oppression is reflected not only in access to material resources but also in their feelings of resentment, anger and despair (Pallotta-Chiarolli & Pease 2014).

Feminist theories, like many of the critical theories we discuss, do not represent one unified theory. Instead, they are informed by diverse standpoints including postmodern, liberal, welfare, Marxist and socialist feminisms. Common to these feminist theoretical orientations, though, is a commitment to the emancipation of women from unequal cultural, material and social relations (Weeks 2003). Feminist critiques challenged the early radical and Marxist approaches for not taking gender (and other dimensions of identity) into account in their analysis of injustice and inequality. These diverse range of theories continue to contribute to critical social work approaches, including feminist social work (Dominelli 2002).

Green theories that focus on the relationship between people and the physical environment and how environmental crises impact on people's lives have had limited impact on social work generally and critical social work in particular until very recently. However, in the last ten years the literature has expanded significantly (Besthorn 2011; Alston 2012; Alston & Besthorn 2012; Gray, Coates & Hetherington 2012a; Dominelli 2012; McKinnon 2012). Gray, Coates and Hetherington (2012b) identify themes in the environment social work literature that are relevant to critical social work, including the critique of modernity and capitalism, the association between critical theory and environmentalism, and the centrality of spirituality and Indigenous perspectives. Dominelli argues for a 'green social work' that addresses 'poverty, structural inequalities, socio-economic disparities, industrialisation processes, consumption patterns, diverse contexts, global interdependencies and limited natural resources' (Dominelli 2012: 3).

Institutional ethnography addresses practices in critical social work. It was first developed as a Marxist, feminist sociology for women by Dorothy Smith (2007) as a method of empirical inquiry that enables people to map the social relations that coordinate and influence the way people perform their work within institutions. This method has been applied in a range of social work contexts (for example, de Montigny 1995; Brown 2006; de Montigny 2011; Hosken 2013) to 'reveal the ideological and social processes that produce experiences of subordination' (DeVault & McCoy 2006: 19). The analysis can be used to understand more about the sites and causes of disconnection between the stated aims of policy, social work approaches and their effects.

While Marxism with its focus on class-based oppression has been marginalised in critical social work since the 1970s, there have been recent attempts to reinvigorate Marxism for radical and critical social work (Lavalette 2011a; Ferguson, I. 2013; Turbett 2014). While those leaning more towards post-structural frameworks will be concerned about its universalising tendencies, we argue that Marxism still provides useful insight into forms of resistance against neoliberalism with its emphasis on free market economics, the privatisation of social services, free trade and user-pay services (Wallace & Pease 2011; Garrett 2013).

We do not accept the argument by some (Ferguson 2008; Turbett 2014) that critical social work is more likely to be postmodernist, while radical social work is more likely to be structuralist and Marxist (see Pease 2013 for the history of critical and radical social work). Nor do we believe, as some postmodernists argue (Fook 2003), that Marxism should be rejected as a foundation for critical social work. Neo-Marxist analysis is still useful in understanding the structural dimensions of social inequality, whereas, post-structural and post-Marxist theories help us understand the cultural dimensions and diverse experiences of inequality.

Ferguson and Lavalette (2007) express concerns about the potential for postmodern approaches as a basis of critical social work practice. Some forms of postmodernism do depoliticise oppression and consequently reproduce patriarchal and capitalist power relations (Morley & Macfarlane 2012). While Gray and Webb (2013b) argue that postmodernism offers nothing to inform social justice struggles, we believe that such approaches, when infused with critical theory, can enrich structuralist approaches to critical practice.

As Baines argues (2011), we also do not believe that postmodern concepts represent such a significant break with Marxism, feminism and other modernist critical theories. We concur with Morley and Macfarlane (2012) that the outright rejection of either modernist critical approaches or postmodern and post-structural approaches, does not provide the most useful strategy for developing critical social work practice. Thus, we locate ourselves in the tradition that draws upon both postmodern and modernist critical theorising in the development of critical social work (Briskman, Pease & Allen 2009; Morley, Macfarlane & Ablett 2014).

We are also mindful that all of the preceding theories are grounded in Western epistemologies. It is important to encourage Indigenous ways of knowing and practising in critical social work (Bennett et al. 2013; Yee & Wagner 2013; Muller 2014; Zubrzycki, et al. 2014). Walter et al. (2013) have pointed out that whiteness is embedded within Australian social work theory and practice and that social work has failed to recognise itself as a racialised profession. Thus, critical social work needs to acknowledge Aboriginal epistemologies and the ways in which Western epistemology has shaped contemporary social work practice.

It is important to recognise the suffering of Aboriginal peoples from social work interventions and the Eurocentric bias embedded in contemporary social work (Yellow Bird & Gray 2008). We do not assume that critical social work discussions in this book will necessarily relate to non-Western contexts or work with Indigenous peoples. For those of us who are white, we can only hope to make culture explicit in our theorising and our practice (Gray, Coates & Yellow Bird 2008).

Theories on race, racism and postcolonial studies have also contributed to critical social work approaches. Early radical, Marxist and feminist social work theories were critiqued for not taking into account 'race' and the experience of racism, imperialism and colonisation in their analysis of inequality and oppression. Postcolonial studies has its intellectual origins in both Marxism and poststructuralism/postmodernism (Ghandi 1998) and is based in numerous diverse disciplines from history to literary studies. Postcolonial and anti-colonial studies contribute to critical social work approaches by exploring the impacts of imperialism and colonisation in society in general and in social work in particular.

Critical theory and mainstream social work practice

We do not regard mainstream social work as being defined by the type of workplace in which social work is practised. Rather, we understand it as a framework for thinking about how to respond to social problems (Baines 2011). Some may argue that the language of critical social work is unnecessary, as mainstream social work promotes human rights and social justice. However, the values of social work are contested and contradictory, and as Banks (2014) notes, not all of social work values are radical.

Social work has been reluctant to commit itself to critical theoretical frameworks. Mainstream social work continues to frame many of the issues that social workers address in conservative theories and models. As Baines (2011) notes, mainstream social work theories still regard economic and social systems as being neutral. Critical social theories provide a useful frame for interrogating the unstated political dimension of traditional theories of social work.

In our brief overview of mainstream approaches to social work below, we acknowledge that those who adhere to some of these approaches may see themselves as being in tune with a critical approach. Furthermore, each of these approaches are written from a variety of perspectives. However, we argue that the main assumptions of these approaches do not match the critical theory premises that we articulate in this book.

Ecological and systems theories that propose all persons, groups, organisations and societies are systems with subsystems embedded within them, provide the foundations of mainstream social work. While they say they are progressive, they have been considerably critiqued over the years. Their premise of fixed boundaries and assumptions about a benign relationship between individuals and the environment is at odds with critical theory understandings of power, conflict and interests (Pease 1991; Wakefield 1996; Payne 2002; Reisch 2013).

Solution-focused social work and strength-based perspectives are also important frameworks in mainstream social work. Solution-focused approaches aim to find solutions and tend to avoid any attention to problems. This avoidance of acknowledging problems results in the inability to recognise injustice and harms caused by social forces. The focus on finding individual solutions can further victimise those who are structurally marginalised (Rossiter 2000). Strength-based models with their optimism about the capacity of people to overcome their problems through greater self-responsibility and lifestyle changes rely on an autonomous self that is consistent with neoliberalism's idea of self-development (Gray 2011).

Task-centred theory which focuses on the achievements of tasks to work towards a goal, can be easily accommodated to managerialist agendas that emphasise efficiency as the primary political value over social justice. These approaches are rooted in behavioural psychology and focus on the identification of problems to be solved within existing structural constraints. While the collaboration and negotiation with the client is emphasised, this aspect of the theory is often overlooked in many agencies in the current environment of separation between those funding the service and those delivering the service. Practitioners are under pressure for goal-directed outcomes within a time-limited framework, and such goals are often co-opted by the agency agendas and performance indicators. Such performance indicators result in the client being seen within an individualist self-responsibility focus, which fails to consider the structural inequalities that bring about personal difficulties.

In recent years, mainstream social work has also embraced evidence-based practice which emphasises empirically supported interventions and randomised controlled trials to construct what is presented as the 'best evidence' to guide social work practice. Critical engagements with evidence-based practice draw attention to the promotion of individualism and behaviourist models of practice with their mechanistic terminology and emphasis on adapting people to their environment. Furthermore, the denial of the influence of social and political forces on people's problems, the lack of attention to consumer perspectives and the close connection of evidence-based practice with neoliberalism and the new managerialism suggest that evidence-based practice is at odds with critical knowledge-informed practices in social work (Webb 2001; McDonald 2006; Pease 2009).

Aside from the limitations of mainstream social work, the concept of critical social work advocated here is not without controversy within the profession. Some argue that theorising about the politics of social work is not helpful for the doing of social work practice (Garrett 2013). Gray and Webb (2013c) refer to the overly academic nature of radical and critical social work, which they believe explains the lack of engagement by social work practitioners. For them, much of critical social work is a critique of practice; not a project of progressive practices. Harry Ferguson (2013) also argues that critical social work has avoided addressing practice in social work.

Carey and Foster (2011) believe that radical social work has been unable to provide practitioners with pragmatic strategies and practices. This, in turn, has contributed to apathy among practitioners about the potential of radical social work. In contrast, Turbett (2014) argues that radical social work has always involved more than just a critique of mainstream social work. While he acknowledges the critique that radical social work was more concerned with wider issues than the detailed politics of practice, he argues that radical and critical social work can utilise the spaces that discretion involves to advance a radical political agenda in social work. In this book, we aim to provide examples of the limitations and potential of such critical practices in social work.

Against neoliberal social work

Singh and Cowden (2009) argue that the denigration of theory by social workers has left it vulnerable to neoliberal reframing of the profession. For them, critical theory provides an important source of resistance to neoliberalism and the development of progressive practice. Many commentators regard the rise of neoliberalism as the most significant challenge to critical social work practice (Garrett 2010; Pollack & Rossiter 2010; Wallace & Pease 2011; Gray & Webb 2013c; Gray et al. 2015). Woodstock (2012), for example, argues that contemporary social work ethics are founded largely on neoliberal ideas.

McLaughlin (2008) argues that neoliberalism has infiltrated the language of contemporary social work. Pollack and Rossiter (2010), for example, note that feminist and progressive language has been co-opted by neoliberalism in many social work fields of practice. Reflecting on social work education in Canada, Yee and Wagner (2013), observe that neoliberalism has co-opted the anti-oppressive framework. This raises questions about the potential co-option of critical social work into neoliberal structures of Australian society (Wallace & Pease 2011).

Yee and Wagner (2013) alert us to the dangers of adopting the language of critical social work without translating the critical theoretical frameworks into progressive practices in social work. This is the challenge we face in developing this book. How do we ensure that the critical practices we advocate contribute to the transformation of the structures within society that reproduce oppression?

Ironically, however, the rise of neoliberal forms of social work has also reinvigorated radical and critical social work in response to the discontent and disillusionment among social workers (Lavalette 2011b). Gray and Webb (2013c) argue that critical social workers can increase people's awareness of the destructive consequences of neoliberal policies and practices. Thus, we argue against the de-intellectualising of social work, for we believe that the critical and radical tradition provides the best bulwark against the incursion of neoliberalism into social work (Singh & Cowden 2009).

Working on the contradictions

Social work is not only an emancipatory profession that is dedicated to human rights and social justice. As the majority of social workers are employed by the state, social workers must address the role of the state in reproducing dominant social relations (Garrett 2014). As Banks (2014) reminds us, the potential for social work to reproduce the existing social order is much greater than its potential to be involved in social change. Jones and Novak (2014a) even argue that social work cannot be a force for progressive social change while it is part of the state.

However, we argue, following Houston (2014), that social workers have some space to reflect on the contradictory nature of both the welfare state structures that employ them and the profession itself. Through the lens of what Houston calls 'the sociological imagination', critical social workers can aim to resist the most harmful effects of state control, while acknowledging that they cannot escape its coercive dimensions completely.

For Wilson (2008), it is important for social work practitioners to interrogate the contradictions inherent within social work practice. These contradictions within social work to some extent reflect the contradictory functions of the welfare state (Abramovitz 2014). This analysis highlights the role social workers play in the defence of neoliberalism. Critical social workers face the contradiction of, on the one hand, resisting and challenging the dominant social order, while, on the other hand, being complicit in reproducing that order (Gray & Webb 2013b). Such an analysis guards against the otherwise likelihood of advocating a form of innocence in social work (Rossiter 2001). Rossiter raises concerns that social workers may delude themselves into thinking that they are doing critical social work if they are not sufficiently aware of the reproductive functions of social work more generally (Rossiter 2001).

Banks (2014) argues that the possibilities for radical social work lies in the use of contradictions to critique the dominant discourses and to develop counter discourses. We argue that the concept of contradiction is important for critical social work practice under the conditions of neoliberalism. Perhaps one of the key functions of critical social work is to work with the contradictions embedded in the context and practice of social work.

Critical reflection as a tool for investigating practice

Effective critical social work practice described so far in this chapter is strengthened by ongoing critical reflection. Many of the contributors to this book engage in forms of critically reflective practice to grapple with the contradictions inherent in the context and practice of social work. Such an interrogation can make visible the opportunities for small acts of resistance against the dominant discourses, which contextualise social work practice (Gray & Webb 2013c).

Taylor (2013) queries, however, whether the placement of the word 'critical' in the front of reflective practice necessarily means that it is informed by critical theories and whether it necessarily leads to emancipatory political practices. While critical reflection aims to create a space for progressive politics at the micro level of service delivery, Taylor raises the question of whether it has really moved beyond the political neutrality of more traditional forms of reflective practice.

Wagner and Yee (2011) argue that critical reflection needs to interrogate social work itself, if it is to challenge practitioners to explore the impact of their own world views on practice. Such a process requires practitioners to acknowledge their complicity with the reproduction of inequalities. In discussing anti-oppressive practice in the Canadian context, Jeffery raises the disjuncture between what she calls 'radical questions and liberal solutions' (Jeffery 2007: 128). She says that in the project of teaching students 'how to do social work', the broader ontological issues underpinning the professional self are neglected. She encourages social workers to become uncomfortable with the tensions and political challenges of the work.

For Rossiter, it is the contradictions embedded within social work in relation to care and control that make it impossible for social workers to avoid their participation in the reproduction of inequalities (Rossiter 2011). In promoting social justice and human rights, critical social work must engage with its complicity with injustice and the violation of human rights. This means that the very process of identifying with social work is problematic when one teaches and practices from a critical perspective. This leads Rossiter to embrace what she calls 'un-settled social work'. Critical social work does not in itself provide a way of avoiding these dilemmas and contradictions.

Doing critical practice, maintaining critical hope

Even within the radical Marxist critique of social work, when it comes to practice, it is small-scale acts of resistance and solidarity that are emphasised (Ferguson, I. 2013). Thus, it is not necessarily traditional political action in the form of protest and social movements where critical social workers will be automatically involved (although of course they may be involved in such movements as well). Rather, it is at the level of small-scale resistance, what Carey and Foster define as 'deviant social work' (Carey & Foster 2011), where the everyday practices of critical social work will be enacted (see also Chapter 4).

Weinstein argues that social workers are the institutionalised conscience of society (Weinstein 2014). Social workers have always been witnesses to the abuse of power in society (Singh & Cowden 2009). Critical social workers have been outspoken critics of society's shortcomings. Wilson, Calhoun and Whitmore (2011) draw upon Gramsci to make the case for social workers as organic intellectuals, as they engage not just in political action but also in the realm of challenging dominant ideas. Jones and Novak (2014b) also reinstate the historical role of social workers as moral witnesses to society's failings. They encourage social workers to speak out about people's suffering that they encounter in practice.

Gray and Webb (2013c) appropriately ask whether such small-scale acts of resistance are sufficient for critical social work. Because the practices available to social workers will only involve micro-level changes at the service delivery level, many radical critics may see such small-scale changes as insignificant (Banks 2014). Solnit (2005), however, who is writing more widely in terms of critical practices, argues that small-scale acts of resistance have historically changed the world. She thus argues for the importance of hope in facing down despair.

Over thirty-five years ago, Peter Leonard (1979) defended the concept of 'critical hope' against the then rising tide of cynicism, fatalism and despair facing social workers. Such hope, for him, arose out of his commitment to the radical tradition of social work at that time. It inspired the courage to develop radical theories and practices in the face of such despair.

Thirty-four years later, Webb (2013) argues that developing a pedagogy of hope is one of the most important challenges for critical educators. Zournazi (2002) says that hope provides sustenance in the struggle against despair. She advocates a philosophy and politics of hope that keeps us committed to social justice struggles.

For Macy (2009), activists must acknowledge their despair and see the importance of it as a capacity to suffer in response to the injustices of the world. She argues that it is important not to block compassion for suffering in the world but to allow ourselves to feel it as a way of moving through it to a different place of agency and commitment.

Van Soest (2012) talks about moving backwards and forwards in relation to pessimism and optimism when facing the challenges presented to social workers. How does one avoid being too pessimistic in the face of the immense issues that social workers engage with, while at the same time avoiding being overly optimistic in the face of these challenges? This movement between pessimism and optimism was evident among us as this book's editors as we discussed our own and other contributors' chapters.

Chapter overview

We have divided the book into five broad sections. Part I addresses the tensions that are experienced in critical social work. Part II explores critical practices in confronting privilege and promoting social justice in social work. Part III considers the development of critical practices within the organisational context of social work. Part IV focuses on doing anti-discriminatory and anti-oppressive practice in social work with particular groups in the community. Part V outlines collectivist and transformative practices in social work and beyond.

Part I begins with this introductory chapter, which explores the historical and contemporary ideas in critical social work. It positions the perspective taken in this book as against neoliberal social work and introduces two key concepts: working on the contradictions embedded in social work and the importance of maintaining critical hope when doing critical social work.

Christine Morley argues in Chapter 2 that critical reflection is a vital component of critical social work because it enhances how critical social work is both theorised and practised. She explores how critical reflection can extend possibilities for critical practice, challenge conservative thinking and practices and improve critical modernist practices.

In Chapter 3, Carolyn Noble argues that by developing a pedagogy that engages with critical reflection, critical thinking and analysis as well as transformative learning, the practice of supervision moves from administrative, supportive and organisational functions towards a position of social resistance informed by social justice and human rights activism.

In Chapter 4, Norah Hosken and Sophie Goldingay explore different approaches to doing critical social work. In particular, through a case study, they acknowledge areas of commonality and difference between modernist structural approaches and postmodern approaches to critical social work. They illustrate the integrity of each approach and show how each strive towards creating more socially just situations, and emancipatory personal and social change.

Part II begins with Chapter 5 by Sharlene Nipperess, which explores how social workers can enact a human rights-based approach from a critical social work perspective. She draws attention to the complex and contested nature of human rights and identifies that commitments to human rights in both social work practice and social work education are ubiquitous but often rhetorical. This chapter outlines a framework that enables social workers to consider how human rights can be used in critical social work practice.

Bob Pease argues in Chapter 6 that social workers who are committed to the radical and critical tradition in social work need to reflect upon their own positioning in systems of inequality. Drawing upon critical studies in the fields of masculinity, whiteness, heterosexuality and other fields of privilege, the chapter explores strategies for social workers to deepen their understanding of their own privileged positioning and ways of engaging members of privileged groups in understanding the benefits that flow from privilege and how they are implicated in the oppression of others.

In Chapter 7, the final chapter in Part II, Norah Hosken invites social workers to explore a poverty and class-awareness approach to practice. In their everyday work, most social workers are witness to, and participants in, the class-based nature of the structural violence of poverty. Hosken focuses on how explanations of class need to always draw on gender and race, and whether people are able-bodied, heterosexual and ageist. The implications of poverty and class for social work are used to suggest a framework for a poverty and class-awareness approach that informs and links social work practice in the day-to-day realities of working with people in organisations to the wider picture of humans living in a society at large where the social is prioritised over the economic.

Part III begins with Chapter 8 by Noel Renouf who argues that in the mental health field, a critical approach to practice closely engages with the actual experiences of people with mental health problems and those around them, including their families. Such a focus moves beyond the dominant approach, which is organised primarily around the 'treatment' of 'illness' alongside approaches to risk management and care that are often fundamentally coercive.

In Chapter 9, Robyn Miller draws on the Best Interests Case Practice Model used for the past five years in Victoria to position critical social work in statutory practice. She challenges episodic, task-focused case management that too often polarises child and family-focused services, and promotes relationship based-practice in contrast to the 'bureaucratisation' of child protection.

Peter Humphries, in Chapter 10, explores critical social work practice in Centrelink. He explores the 'invitations' to a bureaucratised social work practice that strongly influence social workers in Centrelink, and the opportunities that exist for critical social work practice, particularly around the development of the 'worker-client relationship' and in the 'implementation' of often difficult social policy.

In Chapter 11, Sophie Goldingay explores critical social work practice in a prison setting. She argues that while social work is grounded in the values of social justice and human rights, critical social work is further committed to addressing power relations that cause oppression in various contexts. Many social work fields of practice place social workers in positions that present ongoing dilemmas about how to support critical social work values and aims in everyday practice. Prison social work is one such field.

In Chapter 12, the final chapter in Part III, Norah Hosken, Lesley Ervin and Jody Laughton examine how neoliberal influences on staff in universities and the human service sector effect opportunities for social work students to learn, practice and be assessed on their use of critical social work during their placements. A case study frames the chapter, describing the efforts by the authors to enact critical social work practice. The case study introduces and illustrates critical social work practice principles, drawing on critical social work process-orientations as located within the author-developed 'Framework for Critical Social Work Action' (FCSWA). Staff engagement is discussed in relation to the effects of neoliberal ideology, discourses, regulatory documents and practices on students on placement.

Part IV begins with Chapter 13 by Sharlene Nipperess and Sherrine Clark who explore anti-oppressive practice with asylum seekers. Australia's asylum seeker policy is highly controversial and has been roundly criticised by the international community and many within Australia itself, including social workers. The authors reflect on their experiences of working anti-oppressively with asylum seekers over the last fifteen years and explore the challenges as well as the satisfaction of critical practice in different agency contexts.

In Chapter 14, Stephanie Gilbert considers the challenges for Aboriginal and non-Aboriginal workers in the neoliberal context. She notes that in the last decade the field for social workers has changed in the face of an increasingly casualised workforce and identifies that Aboriginal workers are now increasingly contracted to provide services directly to clients. She raises the question of how employing Aboriginality as a skill sits in this context. Taking a critical social work approach in these workplaces requires looking at how professional practice must include challenging structural inequality in workplace operations, and expectations that may work against groups, including Aboriginal and Torres Strait Islander peoples.

In Chapter 15, Ann Carrington discusses some key constraints and practical responses to feminist social work practice within the domestic violence/women's sector. Through a critical reflective process, she identifies five key areas impacted by the neoliberal and managerialist agenda including: collaboration and partnership; keeping gender issues on the agenda; education and training; management; and resilience. Practical responses that may help to inform the practice of other feminist social workers in the field are offered.

Tina Kostecki notes, in Chapter 16 that ageing in Australia is a self-evident experience for each one of us. However, socially constructed notions of ageing adults are mostly negative. Ageism represents systemic patterns of discrimination, social exclusion and negative stereotypes, which are deeply embedded in Western culture. This chapter discusses the need for anti-ageist social work practice and draws upon perspectives from critical gerontology as a guide for practice.

In Chapter 17, Jude Irwin highlights that people from LGBTI (lesbian, gay, bisexual, transgender, intersex) communities have been relatively invisible in the critical social work literature, even though they comprise a significant percentage of the population. This chapter explores how practice is often premised on beliefs and assumptions of heteronormativity (the belief that people have distinct genders, and follow a heterosexual orientation), often unintentionally excluding the life experiences of the LGBTI populations.

Part V begins with Chapter 18 by Mel Gray and John Coates who argue that within the broad environmental movement, social work responds to the social injustices that are the social consequences of environmental destruction, and the social and economic inequalities that are often the cause and consequence. This chapter reviews the development of environmental social work, its contributions to social work and critical social work theory, and raises issues that environmental social work flags for the profession.

In Chapter 19, Jessica Morrison discusses the relationship between activism and critical social work. She argues that it is a core responsibility for critical social workers to bring about social change. The chapter explores three contexts where this can occur: social work practice where social change is the orientation of the organisation; strategic manoeuvring in traditional workplaces to create opportunities for social change; and personal activism outside the workplace.

Russell Shuttleworth, in Chapter 20, explores a critical participatory approach to social work, disability and social change. He provides a critical perspective on social work's minimal engagement with the disability movement and critical disability studies in developing and working toward a progressive disability agenda for social change. He also explores a 'critical participatory' approach to practice with disabled people.

In Chapter 21, José Ramos addresses the need for new strategies in building common ground for common action in the context of contemporary challenges. Globalisation has fundamentally changed the basis for conceiving of community to social-level action and intervention. The chapter challenges the dichotomy between the structural and post-structural perspectives, arguing both are integral to a social and community development.

In Chapter 22, the final chapter of the book, Selma Macfarlane notes that neoliberal, colonialist and social control discourses, which currently predominate in Western societies like Australia, have the potential to reduce social work education to the acquisition of competency-based skills rather than critically reflective, transformative learning. This chapter argues that a critical approach to social work education is vital to social work as an ethical and emancipatory project.

As this chapter overview illustrates, each of our contributors have engaged with the issue of optimism and pessimism differently. They reflect both the opportunities and constraints of their particular workplaces, and their social positioning within them. We hope that this book's diversity of case studies encourage readers to reflect on the relationship between their own practice and the wider context within which their work is situated, and that these case studies provide inspiration to develop practices that extend the emancipatory objectives of critical social work.

References

Abramovitz, M. 2014, 'Which side are we on?', in I. Ferguson and M. Lavalette (eds), *Poverty and Inequality: Critical and radical debates in social work,* Bristol: Policy Press, pp. 27–34

Allan, J. 2009, 'Theorising new developments in critical social work', in J. Allan, L. Briskman & B. Pease (eds), *Critical Social Work: Theories and practices for a socially just world*, 2nd edn, Crows Nest: Allen & Unwin, pp. 30–44

Allan, J, Briskman, L. and Pease, B. (eds) 2009, *Critical Social Work: Theories and practices for a socially just world*, 2nd edn, Crows Nest: Allen & Unwin,

Alston, M. 2012, 'Addressing the effects of climate change on rural communities', in J. Maidment & U. Bay (eds), *Social Work in Rural Australia: Enabling practice*, Crows Nest: Allen & Unwin, pp. 204–17

Alston, M. & Besthorn, F. 2012, 'Environment and sustainability', in K. Lyons, T. Hokenstad, M. Pawar, N. Huegler and N. Hall (eds), *The Sage Handbook of International Social Work*, London: Sage, pp. 56–69

Baines, D. 2011, 'An overview of anti-oppressive practice: Roots, theory, tensions', Baines (ed.), in *Doing Anti-Oppressive Practice: Social justice social work*, 2nd edn, Black Point, Nova Scotia: Fernwood Publishing, pp. 1–24

Banks, S. 2014, 'Reflections on the responses to "Reclaiming social work ethics"' in I. Ferguson & M. Lavalette (eds), *Ethics: Critical and radical debates in social work*, Bristol: Policy Press, pp. 77–83

Bennett, B., Green, S., Gilbert, S. & Bessarab, D. (eds) 2013, *Our Voices: Aboriginal and Torres Strait Islander social work*, Melbourne: Palgrave Macmillan,

Besthorn, F. 2011, 'The deep ecology's contribution to social work: A ten year perspective', *International Journal of Social Welfare*, vol. 21, no. 3, pp. 248–59

Bourdieu, P. 1999, *The Weight of the World: Social suffering in contemporary society*, Cambridge: Polity

Briskman, L., Pease, B. & Allan, J. 2009, 'Introducing critical theories for social work in a neo-liberal context', in J. Allan, L. Briskman & B. Pease (eds), *Critical Social Work: Theories and practices for a socially just world*, 2nd edn, St Leonards: Allen & Unwin, pp. 3–14

Brown, D. 2006, 'Working the system: Re-thinking the institutionally organized role of mothers and the reduction of "risk" in child protection work', *Social Problems*, vol. 53, no. 3, pp. 352–70

Carey, M. & Foster, V. 2011, 'Introducing "deviant" social work: Contextualizing the limits of radical social work whilst understanding (fragmented) resistance within the social work labour process', *British Journal of Social Work*, vol. 41, no. 3, pp. 576–93

Corrigan, P. & Leonard, P. 1978, *Social work practice under capitalism: A Marxist approach*, London: The Macmillan Press

de Montigny, G. 1995, *Social Working: An ethnography of front-line practice*, Canada: University of Toronto Press,

—— 2011, 'Beyond anti-oppressive practice: Investigating reflexive social relations', *Journal of Progressive Human Services*, vol. 22, no. 1, pp. 8–30

DeVault, M. & McCoy, L. 2006, 'Institutional ethnography: Using interviews to investigate ruling relations', in D.E. Smith (ed.), *Institutional Ethnography as Practice*, Rowman & Littlefield Pub Inc., Lanham, pp. 15–44

Dominelli, L. 2002, *Feminist social work theory and practice*, Basingstoke: Palgrave

—— 2008, *Anti-racist social work*, 3rd edn, Basingstoke: Palgrave

—— 'Anti-oppressive practice: The challenges of the twenty-first century', in R. Adams, L. Dominelli & M. Payne (eds), 2008, *Social work: themes, issues and critical debates*, 3rd edn, Basingstoke: Palgrave Macmillan, pp. 49–64

—— 2012, *Green Social Work: From environmental crises to environmental justice*, Cambridge: Polity Press

Ferguson, H., 'Critical best practice' in M. Gray & S. Webb (eds), 2013, *The New Politics of Social Work*, New York: Palgrave, pp. 116–27

Ferguson, I., 'Social workers as agents of change' in M. Gray & S. Webb (eds), 2013, *The New Politics of Social Work*, New York: Palgrave, pp. 195–208

Ferguson, I. 2008, *Reclaiming Social Work: Challenging neoliberalism and promoting social justice*, London: Sage Publications

Ferguson, I. & Woodward, R. 2009, *Radical Social Work in Practice: Making a difference*, Bristol: The Policy Press

Ferguson, I. & Lavalette, M. 2007, '"Dreaming a great dream": Prospects for a new radical social work', *Canadian Social Work Review*, vol. 24, no. 1, pp. 55–68

Fook, J. 2012, *Social Work: A critical approach to practice*, 2nd edn, London: Sage

—— 2003, 'Critical social work: The current issues', *Qualitative Social Work*, vol. 2, no. 2, pp. 123–30

—— 1993, *Radical Casework: A theory of practice*, St Leonards: Allen & Unwin

Fraser, N. & Honneth, A. 2003, *Redistribution or Recognition?: A political-philosophical exchange*, Verso, London

Freire, P. 1993, *Pedagogy of the oppressed*, London: Penguin Books

Garrett, P. 2007, 'The relevance of Bourdieu for social work: A reflection on the obstacles and omissions', *Journal of Social Work*, vol. 7, no. 3, pp. 355–79

—— 2010, 'Examining the "conservative revolution": Neoliberalism and social work education', *Social Work Education*, vol. 29, no. 4, pp. 340–55

—— 'Mapping the theoretical and political terrain of social work' in M. Gray & S. Webb (eds), 2013, *The New Politics of Social Work*, Palgrave, New York, pp. 44–62

—— 2014, 'Radical and critical perspectives on social work with children and families: England and the Republic of Ireland' in I. Ferguson and M. Lavalette (eds), 2014, *Children and Families: Critical and radical debates in social work,* Bristol: Policy Press, pp. 1–32

Garrity, Z. 2010, 'Discourse analysis, Foucault, and social work research: Identifying some methodological complexities', *Journal of Social Work*, vol. 10, no. 2, pp. 193–210

Ghandi, L. 1998, *Postcolonial Theory: A critical introduction*, St Leonards: Allen & Unwin

Gough, I. 1979, *The political economy of the welfare state*, Basingstoke: Macmillan Education

Gray, M. 2011, 'Back to basics: A critique of the strengths perspective in social work', *Families in Society*, vol. 99, no. 1, pp. 5–7

—— 'Hearing Indigenous and local voices in mainstream social work' in M. Gray, J. Coates & M. Yellow Bird (eds), 2008, *Indigenous Social Work Around the World: Towards culturally relevant education and practice,* Ashgate, Farnham, pp. 257–69

Gray, M. & Webb, S. (eds) 2013a, *The New Politics of Social Work*, New York: Palgrave

—— 2013b, 'The speculative left and new politics of social work' in M. Gray & S. Webb (eds), *The New Politics of Social Work*, New York: Palgrave, pp. 209–23

—— 2013c, 'Towards a "new politics" of social work' in M. Gray & S. Webb (eds), *The New Politics of Social Work,* New York: Palgrave, pp. 3–20

Gray, M., Coates, J. & Hetherington, T. (eds) 2012a, *Environmental Social Work*, London: Routledge

—— 'Introduction: Overview of the last ten years and typology of ESW' in M. Gray, J. Coates and T. Hetherington (eds), 2012b, *Environmental Social Work* London: Routledge, pp. 1–28

Gray, M., Coates, J. & Yellow Bird, M., 'Introduction' in M. Gray, J. Coates and M. Yellow Bird (eds), 2008, *Indigenous Social Work Around the World: Towards culturally relevant education and practice,* Ashgate, Farnham, pp. 1–10

Gray, M., Dean, M., Agllias, K., Howard, A. & Schubert, L. 2015, 'Perspectives on neoliberalism for human service professionals', *Social Service Review,* vol. 89, no. 2, pp. 368–92

Hick, S., Fook, J. & Pozzuto, R. (eds) 2005, *Social Work: A critical turn*, Toronto: Thompson Educational Publishing

Hosken, N. 2013, 'Social work supervision and discrimination', *Advances in Social Work and Welfare Education,* vol. 15, no. 1, pp. 91–103

Houston, S. 2013, 'Social work and the politics of recognition' in M. Gray and S. Webb (eds), *The New Politics of Social Work,* New York: Palgrave, pp. 63–76

—— 2014, 'Social work and the sociological imagination' in I. Ferguson and M. Lavalette (eds), *Children and Families: Critical and radical debates in social work,* Bristol: Policy Press, pp. 63–76

Ife, J., 1997, *Rethinking Social Work: Towards critical practice*, South Melbourne: Longman

—— 2012, *Human rights and Social Work: Towards rights-based practice*, Leiden: Cambridge University Press

Jeffery, D. 2007, 'Radical problems and liberal selves: Professional subjectivity in the anti-oppressive social work classroom', *Canadian Social Work Review*, vol. 24, no. 2, pp. 125–39

Jones, C. & Novak, T. 2014a, 'What are we going to do about it?' in I. Ferguson & M. Lavalette (eds), *Poverty and Inequality: Critical and radical debates in social work,* Bristol: Policy Press, pp. 53–8

—— 2014b, 'We don't want to be ashamed tomorrow' in I. Ferguson & M. Lavalette (eds), *Poverty and Inequality: Critical and radical debates in social work,* Policy Press, Bristol, pp. 1–25

Kemshall, H. 2010, 'Risk rationalities in contemporary social work practice', *British Journal of Social Work,* vol. 40, no. 4, pp. 1247–62

Lavalette, M. (ed.) 2011a, *Radical Social Work Today: Social work at the crossroads*, Bristol: The Policy Press

—— 2011b, 'Introduction' in M. Lavalette (ed.), *Radical Social Work Today: Social work at the crossroads*, Bristol: Policy Press, pp. 1–10

Leonard, P. 1979, 'In defence of critical hope', *Social Work Today*, vol. 10, no. 24, pp. 21–4

Lundy, C. 2011, *Social Work, Social Justice and Human Rights: A structural approach to practice*, 2nd edn, Ontario: University of Toronto Press

Macy, J. 2009, 'The global crisis and the arising of the ecological self', *Journal of Holistic Health Care*, vol. 6, no. 3, pp. 5–11

Marston, G. 2013, 'Critical discourse analysis' in M. Gray & S. Webb (eds), *The New Politics of Social Work*, New York: Palgrave, pp. 128–42

McDonald, C. 2006, *Challenging Social Work: The context of practice*, Basingstoke: Palgrave Macmillan

McKinnon, J. 2012, 'Social work and changing environments' in K. Lyons, T. Hokenstad, M. Pawar, N. Huegler & N. Hall (eds), *The Sage Handbook of International Social Work*, London: Sage, pp. 265–78

McLaughlin, K. 2008, *Social Work Politics and Society*, Bristol: Policy Press

Mendes, P. 2009, 'Tracing the origins of critical social work practice', in J. Allan, L. Briskman & B. Pease (eds), *Critical Social Work: Theories and practices for a socially just world*, 2nd edn, St Leonards: Allen & Unwin, pp. 17–29

Morley, C. & Macfarlane, S. 2012, 'The nexus between feminism and postmodernism: Still a central concern for critical social work', *British Journal of Social Work*, vol. 42, no. 4, pp. 687–705

Morley, C., Macfarlane, S. & Ablett, P. 2014, *Engaging with Social Work: A critical introduction*, Melbourne: Cambridge University Press

Mullaly, B. 2007, *The New Structural Social Work: Ideology, theory, and practice*, 3rd edn, Don Mills: Oxford University Press

—— 2010, *Challenging Oppression and Confronting Privilege*, 2nd edn, Don Mills: Oxford University Press

Muller, L. 2014, *A Theory for Indigenous Australian Health and Human Service Work*, St Leonards: Allen & Unwin

Pallotta-Chiarolli, M. & Pease, B. 2014, 'Recognition, resistance and reconstruction: An introduction to subjectivities and social justice' in M. Pallotta-Chiarolli and B. Pease (eds), *The Politics of Recognition and Social Justice: Transforming subjectivities and new forms of resistance*, Routledge, New York, pp. 1–23

Payne, M. 2002, 'The politics of systems theory within social work', *Journal of Social Work*, vol. 2, no. 3, pp. 269–92

—— 2014, *Modern social work theory*, 4th edn, Basingstoke: Palgrave Macmillan

Pease, B. 1991, 'Dialectical models versus ecological models in social work practice', paper presented to the 11th Asia Pacific Regional Seminar on Social Work, Hong Kong, 21–24 August

—— 2009, 'From evidence-based practice to critical knowledge in post-positivist social work' in J. Allan, L. Briskman & B. Pease (eds), *Critical Social Work: Theories and practices for a socially just world*, 2nd edn, St Leonards: Allen & Unwin, pp. 45–57

Pease, B. & Fook, J. (eds) 1999, *Transforming Social Work Practice: Postmodern critical perspectives*, St Leonards: Allen & Unwin

Pollack, S. & Rossiter, A. 2010, 'Neoliberalism and the entrepreneurial subject: Implications for feminism and social work', *Canadian Social Work Review*, vol. 27, no. 2, pp. 155–69

Powell, J. 2012, 'Social work and elder abuse: A Foucauldian analysis', *Social Work and Society*, vol. 10, no. 1, pp. 1–9

Reisch, M. 2013, 'Social work education and the neoliberal challenge: The U.S. response to increasing global inequality', *Social Work Education: The International Journal*, vo. 32, no. 6, pp. 715–33

—— 2005, 'Discourse analysis in critical social work: From apology to question', *Critical Social Work*, vol. 6, no. 1, pp. 1–7

—— 2011, 'Unsettled social work: The challenge of Levinas's ethics', *British Journal of Social Work*, advance access 24 Jan, 2011

Rossiter, A. 2000, 'The professional is political: An interpretation of the problem of the past in solution-focused therapy', *American Journal of Orthopsychiatry*, vol. 70, no 1, pp. 1–12

—— 2001, Innocence lost and suspicion found: Do we educate for or against social work?', *Critical Social Work*, vol. 2, no. 1, retrieved from <www.criticalsocialwork.com>

Singh, G. & Cowden, S. 2009, 'The social worker as intellectual', *European Journal of Social Work*, vol. 12, no. 4, pp. 479–93

Smith, D. 2007, 'Institutional ethnography: From a sociology for women to a sociology for people' in S. Hesse-Biber (ed.), *Handbook of Feminist Research: Theory and praxis*, Sage, Thousand Oaks, pp. 409–16

Solnit, R. 2005, *Hope in the Dark: The untold history of people power*, Melbourne: Text

Taylor, C. 2013, 'Critically reflective practice' in M. Gray and S. Webb (eds), *The New Politics of Social Work*, New York: Palgrave, pp. 79–97

Thompson, N. 2012, *Anti-discriminatory Practice*, 5th edn, Basingstoke: Palgrave Macmillan

Turbett, C. 2014, *Doing Radical Social Work*, London: Palgrave

Van Soest, D. 2012, 'Confronting our fears and finding hope in difficult times: Social work as a force for social justice', *Journal of Progressive Human Services*, vol. 23, no. 2, pp. 95–109

Wakefield, J. 1996, 'Does social work need the eco-systems perspective?', *Social Service Review*, vol. 70, no. 1, pp. 1–32

Wallace, J. and Pease, B. 2011, 'Neoliberalism and Australian social work: Accommodation or resistance?', *Journal of Social Work*, vol. 11, no. 2, pp. 132–42

Walter, M., Taylor, S. & Habibis, D. 2013, 'Walking the journey: The student experience' in B. Bennett, S. Green, S. Gilbert & D. Bessarab (eds), *Our Voices: Aboriginal and Torres Strait Islander social work*, Melbourne: Palgrave Macmillan, pp. 206–29

Webb, D. 2013, 'Pedagogies of hope', *Studies in Philosophy of Education*, vol. 32, pp. 397–414

Webb, S. 2001, 'Considerations on the validity of evidence-based practice in social work', *British Journal of Social Work*, vol. 31, no. 1, pp. 57–79

Weeks, W. 2003, 'Women: developing feminist practice in women's services', in J. Allan, B. Pease & L. Briskman (eds), Allen & Unwin, *Critical Social Work: An introduction to theories and practices*, St Leonards: Allen & Unwin, pp. 107–23

Weinstein, J. 2014, 'Social work and mental health' in I. Ferguson & M. Lavalette (eds), *Mental Health: Critical and radical debates in social work*, Bristol: Policy Press, pp. 1–28

Wilson, M., Calhoun, A. & Whitmore, E. 2011, 'Contesting the neoliberal agenda: Lessons from Canadian activists', *Canadian Social Work Review*, vol. 28, no, 1, pp. 25–48

Wilson, T. 2008, 'Reflecting on the contradictions: Governmentality in social work education and community practice', *Canadian Social Work Review*, vol. 35, no. 2, 187–201

Woodstock, R. 2012, 'Knowing where you stand: Neoliberal and other foundations for social work', *Journal of Comparative Social Welfare*, vol. 28, no. 1, pp. 1–15

Yee, J. & Wagner, A. 2013, 'Is anti-oppression teaching in Canadian social work classrooms a form of neoliberalism?', *Social Work Education: The International Journal*, vol. 32, no. 3, pp. 331–48

Yellow Bird, M. & Gray, M. 2008, 'Indigenous people and the language of social work' in M. Gray, J. Coates, and M. Yellow Bird (eds), *Indigenous Social Work Around the World: Towards culturally relevant education and practice*, Melbourne: Palgrave Macmillan, pp. 59–69

Zournazi, M. 2002, 'Introduction' in M. Zournazi (ed.), *Hope: New philosophies for change*, Sydney: Pluto Press, pp. 14–20

Zubrzycki, J., Green, S., Jones, V., Stratton, K., Young, S. & Bessarab, D. 2014, *Getting it Right: Creating partnerships for change. Integrating Aboriginal and Torres Strait Islander knowledge's in social work education and practice. Teaching and learning framework*, Australian Government Office for Learning and Teaching: Sydney

2

Critical reflection and critical social work

Christine Morley

Introduction

Critical social work is fundamental to any claim that social work as a discipline or profession is emancipatory, concerned with social justice or committed to progressive social change or both. Critical social work is informed by an intricate blend of critical modernist and post-structural theories. These theories are both crucial to critical reflection in this field, despite co-existing in tension. This chapter delineates how this theoretical tension enables critical reflection to further develop the emancipatory potential of critical social work. Critical reflection uses modernist critical theories to expose and oppose conservative thinking and practices. It also draws on post-structural critiques to safeguard against critical practices that are well-intentioned, yet potentially oppressive. Combining critical modernist and post-structuralist thought also enhances the possibilities for critical practice in organisational contexts that are restrictive by empowering practitioners to connect with a sense of agency to create change.

An interpretation of critical social work

Critical social work encompasses a broad area of theoretical approaches. These range from modernist emancipatory perspectives such as structural (Moreau 1979; Mullaly 2010), radical (Fook 1993; Lavalette 2011) and feminist approaches (Marchant & Wearing 1986; Dominelli 2002; White 2006) that privilege materialist understandings of oppression and change. Other approaches extend to the more constructionist and interpretive theories such as post-structuralism (for example, Leonard 1997; Chambon et al. 1999; Pease & Fook 1999). These theories relating to critical social work justify a diverse and contested range of political and ideological positions. At times they are complementary, and at others, they oppose each other. I locate myself somewhere in the middle of this theoretical tension, choosing to draw upon a critically reflexive combination of all of these theoretical frameworks to inform practice. Critical reflexivity involves critically analysing and challenging the impact of dominant paradigms on our world view. This is done in a way that highlights the socially constructed and contested nature of knowledge, and therefore our capacity for agency (Trevelyan et al. 2012).

Critical modernist frameworks provide clear values to guide practice towards contesting, rather than accepting, social inequalities (Holscher & Sewpaul 2006). They also provide a strong analytic basis to understand the structural and institutional dimensions of power and privilege, disadvantage, exploitation and exclusion (Mullaly 2010). In presenting totalising ways of knowing (grand narratives), critical modernist perspectives assist social workers to understand the intimate connection between people's privately experienced problems and the social, political, economic, cultural, gendered, historical factors that shape these problems. Given this link between the personal and the social, critical modernist theories expose injustices that are in dominant power relations and structures. These theories challenge harmful divisions in class, gender, ethnicity and other dimensions of difference (Allan et al. 2009), and orientate practice towards emancipatory goals of social justice, human rights, democracy, equity and progressive social change (Fook 1993; Mullaly 2010; Lavalette 2011). These same goals underpin the model of critical reflection discussed in this chapter and therefore offer 'a broader framework for understanding what critical reflection can and should help achieve' (Fook 2004: 20).

In contrast to these modernist theories are the more interpretive or constructionist theories including post-structuralism. Post-structuralism critiques what it regards as the limiting aspects of modernist critical theories, including their embrace of universal narratives, over-simplified conceptions of power and identity, and binary constructions (Fook 2012). However, post-structuralism can also be used to enhance the way critical modernist theories are applied to social work practice. 'Post-structuralism' literally means 'after structuralism' and it discards the idea that our experiences can be fully attributed to social structures. Post-structuralists reject the universal, grand narratives that characterise critical modernist theories. They interpret 'truth claims' as partial, incomplete, contextually based and what invites multiple understandings based on different individual, cultural and institutional standpoints (Leonard 1997; Chambon et al. 1999; Fook 2012). This displaces the emphasis on analysing and changing social structures as the key strategy for emancipation, which is challenging for modernist thinkers. Critics of post-structuralism have pointed out that it has the potential to be relativist, politically conservative, and nihilistic (for example, Noble 2004; Ferguson 2008). Given these concerns, I would never use post-structuralism without a critical framework to inform practice. Yet at the same time, post-structuralism can be useful in challenging critical modernist theories to think about alternative strategies to achieve emancipatory goals in addition to structural change (Fook 2012; Morley & Macfarlane 2012).

Hence, many social theorists have explored the possibilities of a critical approach to social work that utilises the emancipatory possibilities of both critical modernist and post-structural perspectives (for example, Leonard 1997; Pease & Fook 1999; Healy 2000; Allan et al. 2009; Fook 2012; Morley & Macfarlane 2012; Morley 2014; Morley et al. 2014). On one hand, critical modernist theories highlight oppression and disadvantage caused by social structures (Mullaly 2010). On the other, critical post-structuralism recognises many potential constructions (or understandings of 'reality') that emphasise our capacity for agency to interpret and respond to social structures in a way that can disrupt, resist and challenge dominant power relations (Fook 2012). A critical modernist structural analysis of society can be broadened to include a post-structural interpretive understanding of the ways in which practitioners construct themselves and others, and are constructed by discourses (languages and social practices) that are embedded in their work contexts. Critical reflection, informed by this theoretical combination, aims to unearth discourses about practitioners' sense of agency to envision strategies for change (Fook 2004; Morley 2014). This form of critical reflection is one way to enable 'the emancipatory potential of critical postmodernism to be put into practice' (Morley 2014:68). It enables us to break down accepted world views that reproduce forms of domination and oppression.

Reflection: drawbacks and attributes

It is the combination of critical modernist and poststructuralist theories (collectively referred to as critical) that distinguishes *critical reflection* from reflection. Schon's (1987) reflective model, informed by Dewey (1933), is important for critical social work because it is concerned to uncover gaps between our espoused theory (i.e. the theory we think or say that we are using) and our actual practice, in ways that enable us to match our theorising or practice with our intentions. However, as a concept in its own right, reflection is inadequate for critical social work because if our stated theory is conservative, reflection will only serve to reinforce establishment practice, which 'uncritically accepts existing social inequalities and helps people cope with the impact of injustices instead of challenging them' (Morley et al. 2014: 2). Reflective practice can therefore become a 'political[ly] neutral space' or 'depoliticised view of practice', demonstrating little understanding of the impact of social structures to instead focus on the individual (Taylor 2013: 83). Reflective approaches are important for questioning objectivism and the evidenced-based movement as the only foundation on which to base practice (Taylor 2013), critiquing technical rationality as inadequate for the complexity and messiness of social work practice (Thompson 2011), and exposing professionals as self-interested, self-serving and ineffective because of the powerful elite's influence (Taylor 2013). However, critical social work needs reflection to be *critical* to expand and enhance critical modernist and post-structural theories and practices.

Critical reflection: drawbacks and attributes

Critical reflection can be understood in a variety of contested ways. The model I use largely derives from Fook (2012). Fundamentally underpinned by the critical modernist and poststructural theories outlined above, this model is also influenced by 'reflection,' (Dewey 1933; Kolb 1984) or 'reflective practice' (Schon 1987), which can be a process that aims to improve practice by linking it with theory; as well as 'reflexivity'. This refers to our capacity to look back upon ourselves and examine how our social positioning shapes the way we interpret social phenomena (Taylor 2006). Although more recently developed as a research methodology (for example, Morley 2008; Fook & Gardner 2013), critical reflection is primarily an educational tool to promote professional learning (Fook 2013). As such it is also influenced by critical and experiential pedagogies (for example, Giroux 2011; Brookfield 2013). More recent applications of this model of critical reflection incorporate spirituality (Gardner 2013a, 2014) and Eastern religions (Fook 2013).

As a process, this model of critical reflection includes two phases: deconstruction and reconstruction. Deconstruction interrogates the implicit values and assumptions that underlie our practice to uncover the (often unconscious) ways that we uphold discourses that work against us (Fook 2012). This frees us from static and hegemonic ways of thinking, and then we are open to reconstruction. This is where we review the basis of our practice in ways that engender opportunities for agency and change (Morley 2014).

Taylor differentiates her approach to critical reflection from Fook and Gardner (2007) on the basis of shifting away 'from individual acts of reflection . . . towards a more politically nuanced treatment of social work as collective practice' (Taylor 2013: 86). She is concerned that use of 'poststructuralist thinking about power and subjectivity in order to make sense of, and challenge, the micro-politics of power in every day practice' within critical reflection occurs at the expense of modernist structural analyses of power (Taylor 2013: 86). The key difference, she argues, is that her model focuses on 'analysing and changing the social relations of practice rather than the thoughts and feelings of individual practitioners' (Taylor 2013: 88).

However, a model of critical reflection that draws on both modernist and post-structural aspects of critical theory would seem to address the issues raised by Taylor (2013). From a critical perspective, individual or personal acts of reflection cannot be separated from the social and political realms of social work practice (Fook 1993), and post-structuralism identifies this dichotomous construction as artificial (Fook 2012). Rather than being limited to the individual domain, '[t]he central idea is that the new insight and knowledge gained through [critical] reflection would result in societal changes' (Fook & Askeland 2006: 42). Numerous authors attest to critical reflection's capacity to affect 'very real externalised outcomes' (Fook & Napier 2000: 224; see also, Fook 2004, 2012; Morley 2004, 2011, 2012, 2014; Naudi 2006; Gardner et al. 2006; Pockett & Giles 2008; Thomson 2013) that go well beyond the individual thoughts and reflections of the practitioner. The remainder of this chapter outlines the contribution that this model of critical reflection might make to further developing the emancipatory potential of critical social work.

Extending possibilities for critical practice and helping practitioners create change

The impact of practising social work within globalised, neoliberal contexts, which include the constraints of managerial, bureaucratic, market driven procedures, are now well documented (for example, Ferguson & Lavalette 2006; Holscher & Sewpaul 2006; Wallace & Pease 2011; Rogowski 2010; Madhu 2011; Gardner 2014). Critical modernist theories have helped articulate the challenges created by the 'marketisa-tion' of social work that lead practitioners to feel demoralised and alienated from the means of social change to deal with the 'material and modern suffering that is the only certain consequence of neoliberalism' (Bourdieu et al. 2002:183 cited in Rogowski 2010).

A potential, unintended consequence of this grand narrative about neoliberalism is the sense of fatalism and powerlessness that can emerge for some practitioners. This is due to the determinism (or limited capacity to change the consequences) of the modernist discourses. Associated with the truth of objectivism, critical modernist constructions highlight a selective, universal view of reality. This is quite helpful and appropriate when; for example, highlighting the impact of patriarchal structures in gendered power relations. In some situations, however, one universal view that overlooks other potential interpretations can lock practitioners into a version of reality that disempowers them (Morley 2014). Post-structural theories can counteract the limiting aspects of a singular interpretation by emphasising multiple constructions. These include the theories that highlight the gaps and contradictions within dominant discourses that reveal opportunities for opposition and resistance (Morley 2014). In this way, post-structural theories can support the emancipatory goals of modernist critical practices. Fook (2012) notes that the survival of dominant discourses relies on everyone, even those who are most disadvantaged, to accept the discourse's terms. Rogowski (2010), too, highlights practitioner's responsibility to internalise performance targets, increased bureaucratic procedures and financial limitations for neoliberal discourses to continually dominate. The identification of *responsibility* within a critical framework is never about individualising structural problems or blaming the victim, but aims to highlight one's *ability to respond*. Our ability to respond relies on a critical modernist critique of dominant discourses and their colonising/hegemonic power. This critique also relies on post-structural consideration of the polysemic (many-voiced) possibilities for resistance and change. One study that I was involved with illustrates how critical reflection led to strategies that were set to resist and change dominant power relations (Morley 2004). Critical reflection was used by practitioners to contest the economic priorities that dominated social work service provision in their workplace. By identifying and resisting discourses that devalued their work, colluded with exploitative working conditions and undermined solidarity between practitioners, they created strategies to resist dominant power relations within their organisation (Morley 2004). These strategies included refusing to accept management discourses that devalued or set colleagues against each other, avoiding working through lunch breaks, and not working unpaid overtime (Morley 2004).

Others have used critical reflection to expand possibilities for critical practice in organisations dominated by neoliberal priorities (Ferguson 2013; Gardner 2014). Students too, who felt restricted by managerial policies, have used critical reflection to provide creative alternatives (Morley & Macfarlane 2014). As one student from this study commented: 'I am now more conscious of the way I construct power and this provides me with the confidence to challenge practices that I believe to be unethical within my organisation' (Morley & Macfarlane 2014: 348).

While critical reflection involves individual reflection on practice, it is also well documented as a collective practice process (for example, Ferguson 2013; Gardner 2013b; Baker 2013; Thomson 2013). Thomson (2013), for example, discusses critical reflection within the context of his organisation's peer supervision arrangements.

The shared issues identified by the group included 'immediate concern[s], patterns over time, incidents from the past that have not been resolved, such as conflicts, complaints against a worker, frustrations about support, resources, difficulties with working with other individuals, organisations or sectors, relationships with management, work related depression and anxiety' (Thomson 2013: 47). The critical reflective process generated ideas that effected change at both individual and organisational levels, particularly in relation to strengthening the group's position to respond to organisational issues. The goal was to translate the shared learning from their critical reflection into agency policy and procedures (Thomson 2013). In this sense, as Fook (2013: 241) explains, 'Critical reflection on individual workers' experiences can feed into organisational learning by helping to surface, examine and change the fundamental individual (and shared) assumptions about their organisations and their sense of identity within these.'

Therefore, using post-structural thinking to challenge the 'micro-politics of power in every day practice' (Taylor 2013: 86) does not necessarily abandon structural analyses, but can actually provide *additional* strategies to challenge structural power relations (Morley 2014). Another research project that I was involved in used critical reflection to develop new ways of negotiating complex structural problems with the legal response to sexual assault. This was not limited to dismantling formal structures, but aimed to 'critique received wisdom and agitate for change in multiple ways' (Morley 2014: 1). While the structural problems with the legal response to sexual assault persist, developing new ways to think about them facilitated and helped develop alternative, additional practice strategies to address their impact on victim/survivors. A new practice involved practitioners advocating for themselves to be subpoenaed as expert witnesses in court (rather than being silenced and excluded by formal legal processes). This had very direct outcomes for changing existing power relations and facilitating better legal (and socially just) responses and outcomes for victims/survivors (Morley 2014). Hence, an approach to critical reflection that focuses on the individual practitioner's interpretation of discourse and power 'might potentially unsettle some of our assumed ways of thinking about ourselves in relation to the social structure' and therefore 'provide a means and a site for challenging and resisting different forms of domination' (Fook 2004: 16).

Other writers have similarly discussed extending tactics to work towards structural change 'beyond a narrow focus on the collective activities . . . towards a wider appreciation of resistance as multifaceted' (White 2006: 144–5). It is this multifaceted approach that promotes critical reflection's capacity to analyse and change the thoughts and feelings of individual practitioners as well as, or in ways that contribute to, changing dominant power relations and structures.

Arguably, one of the implications of critical reflective practices that generate agency, is their potential for protecting practitioners from 'burnout.' When practitioners can devise ways to practise critically and in keeping with their emancipatory values, they are likely to feel more purposeful, empowered and sustained in their roles for longer (Ferguson 2013; Gardner 2014; Morley 2014).

Challenging conservative thinking and practices

Another way that critical reflection improves critical social work practice is through identifying conservative assumptions that are embedded in our thinking and practice, and aligning our actual practice to our espoused critical theoretical intentions. Importantly, Tseris (2008: 45) reminds us that 'social workers are not immune to the influences of society, so they need to be constantly assessing and questioning their own views and practices, to ensure that they are not in fact, replicating the very things they so vehemently oppose'. Hence, critical reflection can be helpful in challenging the influence of dominant discourses and power relations in our practice.

Another participant in my research recalled a critical incident in which she was silent when police acted in hostile and dismissive ways towards the young person with whom she was working, leaving him without adequate support (Morley 2014). Initially, she justified her complicity with dominant power relations by asserting that if she questioned the conduct of the police, it would have resulted in adverse consequences for herself, the young person or the relationship between the sexual assault service and the police, or all of these outcomes. Given that critical modernist analyses provide a moral framework to show how critical reflection achievements can improve practice (Fook et al. 2006), critical reflective questions were used to expose power disparities between the young person and the police. This highlighted the need for the practitioner's support and advocacy. Critical reflection thus challenged the practitioner's original construction of the incident, and created possibilities for her to name and resist the inappropriate conduct that she had observed. Therefore she more effectively supported the service user; thus aligning her espoused theory with future practice (Morley 2014). At this point, critical post-structuralism helped position the practitioner's initial account as one interpretation among many, which made other 'truths' possible. Post-structuralist conceptions that view power as something people can exert regardless of where they are situated in a structural hierarchy (rather than viewing power as a commodity to possess) also enabled her to reconstruct her perceived disempowered position in relation to the police, thus creating the possibilities to develop a more critical approach to practice (Morley 2014).

Other practitioners have similarly described critical incidents in which they interrogated and changed practices that have not met with their espoused emancipatory aims (Cosier 2008; Tseris 2008). One child safety practitioner used critical reflection to critique the ways that legal and biomedical discourses had infiltrated her thinking and practice. This resulted in coercive practices to pressure the child into having a forensic medical examination. Deconstruction, using critical modernist theories, enabled her to question the dominant discourse constructing the medical examination as the '"normal" thing to do, and . . . that being examined by the doctor is "good for" or in the "best interests" of the patient' (Cosier 2008: 49). Reconstruction, drawing on post-structuralist ideas about exercising power and multiple identities, assisted her to reimagine the steps to take in her practice that better represented the child's interests (Cosier 2008).

Improving critical modernist practices

Critical reflection can parallel the identification and exposure of conservative thinking and practice. By doing this, it can also pinpoint problematic aspects of critical modernist practices that are well-intentioned, yet experienced as oppressive. As Cosier (2008: 47) notes, 'enthusiasm does not guarantee good practice: even the best intentions can be misguided.'

My own practice has been guilty of this phenomenon when using what I thought were critical practice strategies on consciousness-raising, normalising and validating to resist the individualised, depoliticised, pathology-based understandings of mental health that is entrenched by the medical model. My intent to bring a structural and gendered analysis to my practice with a woman called Suzanne who had been sexually assaulted and diagnosed with a mental illness, fell well below my intentions. In my desire to free Suzanne from the hegemonic oppression that I perceived was being driven by the medical model, and relating her experience to the wider sociopolitical environment, I simply replaced psychiatric orthodoxy with modernist critical theories in a way that became another rigid form of ideological domination. Hence, rather than presenting a critical analysis of mental health and opening a way of conversing with her about options, I simply followed through with the medical/ social hierarchical ideas that denied her choice to define her experience in her own terms (Fook & Morley 2005).

Another example from my practice relates to 'protecting' a recent rape survivor from the bullying behaviour of an aggressive detective. My construction of the detective as oppositional 'other', justified some fairly adversarial practice on my behalf, which means my actions failed to match my intention of being collaborative and respectful with colleagues to achieve the best outcomes for service users. In this situation, the focus of my practice moved away from the victim/survivor's needs towards the power struggle with the detective (Morley 2009).

A related example that demonstrates the limitations of modernist critical theories in practice concerns one manager's enthusiastic attempt to introduce critical reflection into team supervision with his staff. Despite his 'best efforts' to formally observe 'anti oppressive' practice principles, the power-laden divide between managers and workers in the workplace context meant that the model was dogmatically imposed, thus reproducing managerial hierarchies to the detriment of emancipatory goals (Baker 2013: 125). Other examples of practices that intend to be 'critical', but fail to be emancipatory in the process include educators who denigrate other students in quite oppressive ways for not being 'critical' enough. This example is mirrored by the situation where students who refuse to be open to learning become disparaging of field education supervisors who do not espouse a critical position (Morley et al. 2014).

In all of these examples, critical reflection exposes problems in the ways that critical modernist perspectives can set up a form of intellectual elitism that imposes in ways that leads to inequitable power relations. In my work with Suzanne, for example, taking on modernist critical theories as universally applicable led me to think that I knew the 'best' way to empower her. Ironically I favoured my perspective and invalidated hers, while casting myself as the powerful, knowledgeable entity in the relationship, which was completely at odds with my intended practice (Fook & Morley 2005). In focusing on what I perceived to be good outcomes (i.e. Suzanne's rejection of the medical model to recognise her responses to sexual assault as legitimate, rather than as a form of self-blaming, I unwittingly used a 'banking model' (Freire 1970) of education. Also evident in the Baker's (2013) example, the banking model bolsters our power as educators rather than leads to a sense of empowerment for the people with whom we work. The post-structural element of critical reflection thus helped draw attention to the *processes* that we engage in when attempting to enact critical goals in practice (rather than solely focusing on outcomes). Post-structuralist-informed critical reflection also offers possibilities that may result in emancipatory outcomes, rather than assuming there is one singular correct way (Fook 2012).

Such insights were directly relevant for critical reflection on my advocacy with the detective (Morley 2009). The grand narratives of feminism initially led me to assume my perspective was right and that the detective was wrong, given that he had a different viewpoint. This construction of the detective as the enemy, set up oppositional power relations, exacerbated conflict that was destructive, and neglected possibilities for me to align myself with him as a potential ally for the service user's benefit. Reconstruction using post-structuralism to overcome binary thinking allowed me to construct our differences as potentially valuable, rather than necessarily polarised. This construction would have led me to a more conciliatory practice that was less distressing for the victim/survivor, without relinquishing the goal of ensuring that her decisions were respected (Morley 2009).

Conclusion

I have argued that critical reflection, when informed by a critically reflexive blend of both modernist and post-structural theories, can greatly improve the emancipatory potential of critical social work practice. While critical modernist and post-structural theories offer different lenses from which to view the social phenomena, the theoretical tensions often lead to more nuanced and sophisticated understandings of theory and practice. I have explored the potential for critical reflection to enhance critical social work practice, especially in relation to identifying and changing conservative thinking and practices. Also, I have explored how this potential can improve our use of critical modernist theories in practice by drawing on post-structural critiques that scrutinise practices that are well-intentioned, yet potentially oppressive. I have included examples that suggest critical reflection can be a useful educational tool for critical practice in neoliberal organisational contexts by connecting practitioners with a sense of agency to create change. I have also presented examples in which critical reflection has been used to generate new ways of thinking about practice that challenge entrenched structural problems that cause oppressive power relations.

References

Allan, J. Briskman, L. & Pease, B. (eds) 2009, *Critical Social Work: Theories and practices for a socially just world,* 2nd edn, St Leonards: Allen & Unwin

Baker, J. 2013, 'Cringe-ical Reflection?: Notes on critical reflection and team supervision in a statutory setting' in J. Fook, & F. Gardner (eds), *Critical Reflection in Context: Applications in health and social care,* London, Routledge, pp. 117–26

Brookfield, S. 2013 *Powerful Techniques for Teaching Adults,* Jossey-Bass, San Francisco

Chambon, A.S., Irving, A. & Epstein, L. (eds) 1999, *Reading Foucault for Social Work,* New York: Columbia University Press

Cosier, W. 2008, 'What part of "No" don't you understand?: Social work, children and consent' in R. Pockett and R. Giles (eds), *Critical Reflection: Generating theory from practice*, Darlington Press, Sydney, pp. 145–61

Dewey, J. 1933, *How We Think: A restatement of the relation of reflective thinking to the educative process,* Boston: Heath

Dominelli, L. 2002, *Feminist Social Work Theory and Practice*, New York: Palgrave

Ferguson, I. 2008, *Reclaiming Social Work: Challenging neoliberalism and promoting social justice*, London: Sage

Ferguson, I. & Lavalette, M. 2006, 'Globalization and global justice: Towards a social work of resistance, *International Social Work,* vol. 49, pp. 309–18

Ferguson, Y. 2013, 'Critical reflection in statutory work' in J. Fook & F. Gardner (eds), *Critical Reflection in Context: Applications in health and social care,* Routledge, London, pp. 83–92

Fook, J. 1993, *Radical Casework: A theory of practice.* St Leonards: Allen and Unwin

—— 2004, 'Critical reflection and transformative possibilities' in L. Davies & P. Leonard (eds), *Social Work in a Corporate Era: Practices of Power and Resistance*, Aldershot: Ashgate, pp. 16–30

—— 2012, *Social Work: A critical approach to practice,* 2nd edn, London: Sage

—— 2013, 'Critical reflection in context: Contemporary perspective and issues' in J. Fook & F. Gardner (eds), *Critical Reflection in Context: Applications in health and social care,* London and New York: Routledge, pp. 1–11

Fook, J. & Askeland, G. 2006, 'The "critical" in critical reflection' in S. White, J. Fook & F. Gardner (eds), *Critical Reflection in Health and Social Care,* Maidenhead: Open University Press, pp. 40–53

Fook, J. & Morley, C. 2005, 'Empowerment: A contextual perspective' in S. Hick, J. Fook & R. Pozzuto (eds), *Social Work: A critical turn,* Toronto: Thompson, pp. 67–85

Fook, J. & Napier, L. 2000, 'From dilemma to breakthrough: Retheorising social work' in L. Napier & J. Fook (eds), *Breakthroughs in Practice: Theorising critical moments in social work*, London: Whiting and Birch, pp. 212–27

Fook, J. & Gardner, F. 2007, *Practicing Critical Reflection: A resource handbook,* Open University Press, Maidenhead, England.

Fook, J. and Gardner, F. 2013, *Critical Reflection in Context: Applications in Health and Social Care,* Routledge, London and New York.Fook, J., White, S. & Gardner, F. 2006, 'Critical reflection: A review of contemporary literature and understandings' in S. White, J. Fook and F. Gardner (eds), *Critical Reflection in Health and Social Care,* Maidenhead: Open University Press, pp. 3–20

Freire, P. 1970, *Pedagogy of the Oppressed,* New York: Herder and Herder

Gardner, F. 2013a, 'Integrating spirituality and critical reflection; toward critical spirituality' in S. White, J. Fook and F. Gardner (eds), *Critical Reflection in Context: Applications in Health and Social Care,* Maidenhead: Open University Press, pp. 28–43

Gardner, F. 2013b 'Using Critical Reflection to Research Practice in a Mental Health Setting,' in, J. Fook & F. Gardner (eds), *Critical Reflection in Context: Applications in Health and Social Care,* Routledge, London and New York, pp. 68–79.

—— 2014, *Being Critically Reflective,* Houndmills: Palgrave Macmillan

Gardner, F., Fook, J. & White, S. 2006, 'Critical reflection: Possibilities for developing effectiveness in conditions of uncertainty, in eds S. White, J. Fook and F. Gardner (eds), *Critical Reflection in Context: Applications in Health and Social Care,* Maidenhead: Open University Press , pp. 228–40

Giroux, H. 2011, *On Critical Pedagogy,* Continuum: New York.

Healy, K. 2000, *Social Work Practices: Contemporary perspectives on change,* London: Sage

Holscher, D. & Sewpaul, V. 2006, 'Ethics as a site of resistance: The tension between social control and critical reflection' *Research Report,* vol. 1, pp. 251–72

Kolb, D.A. 1984, *Experiential Learning,* Englewood Cliffs: Prentice Hall

Lavalette, M. (ed.) 2011, *Radical Social Work Today: Social work at the crossroads,* Bristol: Policy Press

Leonard, P. 1997, *Postmodern Welfare,* Sage, London.

Madhu, P. 2011, 'Praxis intervention: Towards a new critical social work practice' *SSRN eLibrary* <http://

ssrn.com/paper=1765143>

Marchant, H. & Wearing, B. 1986, *Gender Reclaimed: Women in social work*. Sydney: Hale and Iremonger,

Moreau, M. 1979, 'A structural approach to social work practice' *Canadian Journal of Social Work Education,* vol. 5, no. 1, pp. 78–94

Morley, C. 2004, 'Critical reflection as a response to globalisation?' *International Journal of Social Welfare*, vol. 13, no. 2, pp. 297–303

—— 2008, 'Developing critical reflection as a research methodology' in P. Liamputtong & J. Rumbold (eds), *Knowing Differently: An introduction to experiential and arts-based research methods,* New York: Nova Science Publishers, pp. 265–80

—— 2009, 'Developing feminist practices' in J. Allan, B. Pease & L. Briskman (eds), *Critical Social Work: An introduction to theories and practices*, St Leonards: Allen & Unwin, pp. 145–59

—— 2011, 'Critical reflection as an educational process: A practice example' *Advances in Social Work and Welfare Education: Special Issue—Critical Reflection Method and Practice*, vol. 13, no. 1, pp. 7–21

—— 2012, 'How does critical reflection develop emancipatory possibilities for emancipatory change? An example from an empirical research project', *British Journal of Social Work*, vol. 42, no. 8, pp. 1513–32

—— 2014, *Practising Critical Reflection to Develop Emancipatory Change: Challenging the legal response to sexual assault*, Aldershot: Ashgate

Morley, C. & Macfarlane, S. 2012, 'The nexus between postmodernism and feminism: Still a central concern for critical social work', *British Journal of Social Work*, vol. 42, no. 4, pp. 687–705

—— 2014, 'Critical social work as ethical social work: Using critical reflection to research students' resistance to neoliberalism, *Critical and Radical Social Work,* vol. 2, no. 3, pp. 337–55

Morley, C., Macfarlane, S. & Ablett, P. 2014, *Engaging with Social Work: A critical introduction*, Melbourne: Cambridge

Mullaly, B. 2010, *Challenging Oppression and Confronting Privilege,* 2nd edn, Ontario: Oxford University Press

Naudi, M. 2006, 'Disrupting dominant discourses: Critical reflection and code-switching in Maltese social work' in S. White, J. Fook and F. Gardner (eds), *Critical Reflection in Health and Social Care*, Maidenhead: Open University Press, pp. 118–31

Noble, C. 2004, 'Postmodern thinking: Where is it taking social work?', *Journal of Social Work*, vol. 4, no. 3, pp. 289–304

Pease, B. & Fook, J. (eds) 1999, *Transforming Social Work Practice: Postmodern critical perspectives*, St Leonards: Allen & Unwin

Pockett, R. & Giles, R. 2008, *Critical Reflection: Generating theory from practice: The graduating social work student experience*, Sydney: Darlington Press

Rogowski, S. 2010, *Social Work: The rise and fall of a profession?*, Bristol: The Policy Press

Schon, D. 1987, *Educating the Critically Reflective Practitioner: Toward a new design for teaching and learning in the professions*, San Francisco: Jossey-Bass

Taylor, C. 2006, 'Practicing reflexivity: Narrative, reflection and the moral order' in S. White, J. Fook, & F. Gardner (eds), *Critical Reflection in Health and Social Care*, Open University Press, Maidenhead, pp. 73–88

—— 2013, 'Critically reflective practice' in M. Gray & S. Webb (eds), *The New Politics of Social Work,* Houndmills: Palgrave Macmillan

Thompson, N, 2011, *Promoting Equality: Working with Diversity and Difference,* 3rd edn, Palgrave Macmillan, Houndmills.

Thomson, G. 2013, 'Not beating around the bush: Critical reflection in a rural community health service' in J. Fook & F. Gardner (eds), *Critical Reflection in Context: Applications in health and social care,* London: Routledge

Trevelyan, C., Crath, R. & Chambon, A. 2012, 'Promoting critical reflexivity through arts-based media: A case study, *British Journal of Social Work*, vol. 44, no. 1. pp. 7–26

Tseris, E. 2008, 'Examining these words we use: 'Participation', 'empowerment', and the child protection role', in R. Pockett and R. Giles (eds), *Critical reflection: Generating theory from practice*, Sydney: Darlington Press, pp. 30–44

Wallace, J. & Pease, B. 2011, 'Neoliberalism and Australian social work: Accommodation or resistance?', *Journal of Social Work,* vol. 11, pp. 132–42

White, V. 2006, *The State of Feminist Social work*, London and New York: Routledge

3

Towards critical social work supervision

Carolyn Noble

Introduction

This chapter explores professional supervision informed by a critical analysis. Informing supervision practice with critical analysis can potentially resist the influence of the current oppressive neo-conservative climate. This critically informed practice can also potentially counterweigh the devaluing of social work's social justice and human rights principles. Critical social work theory articulates an alternative vision to the existing social, political, economic and cultural institutions and practices that result in the uneven distribution of society's resources and riches, and access to political representation and power for a large majority of the population. Critical social work theory is underpinned by a commitment to social justice where the naming and elimination of injustice is its central concern (Mullaly 2010; Barnes 2011). When applied to supervision, critical social work theory requires both supervisors and those being supervised to question how social work's policy, research, education and practice responses are constructed by the current sociopolitical, cultural and economic context and to review their impact on people's lives and societal and organisational arrangements. By developing an approach to practice that engages with critical theory, the structure of supervision moves from administrative, supportive, organisational and mediative functions towards a more pivotal site of social resistance informed by a social justice and human rights activism. This is an essential aspect of critical social work theory.

Social work supervision in context

The gradual dismantling of the welfare state and the reduction of social services, resources and welfare programs that have accompanied the rise in neoliberalism, managerialism and fiscal restriction on state spending in favour of the 'market' is receiving a much welcomed critique. This is especially from scholars and practitioners who are interested in promoting a socially just, inclusive and more equal society (Noble 2004; Jamrozik 2009). The gradual move towards almost full privatisation of public assets and services, contracting out of services to market operators, introducing competition between service providers and reducing overall funding for government programs has created an unfamiliar landscape for social work practice to work within its moral and philosophical mandate (Jamrozik 2009). National and state governments are no longer defining themselves as major service providers for individuals' wellbeing through organised social intervention (Jamrozik 2009). Concurrently, public confidence in social workers has diminished as highly publicised cases of poor professional practice, evident in child protection, mental health, domestic and family violence, paedophilia, the treatment of asylum seekers, the elderly and people with disabilities, have further challenged the probity of social work practice (Dominelli 2009).

The integrity, or probity, in social work practice is also being challenged by the rise in discontent led by service users about the lack of their voice and resulting invisibility in the sociopolitical and cultural landscape, and the lack of opportunity to lobby for their rights as citizens. This is despite the field of social work's commitment to empowering the less fortunate in the way that society organises its resources and riches, socially, politically, culturally and economically (Gray & Webb 2012; 2013). Social work is experiencing a crisis in its ability to respond in any meaningful way to the large-scale social problems arising from the sociopolitical, cultural conservatism and associated marketised, risk-adverse, consumerist society of the neoliberal philosophy (Jamrozik 2009; Wallace & Pease 2011) This neoliberal culture, which is increasingly shaping the Australian welfare sector, provides a challenge for social work's emancipatory stance to resist oppression and discrimination and undo privilege (Pease 2010). To meet this challenge, Gray and Webb demand a rethink of a critically theory-informed political practice, a new politics for social work 'in the belief that it bears a public responsibility to confront injustice while seeking justice for all' (Gray &Webb 2013: 3).

It is in response to this clarion call to action, that professional supervision can be pivotal in re-engaging practitioners and their clients with a critical framework. They can play an integral part in a reinvigorated critical social work practice. As an essential component of social work practice, supervision can lead practice in new and effective ways to ensure the needs of the service users remain at the centre of the interaction (Wonnacott 2012). At the same time, it is important to re-engage with a theory and practice that challenges the inequalities and structural barriers based on class, gender, ability, sexual preferences, cultural and religious affiliations, and the way sociopolitical, economic and cultural relations are formed and supported by those who are the power elites and have vested interests (Noble 2011a; Hosken 2013).

Professional social work supervision

Traditionally, supervision has been discussed as providing a supportive, educational, administrative and mediative function for effective practice where supervisors are regarded as expert overseers of social workers at the start of their careers. Also, supervisors are expert practitioners who provide personal, administrative, organisational, and professional development for those being supervised in order to make connections between events and action, theory and practice and organisational management (Kadushin & Harkness 2002). Cooper (2002) suggests that supervisors can have an advocacy role and a responsibility to make sure they know their rights and responsibilities towards the person being supervised. Tsui (2005) argues that supervision should model the field education practicum, with allocated regular time and set agendas so that both parties are prepared and follow a set framework. The content should be comprehensive and cover practice, policy, skill development, and the integration of theory with practice and vice versa. Importantly, there should be time allocated for reflection and review, and to link discussions about cases, issues and workplace dilemmas with practice standards and contemporary intellectual endeavours. These discussions should also be linked to discoveries of interest and relate to a critical approach to practice and policy debates (Tsui 2005; Noble & Irwin 2009; Carroll & Gilbert 2011).

The practice of supervision, according to Hair and O'Donoghue (2009), has to be culturally sensitive, contextually specific and also pursue a social justice agenda. O'Donoghue (2003) argues further that social work needs a restoried practice for supervision; one that would not only pay more critical attention to the issues, dilemmas and concerns discussed in supervision but focus on how these issues, concerns, dilemmas are influenced by the personal, local and global influences, already hinted at earlier in this chapter. Noble and Irwin (2009) are concerned that current practices in supervision prevent supervisors and those being supervised from tapping into new knowledge and research and from reflecting on how they manage the tensions between the 'new' management and a desire for client empowerment and societal change. Hosken (2013) argues that if the goal of supervision is to mini-mise or challenge discrimination, oppression and privilege then it needs to be shaped by a degree of humility rather than competence. This can be done by focusing on the experience of the least privileged, which are usually the clients or those being supervised or both (Hosken 2013). I believe supervision should be used as a means for practitioners to fully engage with a critical theory–informed practice as current policies, rituals and methods continue to focus more on social control and support for the status quo rather than human rights and social justice outcomes for service users and individual practitioners alike (Noble 2011a; 2012).

An overview of critical theory

Critical theory for the helping professions is most comprehensive in the social work literature, where many scholars have conceptualised, extended, analysed, reconcep-tualised and debated its efficacy and relevance for many years now (Allan et al. 2009; Dominelli 2009; Mullaly 2010; Barnes 2011; Lundy 2011; Gray & Webb 2013). As a meta-narrative, (or explanation of social order and social change) it takes its stating point that assumptions about reason, order, predictability and human nature are just that, assumptions. These assumptions need to be critically interrogated with a variety of lenses such as gender, age, ethnicity, ability, sexuality and class. Cultural, historical and ideological heritages are to be questioned as well as the impact of these heritages on both the individual and the social, political, economic, cultural and environmental systems that are assumed as given, inevitable and part of the 'natural order'. Many frameworks are available for this questioning from feminist, Marxist/socialist, anti-oppressive, anti-adultist and critical 'race' theories, including an analysis of whiteness and power and privilege as well as increased political agency around social change and social collective/movement action. Critical theorists high-light the centrality of people's agency, that is, their capacity to be actively involved in the process of social change. Linking personal experiences with experiences of domination encourages those affected by oppressive ideologies and social practices to take action, resist and eventually transform social conditions (Noble 2007; Mullaly 2009; Barnes 2011; Lundy 2011; Gray & Webb 2012).

Forming a critical approach to social work supervision

A critical theory–informed supervision framework has the potential to identify the individual, organisational and societal challenges in the context of practice (Noble 2012). A good place to start this process is by replacing current administrative, managerial and functional processes associated with supervision with a critical gaze that names, identifies and explores the contradictions and cultural complexities in the daily work of practitioners. By linking personal struggles within the context of public systemic constraints, the complexities and uncertainties associated with the new economic order (and how practice scenarios and social problems reflect them) can be more readily addressed. Exploring the influences of diversity and enhancing both the supervisors' and supervisees' responsiveness to cultural scripts (patterns of interaction unique to a particular culture) is also an important aspect of this work (Hair & O'Donoghue 2009). Hosken (2013) argues that supervisors should explore the notion of cultural humility when interrogating one's sense of privilege and, for Australians with Anglo-Celtic backgrounds, they should explore the impact of whiteness on the creation and perpetuation of discriminatory practices. In addressing the issues within a reworked critical theory framework, supervision might be where social change strategies and theories can be modelled, and thus create the much-needed opportunity for a critical approach to supervision to emerge (Noble 2011a; 2011b).

By deconstructing societal and personal beliefs, ideas, histories, meanings, cultural scripts, cultural biases and stereotypes, the underlying intentions and the various social ideas, and power influences are named and challenged, thus fostering a critical capacity to resist these oppressive structures and practices. Underlying this critique is a clearly defined philosophical and value-based stance that includes a social justice and human rights perspective, where developments in critical postmodernist theory and critical race theory extend the critique (Mullaly 2010; Baines 2011; Lundy 2011).

Critical social work theory and social work supervision

A critical social work theory is one that aims to eliminate domination, exploitation, oppression and all undemocratic and inequitable social, political and economic relations that marginalise and oppress many groups in society; that offers privileges for a few, while oppressing many (Mullaly 2010; Baines 2011; Lundy 2011). Significantly, critical social work theory challenges and names the more complex interaction (intersectionality) of class, gender, ethnicity, race, caste, sexuality, and physical and mental health norms (to name a few). These operate on multiple, and often simultaneous levels, and reinforce systemic inequality and oppression. By fostering discussion between various marginalised voices oppressed by this intersectionality (Kincheloe 2008; Giroux 2011), connections with the lived experiences and the making of reality are to be explored and challenged. The task of unmasking these connections are a collective, shared social enterprise in which all the participants' voices are heard equally and where a more socially-just world is envisioned (Kincheloe 2008; Giroux 2011).

Marston, McDonald and Bryson (2014) make a strong case for supporting a politics of resistance, as they argue that politically frontline social workers are traditionally disorganised, citing lack of time, energy, resources, assertiveness, political verve and or conviction to take up active politics. This exposes the weakness of social work as a professional pressure and advocacy group, which is unable to tackle issues that impact on them and their clients from different forms of subordination and discrimination (Marston et al. 2014).

While supervision can use many forms: individual, peer, group and communities of practice, it is primarily aimed to provide both the supervisor(s) and those being supervised with an opportunity to develop, explore, enrich and integrate theory and practice while in the process of 'doing' (Noble 2011b). Applying a critical lens to supervision work will help scrutinise the dominant ideologies in social work practices and workplace relations, and pinpoint local problems in the larger sociopolitical, economic and cultural framework. The aim is to take critical social work theory seriously and self-reflect while engaging with this approach. A reframed supervisory relationship and practice is where practitioners, students and workplaces can, by using critical reflective tools, address the tensions, contradictions, ambiguities and conflicts that result from this exploration (Noble 2011). It is also a site for possible resistances that Marston et al. (2014) and Gray and Webb (2013) argue for to reject the defeatism that prevails in the profession. It is an opportunity for the pressing issues associated with current practice concerns to be discussed, where social work professionals can reflect personally and professionally, and act as required (Noble 2011b).

Developing a critical focus in terms of critically reflective processes

Critical theory applied to social work supervision can draw some ideas from the literature on critical pedagogies, which is most extensively discussed by the critical educationalists such as Friere (1974). Kincheloe (2008), hooks (2009), Giroux (2011) and Freire (1974) argue that education can be used as either an instrument to help learners deal critically and creatively with reality to transform it through participatory action or integrate learners into the oppressive current system by means of conformity and social control. For Kincheloe (2008) and Giroux (2011), pedagogy in the critical sense illuminates the relationship among knowledge, authority and power. Hooks (2009) specifically focuses on 'white' people's ways of being, feeling, seeing and knowing as the basis informing the Westcentrism in the Western curriculum which privileges students from more mainstream societal cultural norms, while alienating students whose cultural histories and traditions are subordinated or excluded or both. Its practice, then, is embedded in notions of social justice, democracy, human rights, empowered citizenry, democratic relations, emancipation, academic freedoms and alternative discourses to the neoliberal status quo and cannot be understood outside the framework of critical theory. Critical pedagogy leaves no possibility for a neutral educational process; it is a politicised methodology and it takes us into deep waters with its provocations.

Developing a critical focus means concentrating on the interactive aspects of practice experiences and situations in the sociopolitical, economic and cultural relations of power by applying critically reflective processes. For supervision, it would include reflecting on the particular interpretations of:

- the relationship
- the 'work' of the supervision; that is, what is discussed and what is left at the door
- the structure, context and associated tasks, discussion and reflections that are undertaken in the sessions. This is by way of making explicit the interpretations, assumptions, knowledge, behaviours in oneself, organisation, and communities of practice, and the work with clients, policy and research practices.
- how these methods are mediated by language, discourse and power relations.

In this sense, supervisors are responsible for maximising the supervisory experience and encouraging those being supervised to learn, reflect, then learn and reflect again; that is, participate in the circle of learning that leads to transformative and teachable experiences. The supervisor also plays a key role in this cyclical learning process as partner in the learning experience. This exploration can cover such aspects as: linking critical theory, critical thinking and critical practice; uncovering underlying beliefs and assumptions in all practice situations about how social problems and issues are experienced, discussed and addressed. This includes asking what was done in the practice, policy or research context, why, by whom, to what end and for whose purpose in order to challenge and change its impact. Other aspects of the cyclical learning process include the structural effects on knowledge construction, and sociopolitical and cultural behaviour, and how to maximise the supervision relationship to develop skills for lifelong learning and make critical reflections an essential part of social work practice beyond the supervision sessions (Noble 2011a; 2011b).

This also means democratising the supervision process and valuing differences in interpretations, experiences, and learning. It also requires a critique of the hierarchal nature of the relationship and the difference in power and authority (Jones 2004; Noble & Irwin 2009). These restrictions place strict boundaries around the use and purpose of supervision, inhibiting new and challenging discussions to emerge. Critical reflection demands that supervision sessions confront differences in power, gender and ethnicity, as well as cultural and other structural barriers and how they impact on service delivery, and make service users' lives and opportunities more explicit and conscious in the supervisory process (Fook & Gardner 2007 Taylor 2014). For example, discussions should address the following issues:

- How are gender, class, ethnic positions as well as sexual preferences and ability incorporated and discussed in the supervision relationship and in the organisational logic and function of the workplace?
- What counts as legitimate knowledge in social work?
- How are power issues addressed in supervision where the preferred model is one-on-one sessions with a supervisor who is also the person who holds power (administrative and managerial authority) of the supervisee?
- How can supervision be equal and encompass a shared experience if the supervisor is the acknowledged expert in the relationship and that this expertise is the basis on which the relationship is formed and developed? Explore what would hinder a democratic relationship and collegial professional interaction.
- How is social work's aim to address disadvantage and abide by oppressed and marginalised people who are mediated in the context of managerial control and evidence-based imperatives of a new conservative order?

Social work supervision: building a critical framework

There are many pedagogical methods that can be adapted from the literature that is quoted in the previous section to aid how critical analysis can be used effectively to build a critical framework for use in social work supervision. Methods include issue-based learning, problem-based learning; critical reflection, critical incident analysis, constructive and transformative learning techniques which include the use of narratives, autobiographical texts, journalling, storytelling, memoir, diaries, blogs and other creative endeavours that emphasise process and authorship as a means of social change and empowerment. Importantly, incorporating supervisees' experiences is also crucial to the process. The reflection and articulation of their lived experiences such as personal confessions, testimonies, and the exploration of different experiences can present a knowledge base from their viewpoints and develop an alternative approach. That is, they can articulate a critical theory informed-practice stance (Noble 2011; 2012). Hosken (2013) has developed what she calls a mutual inquiry approach to supervision to reduce discrimination that is based on humility, using concepts and practices drawn from experience, intersectionality and institutional ethnography.

In the next section I will explore two approaches that are inextricably linked to critical theory that can be used in social work supervision: critical reflection and transformative learning.

Critical reflection

Critical reflection is created by the continual cycle of questions; answers and reflection; reflections on what was done, why, to what effect, and who are the beneficiaries. It is a practice that deconstructs the social, cultural and political structures that shape current content, context and relationships that are embedded in the issues to enable a critical stance to emerge (Fook & Gardner 2007; Taylor 2013. Kincheloe (2008) likens it to creating a three-dimnesional vision that sees through the masks that hide vested interests, power monopolies, inherited and 'white' privilege, gender bias and elitist practices. It involves thinking about and critically analysing the supervisee's work, experiences, thoughts and actions with the goal of improving professional practice towards socially just outcomes.

Critical reflection, both as a process and a technique, is about improving practice, challenging the teaching of technologies and competency-based criteria that is currently dominating the acquisition of professional practice knowledge and skills (Australian Association of Social Workers, AASW, 2012). Reflective work also addresses the separation of theory from the experience of practice. The push for a more critically reflective pedagogy comes from the belief that supervisory processes should be linked to the social justice and human rights principles of critical social work practice. Emphasising the capacity to identify then challenge existing power relations that discriminate and exploit marginalised groups within a self-reflective framework, critical reflection focuses directly on the teaching and learning from inside the professional supervision relationship (Giroux 2011; Noble 2011a). Critical reflection is a useful tool to assist oppressed groups in challenging existing institutions, dominant ideology, and oppressive practices and power relations to resist their overwhelming influence and control. Social workers need to be aware of the ways that their position may embody class, race, gender and sexual privilege (Pease 2006).

Critical reflection is not for the faint-hearted, for embedded in its practice is the expectation that the supervisor and supervisee are willing to make public their assumptions, values, biases, uncertainties, frustrations, stereotypes and dilemmas that underpin their actions and decision-making. It requires practitioners to reflect upon their complicity in reinforcing dominant power relations and their role in reproducing privilege and inequality (Pease 2006). In so doing, this practice uncovers subjugated knowledges, to explore what has been hidden from view by the dominant culture. In making visible other forms of knowledge, experience, cultural artefacts and traditions, a new vision of themselves can be created, including their practice and new ways of acting in the world (Noble 2011a). The linking of old knowledge with new knowledge leads to deeper understanding of issues and skills, and change in a meaningful way by what is learnt (Fook & Gardner 2007; Giles et al. 2010). There is no end point to this process, but a neverending journey of reflection, action and ongoing analysis. However, what is learnt can be used in unfamiliar situations and the complexities and changing nature of the current social work setting (Giles et al. 2010). Critical reflective questions include the following:

- Can you say what previous experiences or knowledge informed your actions?
- What was the source of that knowledge and how is such knowledge produced and disseminated?
- What other ways of looking at the situation can you imagine?
- Can you articulate the particular theories that you used?
- Can you identify the values that underpin your action?
- Can you make explicit your feelings and the meaning of what you did? Why? To what effect?
- Who benefitted from your actions? How?
- Who was disadvantaged by your actions? How?
- What were the consequences?
- Were there alternatives? What were they?
- Were there any constraints on your action? (for example, time, resources, agency policy, agency culture, your own skills)
- What, if anything, would you do differently?
- Was there a desired outcome that was different from the actual outcome?
- On reflection, would you act the same way again?

Transformative learning

Transformative learning is interlinked with the practice of critical reflection. In many ways it is the outcome of this process that is of value to this discussion. It is about shifting attitudes, life meanings, personal and professional consciousness in ways that change the person's world view; that is, it moves surface learning to deep learning (Giles et al. 2010). Deep learning occurs when links are made between the private and the public, the ideal and the reality, the obvious and the hidden, and when conclusions as to the authenticity of the presented claim are reviewed (Noble 2011a). The subject matter or experience being explored is put under the microscope; so too are the assumptions, biases and stereotypes, and the power of symbols and discourses that are embedded in the language used, as well as the very nature of knowledge itself (Giles et al. 2010). Its links with critical theory are further explored when how class, gender and race, as interlocking structures, are analysed and defined as to who has power and how that power is exercised. Another aspect is reflecting on how emotions are constructed and manipulated for certain responses (such as anger, guilt, despair, fear) in the private and public setting. The outcome and process are linked. Transformative questions include the following:

- What constitutes knowledge?
- Whose knowledge is privileged?
- How is such knowledge produced and disseminated?
- What strategies are available for challenging the basis of knowledge?
- Why is this important for the theory and practice interrogation and integration in supervision?
- How does socioeconomic and cultural inequality along the lines of race, gender, class, sexuality, religion, and language influence the answers to these questions?

Conclusion

This chapter explores social work supervision that uses critical reflection and transformative learning that engages with critical theory. Applying a critical theory-based approach to social work supervision means that social problems and issues are analysed as public concerns, which are structurally produced. The challenge is to deconstruct the walls of power that mask these advantages, disadvantages and oppressive acts to create a socially just and democratically informed citizenry that is based on human rights and social change strategies. If social work is serious about committing to a critical theory stance, then a critical lens needs to focus on its supervisory practices as a means of changing the world towards its emancipatory aims.

References

Allan, J., Briskman, L. & Pease, B. (eds) 2009, *Critical Social Work: Theories and practices for a socially just world,* 2nd edn, St Leonards: Allen & Unwin

Australian Association of Social Workers (AASW). 2012, 'Australian Social Work Education and Accreditation Standards', *AASW*, <http://www.aasw.asn.au/document/item/3550>, accessed 10 May 2014

Baines, D. (ed.) 2011, *Anti-Oppressive Practice: Social justice social work*, 2nd edn, Halifax: Fernwood Publications

Carroll, M. & Gilbert, M. 2011, *On Being a Supervisee: Creating leaning partnerships*, 2nd edn, Melbourne: PsychOz Publications

Cooper, L. 2002, 'Social work supervision: A social justice perspective' in M. McMahon & W. Patton (eds), *Supervision in the Helping Professions: A practical approach*, Sydney: Pearson Education, pp. 185–95

Dominelli, L. 2009, *Introducing Social Work*, Cambridge: Cambridge University Press

Fook, J. & Gardner, F. 2007, *Practising Critical Reflection: A resource handbook*, Maidenhead: Open University Press

Freire, P. 1974 (reprinted 2013), *Education for Critical Consciousness*, London: Bloomsbury Academic

Gray, M. & Webb, S. (eds) 2012, *Social Work Theories and Methods*, London: Sage

—— (eds) 2013, *The New Politics of Social Work*, London: Palgrave MacMillan

Giles, R., Irwin, J., Lynch, D. & Waugh, F. (eds) 2010, *In the Field: From learning to practice,* South Melbourne: Oxford University Press

Giroux, H. 2011, *On critical pedagogy*, New York: The Continuum International Pub. Co.

Hair, J. & O'Donoghue, K. 2009, 'Culturally relevant, socially just social work supervision: Becoming visible through a social constructionist lens', *Journal of Ethnic and Cultural Diversity in Social Work*, vol. 18, no. 1, pp. 70–88

hooks, b. 2009, *Teaching Critical Thinking: Practical wisdom*, London: Routledge

Hosken, N. 2013, 'Social work supervision and discrimination', *Advances in Social Work and Welfare Education*, vol. 15, no. 1, pp. 92–104

Jamrozik, A. 2009, *Social Policy in The Post-Welfare State: Australian society in a changing world*, 3rd edn, Sydney: Pearson Education Australia

Jones, M. 2004, 'Supervision, learning and transformative practices' in N. Gould and M. Baldwin (eds), *Social Work, Critical Reflection and the Learning Organisation*, Aldershot: Ashgate, pp. 11–22

Kadushin, A. & Harkness, D. 2002, *Supervision in Social Work,* New York: Columbia University Press

Kinocheloe, J. 2008, *Critical Pedagogy Primer*, New York: Peter Lang Publications

Lundy, C. 2011, *Social Work, Social Justice and Human Rights: A structural approach to practice*, Ontario: University of Toronto Press

Marston, G., McDonald, C. & Bryson, L. 2014, *The Australian Welfare State: Who benefits now?*, Melbourne: Palgrave Macmillan

Mullaly, B. 2010, *Challenging Oppression, Confronting Privilege,* 2nd edn, London: Oxford University Press

Noble, C. & Irwin, J. 2009, 'Social work supervision: An exploration of the current challenges in a rapidly changing social, economic and political environment', *Journal of Social Work,* vol. 9, no. 3, pp. 345–58

Noble, C. 2004, 'Postmodern Thinking: Where is it taking social work?', *Journal of Social Work*, vol. 4, no. 3, pp. 289–304

—— 2007 'Social Work, collective action and social movements' in L. Dominelli (ed.), *Revitalising Communities in a Globalising World,* London: Ashgate, pp. 95–106

—— 2011a, 'Field education: Supervision, curricula and teaching methods' in C. Noble & M. Henrickson (eds), *Social Work Field Education and Supervision across Asia Pacific,* Sydney University Press, Sydney, pp. 3–22

—— 2011b, 'Ways of thinking about field education and supervision: Building a critical perspective' in C. Noble and M. Henrickson (eds), *Social work field education and supervision across Asia Pacific*, Sydney: Sydney University Press, pp. 299–320

—— 2012, 'Social work and the Asia-Pacific: From rhetoric to practice', in C. Noble, M. Henrickson & I.Y. Han (eds), *Social Work Education; Voices from the Asia-Pacific*, 2nd edn, Sydney: Sydney University Press, pp. 343–66

O'Donoghue, K. 2003, *Re-storying Social Work Supervision*, Palmerston North: Dunmore Press

Pease, B. 2006, 'Encouraging critical reflection on privilege in social work and human services', *Practice Reflections*, vol. 1, no. 1, pp. 15–26

—— 2010, *Undoing privilege: Unearned advantage in a divided world*, London: Zed Books

Taylor, C. 2013, 'Critical reflective practice' in M. Gray & S. Webb (eds), *The New Politics of Social Work*, New York: Palgrave Macmillan, pp. 79–97

Tsui, M. 2005, *Social Work Supervision: Contexts and concepts*, Thousand Oaks: Sage

Wallace, J. and Pease, B. (2011) 'Neoliberalism and Australian social work: Accommodation or resistance?' Journal of Social Work, vol. 11, no. 2, pp. 132–142.

Wonnacott, J. 2012, *Mastering Social Work Supervision,* London: Jessica Kingsley

4

Making sense of different theoretically informed approaches in doing critical social work

Norah Hosken and Sophie Goldingay

Introduction

Historically, there have been tensions between modernist structural approaches and postmodern approaches to critical social work. Despite commonalities, modernist and postmodernist critical social work academics and practitioners have been cautious of what their counterparts have to offer. Some of this tension relates to a range of subtle, and more fundamental, differences regarding (among other things) views on truth and reality, power, agency, normative morals, collectivity and universality.

This chapter explores a practice case example with responses from a modernist tradition (Norah Hosken) and from a postmodern tradition (Sophie Goldingay). Areas of commonality and difference are acknowledged as modernist structural and postmodern approaches to critical social work. Both approaches strive towards creating more socially just situations, and emancipatory personal and social change.

Critical social work

The authors share an understanding of critical social work that includes a range of social work practice approaches that are primarily informed by critical theories (Allan, Briskman & Pease 2009). Both authors desire social justice involving social equality that is informed by feminist theories. They see critical social work as focused on emancipatory personal and social change (Allan 2009). There are differences in how the authors place themselves in terms of the degree of influence of postmodern insights for the practice of critical social work.

One of the hallmarks of ethical social work practice is developing critical aware-ness of our social location and 'use of self' during practice (Marlowe, Appleton, Chinnery & Van Stratum 2015). An ability to understand our own positioning, values, beliefs and perceptions and those of others, and how these influence how we practise is integral to ethical social work practice. In the next section we explore how each of our theoretical understandings have been shaped by our own personal biographies and professional experiences.

Socialist-feminist-informed social work: Norah's perspective

Working and learning with co-workers and service users in women's refuges and community legal centres in the early stages of my paid work fundamentally shaped how I understand power, oppression, diversity, resistance and hope. My under-standing is that the problems that social workers and service users experience are primarily caused by hardships that are entrenched in relations of inequality and exploitation. These are inherent in different forms of capitalism, patriarchy, coloni-alism, and other systems of inequality.

My critical social work practice is based on a socialist-feminist understanding that the inequities, particularly the structural violence of poverty (primarily gener-ated by the capitalist market system), underpins much social work practice (see Chapter 7). Socialist-feminist social workers advocate the necessity to consider and challenge the way economic, gender, colonial and other stratifying processes cause injustice and poverty (Noble 2004), that recognises different social locations but works towards a common feminist emancipatory political vision around shared values such as egalitarianism, publicly funded welfare and human rights to achieve transformative change (Yuval-Davis 2016; Dominelli 2002). From this perspective, service users' and social workers' opportunities to control or change things are best understood as 'agency within structure' (Orton 2009: 496) as 'generally, constrained or enabled within people or groups' positions in the relations of structural inequality.

This constraint on the individual agency of workers and service users is one reason why working in solidarity with others is so important.

Challenging and transforming the inequalities that underpin social work practice entails fundamental change to reverse economic dominance over the social sphere. The socialist-feminist position taken here matches Nancy Holmstrom's arguments that although the capitalist economic, political and cultural system has enabled some important gains for some women, capitalism inherently requires a 'pyramid of inequality' (Cudd & Holmstrom 2011: 298).

Socialist-feminist social work is committed to a feminist emancipatory politics that relies on shared value judgements about the causes of material and discursive inequalities and oppression. These judgements need to be formed and critiqued from the position of collaborative inquiry, particularly from the standpoints of those most marginalised (Smith 2005). Critical social work from this perspective is done in solidarity with others in local and global social justice movements who share visions for social justice to prioritise social values over economic ones to create 'socialism from below' (Cudd & Holmstrom 2011: 254).

This approach accepts change towards the greater economic and social equality that is a major part of social justice will involve conflict as corporate owners, leaders and others benefitting most from capitalism's 'pyramid of inequality' (Cudd & Holmstrom 2011: 298) resist giving up, or sharing, power, wealth and privilege. From this approach, I share concerns (for example, Houston 2001; Noble 2004) that 'pure' post-structuralism implies conservatism for social work where:

> deconstruction, to the point of denying commonalities, is not theo-
> retically or politically useful ... because this ... withdraws the tools
> for recognition ... of the ways in which factors such as social class,
> race or gender can impact upon one's life and access to power (Archer,
> Hutchings, & Leathwood 2001: 46).

In terms of acknowledging and respecting diversity of experiences with emancipa-tory politics, I agree with Yuval-Davis (1994) and see more potential for social justice in a political environment based on common aims that endeavour to maintain the 'situated viewpoints of all involved', as compared to a politics solely based on the identity of who we are' (Archer et al. 2001: p. 57).

Postmodern/post-structural informed social work: Sophie's perspective

My background is practising social work in institutionalised environments, such as the forensic psychiatric service, community mental health, and the public prison service, over a 22-year period. In these environments, social work has not been the core business of the agency that has employed me. Rather, the goal of each of these services could be described as containment or management of the client group, with allied professionals having a discrete role within this service. As discussed in Chapter 11, a critical approach to social work using a postmodern approach aims to enable workers to transform what is oppressive to both workers and clients through a localised, flexible, pragmatic and contextual approach to critical social work practice (Allan 2009; Fook 2012).

A critical postmodern approach is characterised by embracing multiple perspectives on what constitutes truth, which is seen as context dependent and contingent (Burr 2003). In addition, a critical postmodern approach as influenced by post-structuralism, focuses on the role of language in the construction and maintenance of power relations. The meanings we give to reality are based on our discourses about it (Fook 2012). As such, the discursive context is the site and target of intervention. The process of intervention involves examining the discursive context to unpack the process, which leads to limiting versions of what constitutes legitimate truth and its effects. After deconstruction, creative strategies to transform the discursive context can begin (Fook 2012).

My experience of working in mental health and prison settings has strongly influenced my connection with a critical postmodern and critical post-structural approach, as have my personal experiences. During my childhood I observed that those who were able to exercise power and influence in my family and beyond were the ones who were able to make their truth claims stick—the ones who were able to say which version of events or character constructions were 'true'. I observed the ways people were talked about by those who took control of the discourse had a direct impact on the treatment of those being talked about.

When I began to practise social work in institutional settings, I observed a similar pattern where those in powerless positions, such as clients, prisoners or some allied health staff, were 'defined' in negative ways by those with more power, such as nurses, doctors or correctional staff. Such definitions appeared to justify a wide range of abuses of power such as bullying and demeaning comments. For clients or prisoners, this could mean harsh punishments, withholding required services and treatments, or in many cases, the delivery of services or treatments which were inappropriate or unhelpful. From this, and through my doctoral studies, which introduced me to writers such as Michel Foucault, Bronwyn Davies and Nancy Fraser, I explored and embraced the potential for critical post-structural perspectives for emancipatory social change.

The critical aspect of critical postmodern approaches is important for me, as many writers have critiqued postmodern approaches for their potential relativism (for example, Ife 1999; Ferguson 2008). In my view, a purely postmodern approach would not fit the values of the social work profession. A critical postmodern approach holds the ideals and values of critical theory, which means that the voices and perspectives of those who hold the least power in a situation, or are experiencing oppressive power relations, are placed at the forefront. Postmodern ways of thinking enable me to put these ideals into practice in ways that take into account nuance, complexity and diversity in localised settings. Thus, critical postmodernism has a moral and directional element that enables me to act on my values.

The focus of practice is therefore to work to influence those ways of talking about clients, workers and the purpose of the organisation which cause oppressive power dynamics in order to reduce oppressive practices. As the approach is designed to develop new discourse and shared understandings to benefit service users, the work involves building alliances with all involved, and not taking an oppositional stance.

Now that we have explained our theoretical and personal viewpoints, the next section in the chapter outlines how processes are orientated within a socialist feminist approach and a critical postmodern approach to social work practice.

Process orientations for modernist and postmodern approaches to critical social work

This following list outlines some shared process orientations that are underpinned by both critical postmodern and socialist feminist theories.

- Dialogical praxis (Ife 2012)—an acknowledgement of both the worker and those with whom they are working, as having expertise and opportunity to learn from each other. This collaboration involves the continuous cycle of critically assessing the value of practice and theories as they inform and are understood in the work with service users, communities, policies or organisations.
- Mutual consciousness-raising—this is used rather than consciousness-raising to acknowledge that social workers and service users have much

to teach and learn from each other, as both are impacted in similar and different ways by social structures.

- Cultural humility— this involves '. . . a lifelong process of self-reflection and self-critique' (Tervalon & Murray-Garcia 1998: 117) aimed at developing respectful relationships with service users and co-workers. Cultural humility is preferable to requiring cultural competence that can unwittingly invite unwarranted arrogance, particularly from people with settler majority culture backgrounds, who often presume an ability, and right, to learn and become competent in another's culture (Hosken 2013). As such this approach aims to acknowledge and embrace multiple ways of knowing.

- Culturally friendly attitude—service users value social workers who can convey warmth and friendliness (Buckley, Carr & Whelan 2011). Social workers can invite interest in a reciprocal, although often structurally unequal, relationship with service users, families and communities, using a culturally friendly attitude (Engelbrecht 2006). Similarly, social workers can enlist a culturally friendly approach with colleagues to build alliances and shared multidisciplinary understandings to ensure the entire team can better respond to the service user's needs (see Chapter 11).

- Deep, respectful ethical listening and stillness—this aims to actively signal respect through demonstrating the listener's receptivity and interest to hear and learn from another's experience as contained in the values, cultural orientations, and feelings conveyed in the acts of being, speech, silence and listening. It is in listening that others can say what they want to say and the listener has the opportunity to learn (Ratcliffe 2005; Bennett, Zubrzycki & Bacon 2011).

- Universalising, individualising and externalising—universalising is focusing on the links between experiences that the service user sees as unique and specific to them, and the experiences of others in similar situations. This involves social and personal empathy. It can be important to individualise, or notice features that are unique to the service user's situation that makes their feelings, thoughts and behaviours unlike those of others. Externalising sees problems as socially created relations of economics, politics, culture and history rather than the individual's inadequacies (Carey & Russell 2002).

- Witnessing, validating and resisting—witnessing means seeing or hearing accounts of service users' experiences, that often involve misrecognition, to confirm and validate their existence, the injuries sustained and impacts on living (Hosken 2014). Validation includes recognising the external, institutional social pressures that condition a person to think, feel and act in a particular way. Social workers and service users are often more able to resist labelling, internalising, stigmatising and pathologising when involved in the social practices of ethical listening, speaking and learning.

- Clear contracting, use of agency and discretion and expanding boundaries—clear contracting refers to openly acknowledging the contradictions and conflicts between what social workers would like to be able to do, what the service user would ideally like and what the agency requires. This involves exposing the social worker's values, biases and limitations. Many social workers push the limits of discretion when working with (and against) the policies and procedures that are expected by the profession and the organisation. Carey and Foster (2011) describe social workers' use of discretion and expansion of boundaries as deviant social work. Use of workers' own agency and discretion may involve finding ways to use aspects of the predominant culture that benefit service users. An example of this might be to draw on the managerialist discourse of consumer satisfaction to advocate for the organisation to get a full understanding of service users' needs and preferences (Jones & May 1992).

- Critical questioning, deconstruction, reflectivity and reflexivity—this involves the social worker engaging in self- and organisational critical reflection, critical questioning and deconstruction to identify, explore, map and challenge the historical, cultural and social functions of particular norms, rules or ideologies that operate in their personal, professional and organisational experience of a situation.

- Critical, deconstructive approach—when engaging in organisational critical reflection, a critically deconstructive approach (Fook 2012) can involve a social worker naming the discourses operating in the organisational context, where they consider how their own beliefs fit these discourses and explore what perspectives are not represented or are devalued by these discourses. They would then consider how the practices associated with these discourses reinforce oppressive power relations. Exploring the ways that client identities become polarised into binary or dichotomous categories (for example, compliant/manipulative, independent/dependent, victim/perpetrator and how these become oppressive because they fail to capture nuances and complexities is also important. Exploring and unpacking assumptions is an important part of this process. In addition, considering new ways of constructing the worker's role and that of others through exercising productive power is also key to this approach.

- Reflexivity—when working directly with a service user, the social worker can explore with the service user the historical, cultural and social functions of particular norms, rules or ideologies operating in their personal experience of a situation. Reflexivity is a social worker's questioning of their own biases and how knowledge about service users is created and how power is used in this process (D'Cruz, Gillingham, & Melendez 2007). It is used to think about an interaction or event after it has occurred to consider how the social worker might have done it better. This then enables the worker to improve their practice when they face that situation next time. Reflexivity also refers to the social worker's ability to learn with the service user in the particular situation as it is happening and for the social worker to moderate their own thinking and actions in line with this greater awareness.
- Research, policy analysis and advocacy—user practice and user-led research is applied to work with others to advocate for changes at the levels of individual practice, organisational policy and practice, and government and corporate national and transnational policy.

The next section in the chapter illustrates a socialist-feminist approach and a critical postmodern approach to social work practice by looking at a case study. While Norah positions herself as 'Freda', a non-government child and family support welfare service worker. Sophie positions herself as 'Sam', the referring child protection social worker.

Applying these approaches to a case study

The following case study presents the clients and the situation that is then used to illustrate potential applications of the critical social work's key principles and practices from a socialist-feminist and critical postmodern approach.

Case study: Jane Smith, Alan Jones and their son, George

A social worker in Support-U, a non-government child and family support welfare service, were allocated a case. Ms Jane Smith and Mr Alan Jones were referred to the agency by the state child protection authority. The team leader advised the social worker that this case

---

had been initially assessed as short-term with limited funding. The referral stated that the child protection service investigated a concern where George (aged 13), the eldest of four children, had presented at school with bruising across his back and buttocks from being hit with a belt by the stepfather, Alan. Alan is the biological father of the younger two children. The four children missed 40 per cent of school days in the previous school term. Alan has been unemployed for three years since the factory where he worked had closed down. Jane has a casual job as a night cleaner, but the company has not offered her many shifts lately. The child-protection referral states the non-attendance at school was due to Jane being inebriated and unable to take the children to school. Child protection services were satisfied that George is not currently at risk because Alan agreed to stop using physical discipline, but the service required Jane and Alan to attend Support-U to consolidate the use of non-physical means of discipline, and for Jane to undergo counselling for alcohol abuse. The social worker had several appointments with Jane who told her that the father of her two eldest children, Tony, was violent towards her. Today, unexpectedly, Jane brought George in with her to see the social worker. Jane is worried about George's verbal and physical aggression towards his stepfather, Alan. Jane says that she hopes the social worker can talk some sense into George as she cannot afford any more trouble at home, or with the child protection services. Jane stands up to leave the room. George is sitting there, looking down.

A socialist-feminist approach to the case study involving Freda

Listen ethically and work with individuals, families and communities to help them connect with, or to access, needed resources and to negotiate problematic situations (Wood & Tully 2013).

My name is Freda. I am a social worker at Support-U and have been working with Jane over a number of weeks. I am aware how the 'structural violence of poverty' (see Chapter 7) significantly reduced the opportunities available for the members of this family to live or parent in the ways they wanted. With Jane's permission, knowledge of the family and their context was used to advocate successfully to my team leader that this family should be reallocated to a higher level of service. This enabled access to greater personal and financial supports, including regular food, clothing and taxi vouchers, respite child-care, home help, and materials and tuition needed for school.

Freda's ability to learn from the location and views of those most affected
Although George's attendance was not planned for that particular day, I had hoped to be talking with George during my work with the family. Drawing on dialogical praxis and mutual consciousness-raising I asked for and received ongoing feedback from Jane in our individual appointments to this point. Jane said the approach in our sessions, where I used socialist-feminist and trauma-informed perspectives, were helpful and meaningful in our work together. Through critical questioning, I was able to learn a lot about how Jane lived with poverty and unemployment. Jane and I both learned how her childhood experience of her own social position in terms of class and gender had instilled in Jane an embedded, involuntary, alertness to the needs of men that meant she was to be submissive and self-sacrificing. This included Jane having developed an understanding of men being the structurally dominant group (Worell & Remer 2003) and of mothers having the responsibility to make families work, while fathers gain and manage the family income. Informed by critical feminist psychology, I asked Jane about some of these socialised understandings, and together, we started to question these understandings. This questioning led to changing the gender-role messages to better reflect the actual situation and hopes of Jane and her family.

I explored with Jane the differences in gender power (Teater 2014) experienced when she was a girl. Jane and I both gained insight into the constant devaluing of her and her own mother, because they are female. This was reinforced by Jane's father's control over all family decision-making including money matters and how this had created 'insidious' and 'indirect' trauma for Jane, worsened by the 'direct' trauma (Root 1992 in Richmond, Geiger, & Reed 2013: 442) of abuse that Tony had inflicted on Jane. By hearing that George had witnessed Tony's physical abuse of Jane, and as George was instructed, had often taken his younger brother with him to hide, I was tuned in to placing George as my main focus.

Freda's use of transparency
I created an opportunity to explain my role with the family, the role of the child protection services, and my role in terms of confidentiality with George and Jane together. I asked Jane what she thought would be useful for me and George to talk about and what were Jane's worries. Jane gave George 'permission' to speak about his feelings, his worries and family matters, especially why there was conflict between George and Alan.

I aimed to create a sense of safety in the transition from Jane being present in the shared sessions to a one-to-one session where I talk with George on his own. Jane was invited to sit outside the office where I suggested George could have access to Jane at any time he chose. Maintaining awareness of the rights and many competences of children (Barnes 2012), I aimed to signal to George my commitment to working in partnership with him, and directly addressed issues of power in our relationship by facilitating that George had some freedom and control over the conversation, its pace and length. I asked George if he accepted that I talk with him while Jane waited outside. George remained looking down, nodded his head from side to side and said, 'I fucking suppose I have to'. Using ethical listening to listen through the use of the swear word, I heard the frustration, anger and lack of control, and said to George that it sounded as though he did not feel that he had been provided with many choices. I discussed with George if he did agree to talk with me, that it would be fine for him to leave the room whenever he wanted to take a break, and that George did not have to talk about things that he did not want to. George then said quietly that he would talk with me. After Jane left the room, I continued with a small Lego blocks building project on the table and invited George to help me with this while we talked, thus reducing the need for direct eye contact in our initial engagement.

Freda's use of dominant ideologies, policies and practices and its impact on the worker and the service user

I aimed to build connection and trust with George through ethical listening, cultural humility and dialogical praxis. I explained a getting-to-know-you game called 'three houses' (Weld & Greening 2004) and I asked George if he would work with me by using words and drawings to explore his worries, some things he liked doing, and anything he might like to change for the future. I told George, unless it raised concerns about his safety, I would not show or discuss his 'three houses' to others without his permission. I learned with George that his socialisation into a male gender role had involved watching his biological father, Tony, control his mother through the use of physical, financial, emotional and psychological abuse. At times, George found Tony was fun to be around. George felt painfully conflicted, having wanted attention and validation from his biological father. He also felt frightened and angry when his father hurt his mother, and when George was asked to protect his younger brother. George felt confused; sometimes his father was loving and confided in him about not being able to cope with unemployment, and said that when George grew up, George should be a decent man that brought a good wage home for the family. George was angry he had not been consulted before his mother packed him and his brother up and left his father, the house they lived in and the school where his mates were.

George told me that his mother tried to please his biological father and his stepfather. George felt blamed by his stepfather, Alan, for getting child protection services involved, for shaming them all and for making things even more difficult.

George said although Alan had not used the belt on him again, he made comments about Georges' child protection 'mates'. George said the school and the child protection services had not given him any choices, they had not listened to him. George said it was easier just to take the belt now and then, rather than having to put up with his stepfather's ridicule. George could not wait to be 18 years old when he could make his own decisions about his life.

Freda's consideration of the structural violence of poverty
Aware that the family lived below the poverty line and could not afford basic living necessities, I had tentatively contemplated the impacts of class and the structural violence of poverty (see Chapter 7) on George.

During the discussion, George expressed feelings of shame because his clothes, shoes and haircut were not up-to-date like those of others in his classes. George thought he was the only one without a mobile phone, who did not have money to buy food at the canteen or at the milk bar after school. George avoided making friends, as he did not wish to take anyone home to his shared bedroom in a state-provided rental house with no good computer games to play. George also avoided people meeting his stepfather, who often put him down in front of others. George was pleased his mother was eligible for assistance to secure funding for the family to purchase a mobile phone, clothing, personal items, a computer and games, and home tutoring.

Freda's work to lobby managers, organisations and funding providers to change discriminatory discourses and institutional work processes
I told George how much I had learned from him, including that George really liked basketball but did not play at school. I shared how affected I was by George explaining how he was supposed to be at the centre of a child protection investigation, but he did not feel anyone had really listened to him. I asked George if he might like to join a basketball team with other boys who also had contact with child protection services or who felt different to some of the other students at their schools. There was a team organised by my agency coached by a man who had had contact with child protection when he was a boy. I suggested that if George was interested, I could discuss this with his mother and stepfather. George said he might give it a go.

I asked George for permission to share some of what I had learned with him at an inter-agency team meeting so child protection workers might improve the way they work with boys. I reassured George that I would not use his name and that his teachings would be mixed with a number of experiences from different young people so that it would not be possible to identify him. George said he would like for child protection services to listen more to the children whom they investigate.

I talked with my team members about my concerns that the policy and assessment tools guiding our work were underpinned by values of individualism and competition and that these set unrealistic outcomes of self-sufficiency and self-management for families without providing the resources for these outcomes to be achieved. Most of our client families were poor and unemployed. I worked with service users, my team members, the union and the local service user-led unemployment advocacy group to collate and share life stories, statistics and data to make the case for change to policies and practices.

A critical post-modern approach to the case study involving Sam

My name is Sam, and I work at the Department of Human Services in the child protection division. I've worked here a number of years now and during this time I've noticed some gaps in the way clients and their families are assessed as a result of the way clients, their parents and what constitutes 'risk' are conceptualised and talked about. As child protection is a statutory agency, I realise that decisions made have considerable impact on clients' lives, and decisions made that are based on incomplete information or a lack of understanding of the complex family dynamics could be experienced as oppressive by clients and their families.

A recent follow-up meeting about the Smith family whom I referred to child and family services some time ago has revealed that Ms Smith is worried about George's verbal and physical aggression towards his stepfather and this had not been picked up by child protection services. As this is an organisational problem, a contextual, organisational approach is necessary. The following process orientations described earlier will be employed, with a focus on the staff and the overall child protection agency: critical questioning, deconstruction, reflectivity and reflexivity; culturally friendly attitude; research, policy analysis and advocacy; and use of agency and discretion. An important skill when using these approaches is the ability to 'read' the cultural climate (Fook 2012), or in other words, to begin to notice what the dominant discourses are, who gets to define them, and why?

To provide an idea of some of the discourses operating in a range of child protection contexts, I (Sam) have consulted literature, which presents extracts of interviews with child protection workers. Nevertheless, while many child protection offices may share similarities to the following, it is important to be aware that each context is unique. Therefore, what follows is a guide, rather than a prescriptive list of facts, and there may or may not be similarities in other child protection offices in other towns and countries.

Sam's use of critical questioning, deconstruction, reflectivity and reflexivity.
The first aspect in that child protection setting that I need to deconstruct is the multiple ways that risk is understood (Collings & Davies 2008), and the binary thinking which seeks to position those involved as either 'risky' or 'at risk', victim or perpetrator (Hughes & Chau 2013). Child protection services are under enormous pressure to manage risk and there are powerful mechanisms which govern this risk management including legislation, policy, and public scrutiny (see Chapter 9). While this is a necessary aspect of the role of child protection services, workers like me need to engage in a critically reflective approach to avoid being caught in discursive ideologies that limit our awareness of the complexities of power and risk within human relationships.

I would firstly question my own assumptions that contribute to a limited understanding of power dynamics occurring in families, and the origins of these. I might then investigate if my peers and managers in the office hold similar assumptions and then I would consider the perspectives of clients, their parents and some of the workers who may not be recognised due to the dominant discursive regimes. Examples of these discursive regimes will now be explored.

Firstly, Collings and Davies report that a common discourse among child protection workers is that children are 'vulnerable' and 'innocent' (Collings & Davies 2008: 186). The authors of this article note the conspicuous absence of workers' descriptions of parents, so that workers do not consider that parents might also be at risk from their children. The dominance of the 'innocence' discourse with regards to children at once positions the parents as the perpetrators of violence or harm, and the children as victims. This does not allow for the fact that both children and adults may be both victim and perpetrator of violence, and hence the possibility is invisible and not explored by any risk assessment tool.

While I, Sam, understand why child protection workers might focus on the child's vulnerability, I also see the limitations of this focus. An important dimension of the assessment of care and risk in families is also missed. The focus on the child alone fails to capture the interrelatedness of the whole family system—and the fact that supporting parents and addressing their issues is likely to improve their children's wellbeing if the parents are more able to care for them effectively.

I am aware of the negative ways that parents are often discussed by my peers and managers, and the influence it has on decision-making. I have found myself feeling more favourable towards those parents who cooperate with care plans that I devise as it makes my job easier. I do find myself feeling frustrated and angry with parents who use violence either towards each other or towards their children. Following the work by Hughes and Chau (2013), I need to remember that while I may feel judgement or disgust at a parent's behaviour, I also need to consider the impact of poverty, violence and discrimination on the limited range of choices that parents face. Around the office, there is a range of ways of talking about parents' substance misuse, and these conversations usually focus on their moral failing as parents. Mothers are seen as complete 'no hopers' if they do not show that they are willing to place the needs of their children before their own choices and needs. These ways of talking about parents become the accepted 'truths' about the character and potentials of these parents. It is rarely acknowledged how difficult and limited some women's lives and choices are.

I am aware that we, in a similar way to what Hughes and Chau (2013) found among the workers whom they interviewed, tend to use our own 'common sense' truths outside the tools we are given to practise with, and that we have developed these tools to manage the immense contradiction and anxiety that is present in our roles (Collings & Davies 2008). The following is therefore some alternative practices that I could use. While this does not solve all the inadequacies facing child protection services, they are some small things that I can do within my sphere of influence as a critical social worker in this setting.

Sam's use of agency and discretion, research, policy analysis and advocacy
One alternative practice, which could lead to more nuanced and empathic ways of constructing families that use harsh or physical discipline, or both, could be using my own worker agency and discretion to instigate some policy work that would enable client's voices to be more effectively heard. I could draw on my good relationships with managers to suggest that we broaden the structured decision-making tool to include family needs and dynamics so that we are less likely to miss important risk factors. This would be accompanied by full training and support by managers at the top of the organisation, and hence would be framed in language that they understand. For example, I could demonstrate how this could make our organisation more effective and less likely to be criticised in the media as I know this is a deep concern for managers. I could draw on research from other countries that show how strengthening families can improve the safety of both children and parents, and how this would be in keeping with our mission statement.

Sam's use of a culturally friendly attitude
Another practice I could engage in is to address the limiting 'common sense' discursive constructions about children and parents that we workers tend to fall back on when anxiety is high, and we see children abused and neglected. As discussed earlier, parents are constructed as either cooperative or risky 'no hopers', and children are

constructed only as innocent and vulnerable. Those parents who have addictions are currently constructed as immoral and irresponsible. By evoking a culturally friendly attitude with colleagues, an alternative way of understanding a substance addiction could be developed. For example, talk about research that poses substance addiction as a medical problem, or even as a response to trauma and despair, during formal and informal conversations at all levels of the organisation, could sow the seeds for new discursive possibilities.

Mr Smith and Ms Jones, parents of George, who were referred by me to the non-government child and family agency, were from one of those families regarded as cooperative by my colleagues. Hence their file was closed and they were referred on. I continued to have concerns about them even though they 'ticked all the boxes' from a bureaucratic point of view. Therefore, I see a need to improve the ways we assess risk and really understand what is happening for the families that come to our attention. We also need to carefully monitor the 'common sense' ways in which we characterise clients and their parents in our everyday talk, so that we really hear what clients and parents are saying to us, with an understanding of the immense difficulties and hardships they may be facing.

Conclusion

The purpose of critical social work is to bring about emancipatory personal and social change and greater social justice and equality through working alongside those who are oppressed and marginalised, and to question and change power relations and assumptions (Allan 2009).

Throughout this chapter we have demonstrated different ways of practising critical social work through taking different roles and different approaches to a case study about Mr Smith, Ms Jones and their son, George. There are several overlaps in the ways each worker approached the problems facing the family as each used agency and discretion, a culturally friendly attitude, research, policy analysis and advocacy, and critical questioning, deconstruction, reflectivity and reflexivity. One difference was in the focus of the policy work, since the child protection worker drew on a critical postmodern approach to work within the context to change discursive practices as a route to changing assessment tools. This was done by drawing on language that the managers and policymakers understood. The child and family support worker drew on a socialist-feminist approach, and collaborated with the service user family members, other service users, user groups, statistics and union power to exert pressure on the agency to change the policy and practice.

We believe that both socialist-feminist and critical postmodern approaches are important in critical social work, and suggest that workers draw on the strengths of both approaches. The degree to which this can be done depends on the context of the work and the professional and social location of the worker, their lived experience, and their theoretical orientations.

References

Allan, J. 2009, 'Theorising new developments in critical social work', in J. Allan, L. Briskman, & B. Pease (eds), *Critical Social Work: Theories and practices for a socially just world,* 2nd edn, St Leonards: Allen & Unwin, pp. 30–44

Allan, J., Briskman, L. & Pease, B. (eds) 2009, *Critical Social Work: Theories and practices for a socially just world,* 2nd edn, St Leonards: Allen & Unwin

Archer, L., Hutchings, M. & Leathwood, C. 2001, 'Engaging with commonality and difference: Theoretical tensions in the analysis of working-class women's educational discourses', *International Studies in Sociology of Education,* vol. 11, no. 1, pp. 41–62

Barnes, V. 2012, 'Social work and advocacy with young people: Rights and care in practice', *British Journal of Social Work,* vol. 42, no. 7, pp. 1275–92

Bennett, B., Zubrzycki, J. & Bacon, V. 2011, 'What do we know? The experiences of social workers working alongside Aboriginal people', *Australian Social Work,* Vol. 64, no. 1, pp. 20–37

Buckley, H., Carr, N. & Whelan, S. 2011, '"Like walking on eggshells': Service user views and expectations of the child protection system', *Child and Family Social Work,* vol. 16, no. 1, pp. 101–10

Burr, V. 2003, *Social Constructionism,* 2nd edn, London: Routledge

Carey, M. & Foster, V. 2011, 'Introducing "deviant" social work: Contextualising the limits of radical social work whilst understanding (fragmented) resistance within the social work labour process', *British Journal of Social Work,* vol. 41, no. 3, pp. 576–93

Carey, M. & Russell, S. 2002, 'Externalising: Commonly asked questions', *International Journal of Narrative Therapy and Community Work,* vol. 2002, no. 2, pp. 76–84

Collins, P. 1991. *Black Feminist Thought: Knowledge, consciousness, and the politics of empowerment,* London: Routledge

Collings, S. & Davies, L. 2008, 'For the sake of the children: Making sense of children and childhood in the context of child protection', *Journal of Social Work Practice,* vol. 2, no. 2, 181–93

Cudd, A. & Holmstrom, N. 2011, *Capitalism, For and Against: A feminist debate,* Cambridge: Cambridge University Press

D'Cruz, H., Gillingham, P. & Melendez, S. 2007, 'Reflexivity: a concept and its meanings for practitioners working with children and families', *Critical Social Work,* vol. 8, no. 1, pp. 1–18

Dominelli, L. 2002, *Feminist Social Work Theory and Practice,* Basingstoke: Palgrave

Engelbrecht, L. 2006, 'Cultural Friendliness as a foundation for the support function in the supervision of social work students in South Africa', *International Social Work,* vol. 49, no. 2, pp. 256–66

Ferguson, I. 2008, *Reclaiming Social Work: Challenging neo-liberalism and promoting social justice,* London: Sage

Fook, J. 2012, *Social Work: A critical approach to practice,* London: Sage

Hosken, N. 2013, 'Social work supervision and discrimination', *Advances in Social Work and Welfare Education,* vol. 15, no. 1, pp. 91–103

Hosken, N. 2014, *HSW313-Anti-Oppressive Approaches to Social Work,* Geelong: Deakin University

Houston, S. 2001, 'Beyond social constructionism: Critical realism and social work', *British Journal of Social Work,* vol. 31, no. 6, pp. 845–61

Hughes, J. & Chau, S. 2013, 'Making complex decisions: Child protection workers' practices and interventions with families experiencing intimate partner violence', *Children and Youth Services Review,* vol. 35, pp. 611–61

Ife, J. 1999, 'Postmodernism, critical theory and social work', in B. Pease and J. Fook (eds), *Transforming social work practice: Postmodern critical perspectives,* Allen & Unwin, Crows Nest, pp. 211–23

—— 2012, *Human Rights and Social Work: Towards rights-based practice,* 3rd edn, Melbourne: Cambridge University Press

Jones, A. & May, J. 1992, 'Frontline work: choices, conflicts and contradictions', *Working in Human Service Organisations: A critical introduction,* Melbourne: Longman Cheshire

Marlow, J., Appleton, C., Chinnery, S. & Van Stratum, S. 2015, 'The integration of personal and professional selves: Developing students' critical awareness in social work practice', *Social Work Education: The International Journal,* vol. 34, no. 1, pp. 60–73

Noble, C. 2004, 'Postmodern thinking: Where is it taking social work?', *Journal of Social Work,* vol. 4, no. 3, pp. 289–304

Orton, M. 2009, 'Understanding the exercise of agency within structural inequality: The case of personal debt', *Social Policy and Society,* vol. 8, no. 4, pp. 487–98

Ratcliffe, K. 2005, *Rhetorical Listening: Identification, gender, whiteness,* Carbondale: Southern Illinois University Press

Richmond, K., Geiger, E. & Reed, C. 2013, 'The personal is political: A Feminist and trauma-informed therapeutic approach to working with a survivor of sexual assault', *Clinical Case Studies,* vol. 12, pp. 443–56

Smith, D.E. 2005, *Institutional Ethnography: A sociology for people,* Lanham: AltaMira Press

Teater, B. 2014, *Feminist Theory and Practice: An introduction to applying social work theories and methods,* 2nd edn, Maidenhead: McGraw-Hill Education

Tervalon, M. & Murray-Garcia, J. 1998, 'Cultural humility versus cultural competence: A critical distinction in defining physician training outcomes in multicultural education', *Journal of Health Care for the Poor and Underserved,* vol. 9, no. 2, pp. 117–25

Weld, N. & Greening, M. 2004, 'The three houses', *Social Work Now,* Vol. 29, December, pp. 34–7

Wood, G. & Tully, C. 2013, *The Structural Approach to Direct Practice in Social Work: A social constructionist perspective,* New York: Columbia University Press

Worell, J. & Remer, P. 2003, *Feminist Perspectives in Therapy: Empowering diverse women,* Hoboken: Wiley

Yuval-Davis, N. 1994, 'Women, ethnicity and empowerment', *Feminism and Psychology,* vol. 4, pp. 179–97

PART II

Critical practices in confronting privilege and promoting social justice

5

Towards a critical human rights-based approach to social work practice

Sharlene Nipperess

Introduction

Despite the increasing interest in human rights-based approaches to practice, social workers still appear to find the concept of human rights complex, contested and challenging. In this chapter I help bridge the gap between the rhetoric of human rights commitments and the reality of human rights practice in critical social work. First, I explore the concept of human rights and its relationship with social work practice. Then I argue that in the contemporary context of neoliberalism and economic globalisation, a revitalised human rights approach provides a strong moral, ethical and political basis for critical social work practice. Third, I present an exploratory framework to embed a critical human rights approach in social work practice. This chapter concludes with a discussion of how such a framework can be applied in social work practice. It invites ongoing debate on the complex and contested ideas surrounding human rights and its relationship with emancipatory social work practice.

Human rights and social work practice

Interest in a human rights-based approach for practice is intensifying and there are comprehensive articulations of human rights-based social work practice (Connolly & Ward 2008; Mapp 2008; Wronka 2008; Lundy 2011; Reichert 2011; Ife 2012; Briskman 2014). However, before discussing how social workers can put human rights into practice, it is important to understand exactly what human rights are. Human rights are generally understood in reference to the United Nations Universal Declaration of Human Rights (UDHR) (United Nations 1948). The UDHR was proclaimed in 1948 by the General Assembly of the United Nations. It was developed in response to the atrocities of World War II; in particular, the genocide of the Jewish people, and to ensure that the tragedy of the Holocaust would never occur again. The UDHR contains 30 articles, which articulate a range of civil, political, social, cultural, economic, and collective/solidarity rights. It is the first comprehensive statement of human rights ever made and, even though it was declared over 60 years ago, it still has the power to motivate and inspire people to both protect and promote human rights. As Freeman notes, the Declaration, as well as directly informing numerous international human rights instruments, 'is also the source of an international movement, and of numerous national movements, of political activists who struggle against oppression, injustice and exploitation by reference to this document' (Freeman 2011: 42).

The UDHR is not a list of international laws. It was designed as a statement of principles to which people, communities and nations can aspire. It does not give any specific direction about how to achieve the stated human rights. Two covenants were subsequently declared to address this: the International Covenant of Civil and Political Rights, ICCPR (OHCHR 1966a) and the International Covenant on Economic, Social and Cultural Rights, ICESCR, (OHCHR 1966b). These two covenants and the UDHR have become the foundation of the contemporary international human rights system. When a nation agrees to be bound by a human rights treaty, as Carey, Gibney and Poe note, it is 'committing itself not only to protecting human rights within its own territorial borders, but also to helping to work towards the elimination of violations of human rights, no matter where these take place' (Carey, Gibney & Poe 2010: 31). It is this aspect, Carey, Gibney and Poe stress, which makes the idea of human rights so revolutionary.

Australia has agreed to be bound to the ICCPR and the ICESCR and other significant human rights instruments; many of which are of particular interest to social work (Australian Human Rights Commission, AHRC 2015). These include the International Convention on the Elimination of all forms of Racial Discrimination,

Convention on the Elimination of all forms of Discrimination against Women, Convention against Torture and Other Cruel, Inhuman and Degrading Treatment or Punishment, Convention on the Rights of the Child, Convention and Protocol Relating to the Status of Refugees and Convention on the Rights of Persons with Disabilities. Australia also formally supports the United Nations Declaration on the Rights of Indigenous Persons.

The UDHR and the various conventions and declarations derived from it are significant to the social work profession both in Australia and internationally. The UDHR is referred to in the international Statement of Ethical Principles (International Federation of Social Workers, IFSW, 2004) and in numerous national codes of ethics (Keeney et al. 2014), including Australia's Code of Ethics (AASW, 2010). These documents obligate social workers to commit to the principles of these international human rights instruments. The UDHR and many of the conventions and declarations provide the basis for social workers' explorations of human rights in practice (for example, see Reichert 2011). Indeed McDonald notes that the UDHR, the ICCPR and the ICESCR provide social workers with 'a clear set of foundational documents' from which to practise (McDonald 2006: 177).

While the significance of the UDHR to social work is clear, there is often an uncritical acceptance of the UDHR, which ignores the critique of human rights generally and of the UDHR specifically. As remarkable an achievement as the UDHR is, it is important to interrogate the notion that human rights 'exist' and that they remain fixed and unchanging over time and place (Evans 2011; Ife 2012). The risk of simply referring to human rights in relation to the UDHR is that its complexity and critique are ignored, particularly in relation to the Western (Swenson 1995; Aziz 1999), legal (Freeman 2011), patriarchal (Reichert 1998; Wetzel 2007) and privileged voices (Tascón & Ife 2008) that some argue dominate the human rights discourse (George 1999; Solas 2000; Skegg 2005; Ife 2012). While it is not possible to explore these critiques in detail here, a more nuanced understanding of human rights, one that takes into account the complexity and critique as well as the strengths, will move beyond rhetorical commitments and ultimately strengthen human rights-based practice (Cemlyn 2008).

Defining human rights is therefore a challenge. Ife (2010) identifies that 'human' and 'rights' by themselves are contested ideas but together 'human rights' is a concept that is both abstract and problematic (Freeman 2011). Human rights are often defined in specific terms—in relation to a particular value, such as freedom, or in relation to a particular group, such as refugees. The idea of human rights is that they 'are those entitlements that people possess simply by virtue of their humanity' and they are usually considered to be universal, indivisible and inalienable (Nipperess &

Briskman 2009: 62–3). Human rights practice, by extension, is practice that attempts to both protect and promote human rights, however defined, in social work practice.

Human rights in the context of neoliberalism and globalisation

Since the economic crisis of the early 1970s, many Western governments have become more conservative and neoliberalism has become the dominant ideology. Neoliberalism emphasises individualisation, corporatisation, marketisation, competition, managerialism and privatisation and the focus on economic policy over social policy (Rees & Rodley 1995; Ferguson 2008), and as such, many social workers find themselves working in an environment that is antithetical to their values. It is within this landscape that Ferguson and Lavalette argue that social work has lost its way, that human rights and social justice are far from being at the heart of the profession, that:

> social work practice is increasingly dominated by managerialism, by the fragmentation of services, by financial restrictions and lack of resources, by increased bureaucracy and work-loads, by the domination of care-management approaches with their associated performance indicators, and by the increased use of the private sector (Ferguson & Lavalette 2005: 207).

The consequences of neoliberalism have been exacerbated by globalisation, especially economic globalisation (Falk 1999). Indeed, globalisation has intensified social and economic inequality and worsened environmental degradation (Alston 2012; Dominelli 2012).

The forces of neoliberalism and globalisation contribute to the marginalisation of numerous groups of people with whom social workers work. Ferguson and Lavalette (2006) argue that emancipatory approaches in social work seek to resist these forces and provide an alternative perspective in social work. A human rights-based approach that takes into account the critiques, the complexity and the contradictory nature of human rights, as well as the strengths, has the potential to enhance the emancipatory goals of critical social work. It provides social workers with the opportunity of working with people in ways to protect and promote human rights.

Towards a critical human rights approach to social work

A critical human rights-based approach to social work practice recognises and values the universal commitments to human rights that are expressed in the Universal Declaration of Human Rights (UDHR 1948), and that are reflected in the national and international social work organisations policies as well as the social work literature. These statements are both inspirational and aspirational and provide social workers with a strong moral basis for practice (Ife 2012). Many of these rights have been incorporated into national legislation, and consequently there is a solid legal basis for practice. A critical human rights approach to practice, informed by a range of critical theories, also appreciates the complex, contested and contextual nature of human rights. Drawing on Allan's (2009: 40–1) conceptualisation of critical social work, I argue that a critical human rights approach to practice is committed to:

- working towards greater social justice and equality for those people who are oppressed and marginalised within society as well as the wider non-human environment
- working alongside and with oppressed and marginalised people in a 'bottom-up' rather than 'top-down' approach
- incorporating an analysis of power that helps to explain the oppression and marginalisation of vulnerable groups and nature
- interrogating dominant assumptions and beliefs about human rights
- working towards emancipatory personal, cultural and social change.

Applying a critical human rights-based approach in practice

At the centre of this approach are the lived experiences of those with whom we work. It is informed by knowledge of the ethical, legal, historical, political, organisational, theoretical and practice contexts. The following case study provides an opportunity of considering how a critical human rights approach can be applied in practice. This case study explores the particular experience of a young Muslim woman, Zarah, who experiences vilification due to her wearing the hijab, a personal and public expression of her faith. However, the general principles can be applied to other fields of practice or vulnerable groups.

Case study: Zarah

A social worker works in a community health service in Melbourne, Australia. She has been working with Zarah over the last three weeks in relation to her experience of persistent headaches and difficulties in sleeping. Zarah has a refugee background, she is Muslim, 23 years old and has lived in Australia for three years. On this occasion when Zarah visits you, she appears irritated and expresses anger about an abusive comment that she received on the train while she was on her way to see you, about her hijab, the headscarf that she wears. Zarah indicates that she is receiving comments like these more often and she is finding them extremely upsetting.

Begin with lived experiences

A critical human rights-based approach invites practitioners to start with the lived experiences of the people with whom they are working. At one level, this may be assumed as 'good' social work practice but the voices of the people with whom we work are often ignored or are missing in social work practice. In relation to this case, listening deeply to Zarah's lived experience of being abused for her religious expression is central.

While Zarah's experience as a young Islamic woman from a refugee background is unique, many of her experiences of resettling in Australia may be shared by others, including the experience of being vilified because of her religion. There are other ways of hearing the diverse voices of people with whom we work, for example, biographical and autobiographical accounts, documentaries and other film, historical and archival material.

Beginning with lived experiences means working to ensure that these voices are not only heard but are valued throughout the organisation in which the social worker is employed or self-employed. This can mean providing meaningful opportunities for service users to participate in the planning, delivery and evaluation of social work services, participate in social-work practice research, community education and social action campaigns.

A critical human rights-based approach also invites practitioners to reflect on their own lived experiences. Developing critical self-awareness using the skills of reflectivity and reflexivity (Fook & Gardner 2007) involves asking questions such as 'What do I understand about human rights'?, 'Where was this value developed'?, 'How has my lived experienced shaped my understanding of human rights'?, 'What is my relationship to both oppression and privilege'?, 'What are my assumptions in relation to human rights with people from refugee backgrounds'?, 'What are my assumptions in relation to religion, spirituality and, in particular, Islam'?, 'What values, knowledge and skills do I bring to practice with Zarah?'. These and other critical questions may help the practitioner to critically reflect on their own social positioning and their practice.

An example from my own practice illustrates how I used critical reflection to interrogate some of my values, beliefs and assumptions on religion, spirituality and faith. In my practice as a social worker working with people from migrant, refugee and asylum-seeker backgrounds, I was offered the opportunity of exploring my Anglo-Australian background and some of my assumptions around religion. I was raised in a working-class family, which celebrated some of the Christian rituals such as Christmas and Easter. However, my father was an atheist and, although my mother identifies as Christian, we did not go to church or practise other beliefs or rituals of the Christian church. As such, I was not christened, although oddly, given my family's ambivalent attitude to religion, I attended Salvation Army Sunday school until I was about eight years old. I considered my Christianity as 'nominal', not important, until I started working with people from migrant and refugee back-grounds. I began to reflect on my own social location, in particular my relationship to the dominance of Christianity in Australian contemporary life. I began to under-stand how Christianity permeates daily life in Australia including the public holidays that many Australians take for granted. I also reflected on some of my assumptions about religion and spirituality, and how important it was for many of my co-workers and the people with whom we worked, contrasted to the ambivalence I, and the social work profession generally, had towards religion and spirituality (Crisp 2010). Interrogating my values, beliefs and assumptions was deeply unsettling because I was forced to acknowledge my role in perpetuating the dominance of Christianity and marginalising those who identify with another religion or none.

Explore the ethical context

Post-9/11, people who practise the Muslim faith are particularly vulnerable to discrimination, vilification and human rights violations. The increase of Islamophobia in Australia and other Western countries is well documented (Dunn, Klocker & Salabay 2007; Ferguson & Lavalette 2015) and with this comes an increase in human rights violations. In relation to Zarah's experience of being vilified for wearing a hijab, a social worker using a critical human rights-based approach could explore the commitment to human rights which is outlined in the Australian and inter-national codes of ethics. This would enable the worker and Zarah to move beyond such commitments by exploring what human rights mean to Zarah and others who experience religious discrimination.

Although Zarah may have experienced a number of her human rights being violated in her home country, on the journey to Australia and on arrival in Australia (see Chapter 13), the human right that may be most relevant in this situation is the right to freedom of religion and religious expression. In practice this can mean starting with a human right statement such as Article 18 of the UDHR, 'Everyone has the right to freedom of thought, conscience and religion; this right includes freedom to change his religion or belief, and freedom, either alone or in community with others and in public or private, to manifest his religion or belief in teaching, practice, worship and observance' (UN 1948), and exploring what this means in one's own context. It can mean moving from the universal—the right to religious freedom—to the relative—what does religious freedom mean in my culture, my community, my country at this point in time. For practitioners, it can mean exploring the idea of religious freedom with the people with whom we work to determine how such a right might be promoted and protected in practice (Hodge 2006).

It may also be useful for the social worker to explore human rights and its relationship to other key values of the profession. In the Australian context, the AASW Code of Ethics prescribes a number of general ethical responsibilities including respect for human dignity and worth (clause 5.1.1), culturally competent, safe and sensitive practice (clause 5.1.2) and commitment to social justice and human rights (5.1.3) (AASW 2010). There are also a number of clauses that specifically explore the social work professions' responsibilities for how religion and spirituality relates to our colleagues as well as to those with whom we work (for example, clause 5.1.2.d and 5.1.2.k). Exploring these responsibilities can be a starting point to explore the debates and critiques inherent in these statements. For example, the terms human rights and social justice are often used interchangeably but as Hugman notes, while both principles are equally important, they 'do not connect automatically and unproblematically' (Hugman 2012: 384). Similarly, the idea of cultural competence has been critiqued extensively (Furlong & Wight 2011; Hosken 2013; Fisher-Borne, Montana Cain & Martin 2015).

Explore the legal context
When working with Zarah and other people from refugee backgrounds, it would be helpful to understand the key terminology or definitions used in the literature, policy and legislation. For example, understanding the similarity and difference between the conceptual categories of 'migrants', 'refugees' and 'asylum seekers' in Australian and international policy and legislation, and in human rights instruments such as

the Convention and Protocol Relating to the Status of Refugees (UNHCR 2010) is particularly important. Specifically this means understanding the specific rights and responsibilities that are afforded to people under domestic legislation and international law. It also means understanding the challenge of using such labels (see Chapter 13).

Understanding the legal context would also mean developing knowledge about state, national and international policy and legislation. In the international context, it would be useful to understand how the international Convention and Protocol Relating to the Status of Refugees (United Nations) is reflected in Australia's domestic legislation. The *Migration Act 1958* (Cwlth) is national legislation that specifically relates to migrants, refugees and people seeking asylum. Understanding the legal protections in Australian law in relation to religion would be useful when working with Zarah; in particular, the few protections which are provided under the Australian Constitution and the other protections that are provided under the *Racial Discrimination Act 1975* (Cwlth), the *Human Rights and Equal Opportunity Commission Act 1986* (Cwlth) and in Zarah's particular case the *Charter of Human Rights and Responsibilities Act 2006* (Vic).

Explore the historical context

It would also be useful, when working with Zarah, to understand the historical context, in particular the history of migration and the geographical movement of people both internationally and nationally, the concept of refuge and asylum, and the history of Australia's immigration policy and its racist underpinnings. It would also be helpful to understand the history of Australia's immigration policy in the context of invasion and colonisation. Understanding the development of Australia as a secular nation according to the Australian Constitution and the dominance of the Christian faith in our legal, educational and political institutions would be important.

Explore the political context

Knowledge of the political context would mean understanding the debates that are currently being held at the local, national and international level and the impact that they have on people who come from a refugee background and those who experience religious discrimination, such as Zarah. In Australia, particularly since 2001, political debates about people seeking asylum have been particularly vitriolic (see Chapter 13) and, internationally, the conflict in Syria has resulted in the 'biggest refugee crisis the world has seen since World War II' (UNHCR 2015). International conflicts and the impact on refugees can have far-reaching effects on people in Australia who come from a refugee background. In relation to the political debates about Islam, these have also been occurring in Australia and internationally, particularly since 2001 and 9/11. This has manifested as increasing Islamophobia at a local, national and international level. For example, in regional Victoria, anti-Islam and anti-mosque groups, including the United Patriots Front, have been protesting against a decision to build a mosque in Bendigo (Cowie 2015). There have been numerous anti-Islam rallies held across Australia (Nightingale 2015) and at the federal political level an anti-Muslim party, the Australian Liberty Alliance, has recently been formed (Jones 2014). Internationally the growth of far-right organisations is concerning, many of which express anti-Muslim sentiments (Ferguson & Lavalette 2015).

Explore the organisational context

Understanding the organisational context would mean understanding that social workers work with people from refugee backgrounds and people with diverse faiths in a range of organisations. This includes government and non-government organisations, national and international organisations and a range of faith-based organisations. In Zarah's case, the social worker is working in a community health centre but they would need a thorough understanding of the range of organisations that can support Zarah.

Explore the theoretical context

The theoretical orientation which informs a critical human rights-based approach would assist the social worker, when working with Zarah, to appreciate the oppression potentially experienced by Zarah in relation to class (Ferguson 2011; see also Chapter 7), gender (Penketh 2011; see also Chapter 15) and race/ethnicity (McMahon 2002; Williams & Johnson 2010) and the intersecting nature of such oppression (Mullaly 2010) along with other areas of identity such as age, sexuality and religion. Whiteness studies and scholarship on privilege would assist the worker in examining their own privilege and social positioning (Pease 2010; Walter, Taylor & Habibis 2011; see also Chapter 6). Postmodernist theorising would enable the worker to understand the various guises of oppression (Mullaly 2010) and move between the universal discourses of class, gender and race/ethnicity (as well as human rights) and more relative, diverse and uncertain experiences that do not depict Zarah as necessarily having the same experiences as other Australian women, or other Muslim refugees and so on (Pease & Fook 1999; Allan 2009). This would mean sitting with the contradictions between these positions (see Chapter 1). Finally, theorising with an environmental context reminds the worker that humans are not separate from the environment and therefore social work practice is strengthened by exploring the impact of environmental degradation, from industrial pollution to climate-caused disasters, on vulnerable peoples as well as working towards a more sustainable future (Dominelli 2012; see also Chapter 18). This could mean exploring the impact of environmental issues on Zarah and understanding that, although the term refugee has a distinct meaning according to international law, many refugees are fleeing both political conflict and economic dislocation often caused by climate change.

Explore the practice context

When working with Zarah and other Muslims from refugee backgrounds, it is important to recognise the significant diversity in this group of people on dimensions of identity such as class, gender, ethnicity, language, age, disability or ability, sexuality and national origin. Many Muslim people from refugee backgrounds are vulnerable to further discrimination, disadvantage and human rights violations. It is important to note that the field of social work practice with people from migrant and refugee backgrounds has been somewhat marginal in social work until recently (McMahon 2002) and little attention has been paid to religious discrimination, in particular Islamophobia (Ferguson & Lavalette 2015) in social work practice.

A number of approaches may be useful for practice with Zarah such as anti-colonialist, anti-racist, culturally inclusive social work and anti-oppressive social work. In particular, the personal, cultural, structural approach developed by Thompson (2006) helps social workers to understand that human rights can be violated at each of these levels. It also provides a guide as to where social workers can work with people who experience oppression or violation of human rights. For example, Zarah reports being distressed by what she perceives as increasing verbal attacks on her Muslim identity and, in particular, wearing the hijab. Research demonstrates that Muslim women who wear the hijab experience higher levels of racism than other Muslim women (Australian Muslim Women's Centre for Human Rights, AMWCHR, 2008). While it is important to understand the resilience of the people with whom we work generally and Zarah, in particular, there are groups that are particularly vulnerable to human rights violations. The AMWCHR (2015), for instance, identifies that young Muslim women in Australia are particularly vulnerable to discrimination and this has implications for a critical human rights-based approach to practice.

The vilification that is the result of the intersection between race/ethnicity, gender and religion is experienced at the personal level and therefore workers can work collaboratively with Zarah at the personal level to identify her goals. This may include the provision of, or referral to, a range of services including counselling, in particular, trauma counselling such as that provided by the Victorian Foundation for Survivors of Torture and other torture and trauma services and support groups such as the Young Women's Programs offered by AMWCHR. It may also include the provision of advocacy, information and support to assist Zarah to understand and avail herself of the human rights protections that are offered in relation to religious discrimination at the state and federal levels.

In relation to the cultural level, in the Australian context Muslim people have been stereotyped, and the stigma and discrimination that results from this stereotyping is disseminated at the cultural level through the media and in the political process. As it has already been identified, the phenomenon of Islamophobia is increasing in Australia (Dunn, Klocker & Salabay 2007) and across the world. Social workers can work to ameliorate this oppression by being involved in social action campaigns to challenge these stereotypes and the resulting discrimination, such as the Voices Against Bigotry (2015) campaign, which was started to organise Australians to stand against anti-Muslim bigotry.

Human rights are abused at the structural level through policies, legislation and organisations. For example, in Australia some religious organisations receive exemptions from federal anti-discrimination law to allow them to act in ways that would otherwise be unlawful. Participating in inquiries, such as the recent Rights and Responsibilities 2014 inquiry, which explored the rights to freedom of thought, conscience and religion in Australia (Australian Human Rights Commission, AHRC, 2015b) would enable social workers to present submissions related to this and other issues related to religious discrimination. Social workers could participate in the Religious Freedom Roundtable, which is one of the key recommendations from the inquiry. Social workers can also work at the structural level using such methods of social policy advocacy and research-to-inform policy on such programs as the National School Chaplaincy Program, which has been particularly controversial in recent years. Working at these three levels—the personal, cultural and structural levels—demonstrates the importance of working in all of the domains of practice (Chenoweth & McAuliffe 2014). So while this case study refers to practice at the individual level (individual work with Zarah in a community health setting) social workers should be working across direct practice, social policy, research and education.

Conclusion

This chapter explores the meaning of human rights generally and its relationship with social work in particular. It examines the central role of the UDHR to social workers as well as exploring some of the critiques associated with human rights. Human rights offers a way forward to meet the emancipatory potential of critical social work. Finally, this chapter proposes an exploratory framework to embed a critical human rights-based approach into social work practice and explores how such a framework can be applied in practice. This chapter's central assumption is that although the concept of human rights is highly complex and contested, it provides a strong basis for practice that challenges the inequality, exploitation, domination and oppression that is experienced by vulnerable peoples in Australia and around the world.

References

AASW 2010, *Code of Ethics*, Canberra: AASW (Australian Association of Social Workers)

Allan, J. 2009, 'Theorising new developments in critical social work' in J. Allan, L. Briskman & B. Pease (eds), *Critical Social Work: Theories and practices for a socially just world*, 2nd edn, St Leonards: Allen & Unwin, pp. 30–44

Alston, M. 2012, 'Addressing the effects of climate change on rural communities', in J. Maidment & U. Bay (eds), *Social Work in Rural Australia: Enabling practice*, St Leonards: Allen & Unwin, pp. 204–17

AMWCHR 2008, *Race, Faith and Gender: Converging discriminations against Muslim women in Victoria. The ongoing impact of September 11, 2001*, Northcote: AMWCHR (Australian Muslim Women's Centre for Human Rights)

Australian Association of Social Workers, *see* AASW

AHRC 2015a, 'Human rights explained: Fact sheet 7: Australia and human rights treaties', AHRC, <www.humanrights.gov.au/human-rights-explained-fact-sheet-7australia-and-human-rights-treaties>, accessed 1 September 2015

—— 2015b, *Rights and Responsibilities Consultation Report 2015*, Sydney: AHRC

Australian Human Rights Commission *see* AHRC

Australian Muslim Women's Centre for Human Rights *see* AMCHR

—— 2015, 'Young women's programs', *AMWCHR*, < http://ausmuslimwomenscentre.org.au/2011/young-womens-programs>, accessed 22 September 2015

Aziz, N. 1999, 'The human rights debate in an era of globalization: Hegemony of discourse', in P. Van Ness (ed.), *Debating Human Rights: Critical essays from the Unites States and Asia*, London: Routledge, pp. 3–55

Briskman, L. 2014, *Social Work with Indigenous Communities: A human rights approach*, Sydney: Federation Press

Carey, S., Gibney, M. & Poe, S. 2010, *The Politics of Human Rights: The quest for dignity*, Cambridge: Cambridge University Press

Cemlyn, S. 2008, 'Human rights practice: Possibilities and pitfalls for developing emancipatory social work', *Ethics and Social Welfare*, vol. 2, no. 3, pp. 222–42

Chenoweth, L. & McAuliffe, D. 2014, *The Road to Social Work and Human Service Practice*, 4th edn, South Melbourne: Cengage Learning

Connolly, M. & Ward, T. 2008, *Morals, Rights and Practice in the Human Services: Effective and fair decision-making in health, social care and criminal justice*, London: Jessica Kingsley Publishers

Cowie, T. 2015, 'Bendigo mosque protest: anti-mosque and anti-racism protesters clash', *The Age*, <www.theage.com.au/action/printArticle?id=999867356>, accessed 18 September 2015

Crisp, B. 2010, *Spirituality and Social Work*, Burlington: Ashgate

Dominelli, L. 2012, *Green Social Work: From environmental crises to environmental justice*, Cambridge: Polity Press

Dunn, K., Klocker, N. & Salabay, T. 2007, 'Contemporary racism and Islamaphobia in Australia', *Ethnicities*, vol. 7, no. 4, pp. 564–89

Evans, T. 2011, *Human Rights in the Global Political Economy: Critical processes*, Boulder: Lynne Rienner Publishers

Falk, R. 1999, *Predatory Globalization: A critique*, Cambridge: Polity Press

Ferguson, I. 2008, *Reclaiming Social Work: Challenging neoliberalism and promoting social justice*, London: Sage Publications

—— 2011, 'Why class (still) matters' in M. Lavalette (ed.), *Radical Social Work Today: Social work at the crossroads*, The Policy Press, Bristol, pp. 115–34

Ferguson, I. & Lavalette, M. 2005, '"Another world is possible": Social work and the struggle for social justice' in I. Ferguson, M. Lavalette & E. Whitmore (eds), *Globalisation, global justice and social work*, Routledge, Abingdon, pp. 207–23

—— 2006, 'Globalization and global justice: Towards a social work of resistance', *International Social Work*, vol. 49, no. 3, pp. 309–18

—— 2015, 'Editorial: "Race", racism and anti-racist social work', *Critical and Radical Social Work*, vol. 3, no. 2, pp. 185–7

Fisher-Borne, M., Montana Cain, J. & Martin, S. 2015, 'From mastery to accountability: Cultural humility as an alternative to cultural competence', *The International Journal of Social Work Education*, vol. 34, no. 2, pp. 165–81

Fook, J. & Gardner, F. 2007, *Practising Critical Reflection: A resource handbook*, Maidenhead: Open University Press

Freeman, M. 2011, *Human Rights: An interdisciplinary approach*, 2nd edn, Cambridge: Polity Press

Furlong, M. & Wight, J. 2011, 'Promoting "critical awareness" and critiquing "cultural competence": Towards disrupting received professional knowledges', *Australian Social Work*, vol. 64, no. 1, pp. 38–54

George, J. 1999, 'Conceptual muddle, practical dilemma: human rights, social development and social work education', *International Social Work*, vol. 42, no. 1, pp. 15–26

Hodge, D. 2006, 'Advocating for the forgotten human right: Article 18 of the Universal Declaration of Human Rights—religious freedom', *International Social Work*, vol. 49, no. 4, pp. 431–3

Hosken, N. 2013, 'Social work supervision and discrimination', *Advances in Social Work and Welfare Education*, vol. 15, no. 1, pp. 92–104

Hugman, R. 2012, 'Human rights and social justice' in M. Gray, J. Midgley and S. Webb (eds), *The SAGE Handbook of Social Work*, London: SAGE Publications, pp. 372–85

Ife, J. 2010, *Human Rights from Below: Achieving rights through community development*, Melbourne: Cambridge University Press

—— 2012, *Human Rights and Social Work: Towards rights based practice*, 3rd edn, Melbourne: Cambridge University Press

IFSW 2004, 'Statement of ethical principles', <http://ifsw.org/policies/statement-of-ethical-principles/>, accessed 1 September 2015

International Federation of Social Workers *see* IFSW

Jones, B. 2014, 'The Australian Liberty Alliance and the politics of Islamophobia', *The Conversation*, http://theconversation.com/the-australian-liberty-alliance-and-the-politics-of-islamophobia-24225, accessed 18 September 2015

Keeney, A., Smart, A., Richards, R., Harrison, S., Carillo, M. and Valentine, D. 2014, 'Human rights and social work ethics: an international analysis', *Journal of Social Welfare and Human Rights*, vol. 2, no. 2, pp. 1–16

Lundy, C. 2011, *Social Work, Social Justice and Human Rights: A structural approach to practice*, 2nd edn, Ontario: University of Toronto Press

Mapp, S. 2008, *Human Rights and Social Justice in a Global Perspective: An introduction to international social work*, New York: Oxford University Press

McDonald, C. 2006, *Challenging Social Work: The context of practice*, Basingstoke: Palgrave Macmillan

McMahon, A. 2002, 'Writing diversity: Ethnicity and race in Australian social work', *Australian Social Work*, vol. 55, no. 3, pp. 172–83

Mullaly, B. 2010, *Challenging Oppression and Confronting Privilege*, 2nd edn, Don Mills: Oxford University Press

Nightingale, T. 2015, 'Anti-Islam rallies across the country this weekend could be violent, former right-wing organiser warns', *ABC News: The World Today*, <www.abc.net.au/news/2015-07-17/weekend-anti-islam-rallies-could-be-violent/6628208>, accessed 18 September 2015

Nipperess, S. & Briskman, L. 2009, 'Promoting a human rights perspective on critical social work' in J. Allan, L. Briskman and B. Pease (eds), *Critical Social Work: Theories and practices for a socially just world*, 2nd edn, St Leonards: Allen & Unwin, pp. 58–69

Office of the High Commissioner for Human Rights *see* OHCHR

OHCHR 1966a, 'International Covenant on Civil and Political Rights', *OHCHR*, <www.ohchr.org/en/professionalinterest/pages/ccpr.aspx, accessed 22 September 2015

—— 1966b, 'International Covenant on Economic, Social and Cultural Rights', *OHCHR*, <www.ohchr.org/EN/ProfessionalInterest/Pages/CESCR.aspx>, accessed 22 September 2015

Pease, B. 2010, *Undoing Privilege: Unearned advantage in a divided world*, London: Zed Books

Pease, B. & Fook, J. (eds) 1999, *Transforming Social Work Practice: Postmodern critical perspectives*, St Leonards: Allen & Unwin

Penketh, L. 2011, 'Social work and women's oppression today' in M. Lavalette (ed.), *Radical Social Work Today: Social work at the crossroads*, Bristol: The Policy Press, pp. 45–58

Rees, S. & Rodley, G. (eds) 1995, *The Human Costs of Managerialism: Advocating the recovery of humanity*, Marrickville: Pluto Press

Reichert, E. 1998, 'Women's rights are human rights: platform for action', *International Social Work*, vol. 41, no. 3, pp. 371–84

—— 2011, *Social Work and Human Rights: A foundation for policy and practice*, 2nd edn, New York: Columbia University Press

Skegg, A. 2005, 'Human rights and social work: A western imposition or empowerment to the people?', *International Social Work*, vol. 48, no. 5, pp. 667–72

Solas, J. 2000, 'Can a radical social worker believe in human rights?', *Australian Social Work*, vol. 53, no. 1, 65–70

Swensen, G. 1995, 'Female genital mutilation and human rights', *Australian Social Work*, vol. 48, no. 2, pp. 27–33

Tascón, S. and Ife, J. 2008, 'Human rights and critical whiteness: Whose humanity?', *The International Journal of Human Rights*, vol. 12, no. 3, pp. 307–27

Thompson, N. 2006, *Anti-discriminatory Practice*, 4th edn, Basingstoke: Palgrave Macmillan

United Nations 1948, 'Universal Declaration of Human Rights', *United Nations*, <www.un.org>

United Nations High Commissioner for Refugees *see* UNHCR

UNHCR 2010, Convention and Protocol Relating to the Status of Refugees, *UNHCR*, <www.unhcr.org/protect/PROTECTION/3b66c2aa10.pdf>, accessed 22 September 2015

—— 2015, 'Refugee crisis in Europe', *UNHCR*, <www.unrefugees.org.au/donate/refugee-crisis-in-europe?WT.mc_id=AW0015-37&gclid=CJvS44Lli8gCFUWXvQodzpcGoQ#one-off>, accessed 23 September 2015

Voices Against Bigotry. 2015, 'Stand up, speak out, stop Islamophobia', *Voices Against Bigotry*, <www.voicesagainstbigotry.org>, accessed 22 September 2015

Walter, M., Taylor, S. & Habibis, D. 2011, 'How white is social work in Australia?', *Australian Social Work*, vol. 64, no. 1, pp. 6–19

Wetzel, J.W. 2007, 'Human rights and women: A work in progress' in E. Reichert (ed.), *Challenges in Human Rights: A social work perspective*, Colombia University Press, New York, pp. 162–87

Williams, C. & Johnson, M. 2010, *Race and Ethnicity in a Welfare Society*, Maidenhead: Open University Press

Wronka, J. 2008, *Human Rights and Social Justice: Social action and service for the helping and health professions*, Thousand Oaks: Sage Publications

6

Interrogating privilege and complicity in the oppression of others

Bob Pease

Introduction

Social workers who are committed to the radical and critical tradition in social work need to reflect upon their own positioning in systems of inequality. Social workers are beneficiaries of the systems that oppress the people they work with. They are part of a professional-managerial class that occupy contradictory locations between the two major classes (Pease 2010) and those who are also white, male, heterosexual and able-bodied receive further benefits from the unjust system they oppose.

How might social workers who adopt a critical perspective, unwittingly reproduce systemic oppression, while espousing social justice and human rights? How might they be complicit in the reproduction of patriarchy, white supremacy, class domination and other systems of inequality? Probyn (2004) challenges social work practitioners and academics to consider the connections between the work that we do on social justice issues and the privileged positions that we occupy. This means that social workers will need to be more aware of their complicity and challenge it in others. They will also need to develop strategies and skills for critical practices that encourage responsibility to expose this complicity. In addressing these challenges, social workers need to explore critical studies in the fields of masculinity, whiteness, heterosexuality, ableism and other fields of privilege.

Resistance and epistemologies of ignorance

Experiences of oppression, violence and abuse are not generally acknowledged by members of privileged groups. One of the common practices that reproduces social inequality is the denial of oppression and privilege (Pease 2010). How do we encourage a critical consciousness of privilege and complicity among members of privileged groups?

Increasing people's awareness of the unearned advantages that come from their membership of privileged groups often leads to resistance. Many people express anger and hostility when they are challenged about their privilege. A critical awareness of privilege does not occur without difficult exchanges about what it means to be privileged. Some level of resistance to explore privilege can be expected by members of privileged groups.

One way of understanding the complicity of members of privileged groups with normative and exploitative practices is through the scholarship on epistemologies of ignorance (Sullivan & Tuana 2007). Members of privileged groups, even when they have good intentions, can reproduce social inequalities through various forms of ignorance. The way in which epistemologies of ignorance operate is that members of privileged groups generally do not know the extent to which they do not know (Applebaum 2013).

Thus, it can be argued that there is an epistemology of ignorance in relation to structural forms of privilege. Such ignorance is sometimes systemically reproduced through the attempts of some members of privileged groups to deflect attention away from the social processes that produce privilege. Members of privileged groups can prefer to remain ignorant because it allows them to avoid facing their moral complicity in the reproduction of social inequality (Applebaum 2013).

Therefore we can see that there are various levels of ignorance in relation to privilege and various degrees of conscious agency used to maintain ignorance. While some educational strategies succeed in heightening awareness of privilege among those who are unaware of the extent of their privileged positioning, other strategies are required to address those members of privileged groups who actively deflect and knowingly stay 'ignorant' in the face of such knowledge.

Becoming aware of privilege

One of the strategies to address members of privileged groups is to ask them to reflect on their race, gender, class, sexuality, able-bodied and age privilege (Smith 2013). Ways of being self-reflexive about privileged positioning is important to transform biases among those who are privileged (Pease 2014a).

This reflection often takes the form of a confession to others about their respective privileges. McIntosh's (1998) work has been significant in raising awareness of white privilege and her white-privilege checklist has led to similar lists of male privileges (Schacht 2003), class privileges (Class Acts 2007), heterosexual privileges (Johnson 2006) and able-bodied privileges (May-Machunda 2005). I have used this approach myself when teaching (Pease 2006). However, this way of addressing privilege has been criticised. Many of those who have used McIntosh's seminal article in teaching have reported that the discussion of the checklist did not lead to anti-racist action (Lensmire et al. 2013).

Lensmire et al. (2013) argue that McIntosh's understanding of privilege seems to be premised on the idea that privilege is individual rather than systemic. Understanding one's own privilege does not necessarily lead people to struggle to overcome systemic oppression. Applebaum (2010) suggests that the admission of privilege can prevent members of privileged groups from recognising their complicity in the structures that reproduce oppression. For Applebaum (2010), members of privileged groups must see themselves as having privileged group membership rather than simply seeing themselves as individuals. Otherwise, they will be unable to differentiate between individual suffering (possibly involving harm) and systemic suffering, which is oppression.

Ironically, when people acknowledge privilege, it can lead to them avoiding the recognition of their complicity in the structures that maintain privilege. Levine-Rasky (2010) believes that teaching about privilege as something that individuals possess can obscure the links between the benefits of privilege and the practices by members of privileged groups that reproduce structures of privilege. Thus, the focus should be on the advantages received by privilege and the processes by which privilege is appropriated (Leonardo 2004).

Towards a pedagogy of the privileged

One of the key issues in this emerging area of pedagogy for the privileged is developing models and practices to encourage members of privileged groups to acknowledge their privilege and their complicity in the oppression of others.

Curry-Stevens (2007) has developed a six-step transformational model of the cognitive changes that members of privileged groups should move through to become aware of their privilege:

- Step 1: Awareness of oppression. Members of privileged groups must be convinced that oppression still exists today.
- Step 2: Awareness of oppression as structural and therefore enduring and pervasive. Members of privileged groups must develop a structural analysis of power relations and oppression.
- Step 3: Locating oneself as oppressed. Members of privileged groups must first identify themselves as oppressed before they see themselves as being privileged.
- Step 4: Locating oneself as privileged. After recognising their oppression, members of privileged groups recognise their privileged positioning.
- Step 5: Understand the benefits that flow from privilege. Members of privileged groups understand how their life experiences have been shaped by their privileged position.
- Step 6: Understanding oneself as implicated in the oppression of others and understanding oneself as an oppressor. Members of privileged groups understand the role that they play in upholding systems of oppression and how they are culpable for, and implicated in, oppression.

In Curry-Stevens' (2007) view, these stages are necessarily sequential and members of privileged groups must engage with the earlier stages before they can accept their privilege and complicity in the oppression of others. In her view, members of privileged groups will reject attempts to challenge them about their complicity if they have not slowly moved through the earlier stages of awareness. Thus there is a focus on people locating themselves as oppressed before exploring their privilege.

However, in relation to Step 3, while one can focus on relative forms of oppression if the privileged group participants are also members of oppressed groups, it raises questions about how you challenge privilege with white, heterosexual able-bodied upper-class men. Also, some critical educators (Leonardo 2004; Mayo 2004) argue that staging levels of awareness to fit in with the learning needs of members of privileged groups can reinforce their privileged positioning. These educators argue that we begin by recognising ourselves as being privileged and implicated in the oppression of others rather than seeing this as the end point of the transformation process. For Smith (2013), the starting point for change should be the presumption that all members of privileged groups are complicit in the structures of dominance.

By recognising this complicity, we then explore how to transform our practices to address this complicity.

One way for social workers who are committed to the critical and radical tradition in social work to address their complicity is to consider themselves as a potential ally for the oppressed (Curry-Stevens 2007). Members of privileged groups who see themselves as good allies, however, are often not reflective about their own complicity in systems of oppression. If we do not see ourselves as being prejudiced, then it is easy to avoid recognising the ways in which we can be complicit in reproducing structures of oppression (Applebaum 2010); complicity does not rely on intention.

Ahmed (2006) argues that we should be careful not to respond too quickly with answers to the question about what are members of privileged people to do. If people act too quickly, she suggests, they can avoid hearing the message about their complicity. Mayo (2004), for example, draws attention to the resentment expressed by anti-sexist men who are opposed to rape but who demand a place in Reclaim the Night marches. They need to be acknowledged by feminists that they are not part of the problem, when the feminist critique is that all men are implicated in men's violence against women. More listening with an awareness of privilege on the part of these men about women's experiences might have avoided this outcome.

Overcoming complicity in the oppression of others

According to Blum, a person is 'complicit in injustice if she benefits from it (even if she did not seek that benefit)' (2008: 311). Applebaum defines complicity as involving 'participation *without* intention' (Applebaum 2006: 350). Systemic oppression does not require the intent of individuals. It is through systemic patterns that are naturalised, normalised and appear to be invisible (Applebaum 2006).

Because the structures of privilege are so deeply embedded in Australian society, it is almost impossible for members of privileged groups to avoid receiving unjust benefits. As Trepagnier notes: 'No one is immune to the ideas that permeate the culture in which he or she is raised.' (2006: 15).

Much complicity by members of privileged groups is lawful and manifested, for example, in the forms of everyday sexism and everyday racism that aggravate harm but are not criminalised. As Card (2010) notes, these forms of everyday oppressive practices allow for physical violence against women, gays and non-white people to be legitimated and excused. Card (2010) uses the language of 'enablers' to describe those men who are not physically violent but are connected to men who are violent without challenging them.

All men are complicit to varying degrees in the reproduction of patriarchy. Because men benefit from patriarchy (although not equally), they are less motivated than women to be aware of the costs associated with it. If men do not notice how patriarchy advantages them and disadvantages women, they are likely to regard the distribution of rewards as normal and natural (Card 2010).

Applebaum (2013) refers to two types of complicity. One form of complicity is seen as the outcome of unconsciously negative attitudes and beliefs that privileged-group members hold about marginalised people that shape their practices. The second form of complicity is more focused on practices and habits of doing whiteness, or gender or class or other forms of privilege.

Applebaum (2010) argues that if white people (and by extension, all members of privileged groups) want to be allies to challenge systemic racism and other forms of structural inequality, they have to acknowledge their complicity. She doubts allies who espouse their commitment to social justice but avoid recognising their own culpability for perpetuating oppression. In her view, acknowledging complicity is the first step to opening discussion, rather than the final step as Curry-Stevens (2007) argues.

Thus it is important to ask the question: 'How might I be complicit in sustaining rather than challenging systemic oppression and white privilege?' (Applebaum 2006: 353). Barton argues that 'I can only become part of the solution when I recognise the degree to which I am part of the problem, not because I am white but because of my investment in white privilege' (Barton 2010: 1). The enormity of this realisation can be daunting and it begs the question of 'What happens now?' In the remainder of this chapter I explore some of the efforts required in taking responsibility to challenge complicity. As part of this, I need to acknowledge my own positioning as a white male class-privileged social work academic (Pease 2015a).

Beyond neoliberal frameworks of responsibility

Payson (2009) makes the point that because a person was born into systems of privilege and oppression does not mean that they have no responsibility to challenge them. The structures of inequality are not self-perpetuating; they are reproduced by individual participants, especially those who are members of privileged groups. The burden of responsibility to promote social justice should fall more heavily on those who benefit most from their complicity than on those who are non-beneficiaries (Young 2011).

The most common understanding of responsibility is that based on the assumption that society consists of individuals who are disconnected to their historical and social contexts. In this view, perpetrators of racism, or violence against women or other abusive practices are prejudiced and ignorant individuals. The approach focuses on the individual perpetrator's mind. Applebaum (2006) argues that we need to develop new responsibilities that are less focused on the acts of individual perpetrators and more focused on the contribution that members of privileged groups make to the structural patterns of privilege and oppression.

Boyd (2004) queries whether the conception of the subject that underlies the notion of the liberal individual (who has moral responsibility for individual actions) obscures systemic oppression and protects members of privileged groups because the focus is on individual intention. In the liberal concept, the individual is isolated from others, exercises rational choice and is able to transcend structural constraints in the exercise of their agency, or capacity to act in the world (Boyd 2004).

The responsibility model that is based on the premise of the liberal individual conceals the complicity of members of privileged groups in the perpetuation of privilege and oppression (Boyd 2004). There is a need to challenge this concept of the liberal individual to encourage people to recognise their complicity. This means that it is important to focus less on individual responsibility and more on collective responsibility to challenge the structural dimensions of inequality.

Crowe (2011) has noted the defensive responses of many men in regards to feminism. In addressing such defensiveness, it is tempting for feminists to say to men that it is not their fault and that they are not personally responsible. However, men in general are complicit in the continuing oppression of women. If they are unable to understand their complicity, they will not be able to engage constructively with feminism.

Engaging men emotionally in terms of violence against women: An exercise from practice

Encouraging members of privileged groups to recognise their complicity in the perpetuation of injustice is notoriously difficult. Below, I provide an example of a workshop exercise that I have used to encourage men, who have not been identified as violent, to recognise their complicity in the oppression of women.

I am sitting with a group of men in a circle and I roll out a long sheet of paper, which has a timeline from 5000 years BC to the present day. I scatter some felt-tip pens across the paper and I say to the men: 'What I would like you to do is to think about ways in which men have used their power over women. This may be in the form of violence, discrimination or unequal treatment. It can include something that impacts on all women or just some women or just one woman. It can include an event that you remember from history or a recent or contemporary event that you remember being reported in the media. It can also include something that impacted on a woman in your life. You may also want to consider whether there is anything that you do not feel particularly proud of in terms of your own behaviour in relation to a woman in your life. You may not choose to disclose this. But I want you to think about it.'

I give the participants a few minutes to think and then I invite them to come forward and name the event they want to record on the timeline, and the date on which it occurred. After recording the event on the timeline, they return to their seats. Participants come forward as many times as they want, until there is nothing more they want to record. I do not allow for any discussion during the exercise. At the end of the exercise, the timeline is covered with numerous incidents of violence and abuse against women, including personal disclosures about women in their own lives who have been affected by violence and it sometimes includes the men disclosing their own complicity in the abuse of women.

When the timeline is completed, we sit silently to reflect on the events that the participants have recorded. From my experience in running the workshops over a number of years, the exercise always evokes emotional responses in many of the men, ranging from sadness and distress to anger as they reflect on the extent of the processes of victimisation and violence against women throughout history, in contemporary society and in their own lives and the lives of women whom they love.

This exercise provides an example of how men's emotional investments in privilege can be disrupted, even if momentarily. If men are to be engaged in promoting gender equality, they need to recognise the role that emotions play in sustaining their privilege and address the barriers that inhibit them from experiencing compassion, empathy and sadness in response to the suffering of others. When men are emotionally engaged in the injustices experienced by women, they are more likely to interrogate their own complicity in women's oppression and to recognise their responsibility to challenge their own unearned advantages (Pease 2012). This is only one small step in engaging men in violence prevention and it is used here to illustrate some of the pedagogical issues in engaging one particular group of participants about their privilege. I have written elsewhere about the wider issues involved in violence prevention (Pease 2008, 2014b, 2015b).

Since the 1990s, I have facilitated hundreds of these workshops as both part of gender awareness and gender equality training within workplaces (including local councils, church-based organisations, schools, universities and the corporate sector), and as interventions in community-based and social movement organisations, and political parties. In all cases, the participants are recruited from the ranks of the respective organisations. Often the workshops are required by the workplace as part of professional development and hence there is sometimes a level of resistance by the men who attend. While some men may be motivated in becoming more aware of their male privilege, other men are initially resistant to the intervention. Even the latter group of men sometimes shift their perspective as a result of these workshops.

In evaluations I have conducted, and from feedback received from participants and the participants' female colleagues, these emotional responses by men to men's violence against women seem to shatter some of the men's complacency about violence against women. Because the timeline is constructed from their own observations and experiences, they begin to see connections between the impact of violence on women in their lives and the wider systemic mistreatment of women throughout history. As a man facilitating these workshops, I always gain new knowledge about forms of discrimination and violence against women. Although I have run these workshops many times, I never fail to be emotionally affected by the participants' observations and experiences of men's violence against women.

I argue that this strategy of engaging men emotionally in addressing violence against women applies to other privileged groups in relation to, for example, racism, homophobia and class elitism. In the latter part of this chapter, I explore other dimensions of this argument in relation to engaging with discomfort, dealing with guilt and shame, and addressing the losses that are associated with relinquishing privilege.

Towards a pedagogy of discomfort?

Many attempts to engage members of privileged groups in addressing various forms of inequality try to avoid inducing shame or guilt among those who benefit from unjust systems. Applebaum (2010) says that in understanding complicity in the oppression of others we should avoid immobilising guilt. This approach suggests that educators tone down their critiques of structural oppression and encourage members of privileged groups to feel more comfortable.

Those in privileged groups have the most to lose in terms of resources and status in struggles for equality. Many attempts at engaging members of privileged groups in struggles for social justice avoid threatening them so their resistance is minimised. In a discussion of anti-racist practice, Leonardo (2004) talks about the limitation of framing racism as a problem perpetuated by 'bad' whites who are challenged by 'good' white allies. Constructing racism as the 'other', which does not implicate 'good whites', creates a sense of comfort for white allies. Leonardo (2004) argues that if whites do not feel a sense of discomfort they will be unable to empathise with the pain and suffering of those who are oppressed by racism. I have argued elsewhere that the same applies to engaging men in campaigns against violence against women (Pease 2015b).

Guilt can be paralysing and it can inhibit critical reflection (Leonardo 2004). However, I argue here that if one is complicit in perpetuating inequalities, one should feel guilty (Payson 2009). Smith (2013) similarly argues against the notion of creating 'safe spaces' for dialogues between members of privileged groups and members of marginalised groups. Even when members of privileged groups are aware of their privileges, they do not disappear in these dialogues. Like Smith, I am concerned that the accusation of 'unsafe' can be used against marginalised people who may express their anger at exploitation and oppression. The question is whether a safe space is possible in the context of enduring structural inequalities.

Challenging privilege and complicity should involve emotions as people connect to their responsibility and culpability in the perpetuation of oppression. Many commentators argue that learning about privilege is painful. Allen and Rossatto (2009) argue that members of privileged groups can only come to understand their privileged positioning through significant emotional experiences.

Members of privileged groups may never be fully able to understand their privileged position. While it may be impossible to bridge the gulf that separates members of privileged groups from those who are marginalised, the recognition that one's understanding can only be partial enables a more respectful encounter (Ang 1997).

The politics of privileged identities

Within the studies of dominance and privilege, there are two different strategies for educating members of privileged groups about their privileged positions. One approach involves articulating a positive and progressive identity associated with whiteness, masculinity, class and so on. Allen and Rossatto (2009) argue that critical pedagogy must encourage the development of positive identities for members of oppressor groups.

In relation to anti-racism, those that emphasise a positive identity focus on the importance of white participants feeling pride in being white (Levine-Rasky 2010). These strategies are premised on the notion of needing to build a sense of identity in white people to encourage them to engage in anti-racism work (Mayo 2004). The aim is to encourage white people to be comfortable in their anti-racism work. To be able to do this, it is argued that white anti-racists have to be able to see themselves as being outside the critique of whiteness as racism (Mayo 2004).

In relation to engaging men in gender equality and anti-violence work, Katz (2006) emphasises that he is careful not to adopt an accusatory tone in working with men about violence against women. Flood adopts a similar invitational approach when he comments: 'Most men are not violent and most men treat women in their lives with respect and care' (Flood 2009: 17). In this view, men are positioned as being either violent or non-violent. Non-violent men are encouraged to challenge the violence of other men. Such men are framed as 'good men' who will protect women from 'bad men'.

The question is whether people can understand their privilege and then develop a positive identity based on whiteness, being a man or being heterosexual or so on and then relinquish their association with that privilege. I argue that members of privileged groups are always caught up in systems of privilege and that they cannot escape their complicity (Applebaum 2010). In my view, people must renunciate their identification with whiteness, masculinity, class elitism and other forms of privilege. People do this by developing a traitorous identity in relation to the privileged groups to which they belong. Developing a traitorous identity entails challenging internalised moral superiority and rejecting the sense of entitlement that so many members of privileged groups are socialised to have. The following examples from privilege studies illustrate the rationale for such politics (see also Pease 2010 for an outline of practical strategies for challenging the reproduction of privilege from within).

In relation to whiteness, for example, anti-racist abolitionists focus on moving beyond whiteness (Manglitz 2003). Mayo (2004) talks about anti-racist white people wanting to exceptionalise themselves so that they are not seen as the average white person. In her view, the identity of the ally is not as important as the commitment they have to challenging some form of privilege. She argues against the practice of attempting to remake white identity as part of challenging institutionalised racism. Rather than engaging in a project of white identity development, she argues that it is more politically appropriate to unsettle the certainty of white privilege and to form alliances against racism that do not involve the reconstruction of white identity.

In relation to masculinity, Connell (1995) proposes a strategy of 'exit politics' to oppose patriarchy and try to exit from dominant masculinity. She identifies this strategy as the only path that has any potential to challenge the gender order. Stoltenberg (1989) similarly argues that men should 'refuse to be a man' and construct a subjectivity based on moral selfhood. In this view, we have to destabilise men's identities and encourage them to create solidarity with women on the basis of respect for difference.

The above debates about strategy reflect different notions of identity. The creation of identity is intrinsically connected with social processes and the relations of ruling (D. Smith 1989) which is the system of dominating others. Following Andrea

Smith (2013), I argue that allies should be less concerned with constructing a new form of identity for themselves and more focused on creating new forms of social relations.

The other side of privilege

Those who have been involved in transforming the subjectivities of members of privileged groups often talk about the challenges and discomforts involved, where one's world view and identity is shaken and destabilised (Curry-Stevens 2007). In such models, little attention is given to the benefits that come to those with privilege as a result of their transformation.

One strategy is to suggest that privilege is not entirely or unilaterally beneficial (Logue 2005). Logue develops what she calls a contrapuntal approach to deconstructing privilege (Logue 2005), which involves recognising the perils as well as the benefits of power and privilege. She argues that not all privileges are desirable or even beneficial. Thus, she is interested in the costs of privilege for those in privileged groups. This includes the dehumanisation of those with privileges. Logue's argument is that those involved in social justice struggles should not be primarily motivated by doing something for 'them' as it can position members of oppressed groups as powerless (Logan 2005). Rather, they should be more concerned with addressing their own issues embedded in the social relations of exploitation (Mayo 2004).

Mayo (2004) acknowledges that there are risks involved in exploring how members of privileged groups suffer. There is the danger of re-centering privilege, and failing to differentiate between the harms caused by the psychological consequences of having privilege, as well as the systemic oppression of those who are on the receiving end of structurally-based inequalities. I have also argued elsewhere that emphasising the positive outcomes for men being involved in gender equality and anti-violence work can fail to address the resistances that men have to relinquishing their privilege and acknowledging their complicity in the reproduction of gender inequality (Pease 2015b).

While it can be important when working with members of privileged groups to draw attention to the personal benefits for them of relinquishing privilege, it is also important to emphasise the moral, ethical and political reasons why they should change. We should not underestimate the level of resistance that many people have to acknowledge and surrender their privilege.

Conclusion

In this chapter I have explored the limits and potential of various practices in facilitating a critical consciousness of people's privileged positioning. Good intentions are not enough to exclude progressive social workers from the perpetuation of forms of injustice. Social workers who are committed to the radical and critical tradition need to be open to the many ways in which they may be part of the problem, even as they espouse a social justice and human rights approach to practice. They need to understand the social and political processes that produce various forms of social inequality. If they do not understand how the structures of privilege and oppression are reproduced, they will not know how best to challenge them (Blum 2008). A key issue is unsettling the moral certitude, which inhabits the subjectivity of those who are privileged. In place of moral certitude, we should strive for a more humble, fallible and vulnerable sense of positioning (Appelbaum 2010).

Social workers cannot simply transcend the structures of privilege in which they are embedded. Their responsibility lies in continually challenging the systems that privilege them. No one is innocent when it comes to complicity. We need to develop a critical awareness of how we are implicated in the perpetuation of inequality through our social work practices. This chapter has started to explore how to challenge those practices in ourselves and in others.

References

Ahmed, S. 2006, 'The nonperformativity of antiracism', *Meridians: Feminism, Race, Transnationalism*, vol. 7, no. 1, pp. 104–26

Allen, R. & Rossatto, A. 2009, 'Does critical pedagogy work with privileged students?', *Teacher Education Quarterly*, vol. 36, no. 1, pp. 163–80

Ang, I. 1997, 'Comment on Felski's "The doxa of difference: The uses of incommensurabililty"', *Signs*, vol. 23, no. 1, pp. 57–64

Appelbaum, B. 2006, 'Race ignore-ance, colortalk and white complicity: White is . . . white isn't', *Educational Theory*, vol. 56, no. 3, pp. 345–62

—— 2010, *Being White, Being Good: White complicity, white moral responsibility, and social justice pedagogy*, Lanham: Rowman & Littlefield

—— 2013, 'Vigilance as a response to white complicity', *Educational Theory*, vol. 63, no. 3, pp. 17–34

Barton, A. 2010, 'Going white: Claiming an identity of white privilege', paper presented at the Symposium: Future Stories/Intimate Histories, Australian Critical Race Studies and Whiteness Studies Association Conference, Adelaide, South Australia, 10 December

Blum, L. 2008, 'White privilege: A mild critique', *Theory and Research in Education*, vol. 6, no. 3, pp. 309–21

Boyd, D. 2004, 'The legacies of liberalism and oppressive relations: Facing a dilemma for the subject of moral education', *Journal of Moral Education*, vol. 33, no. 1, pp. 3–22

Card, C. 2010, *Confronting Evils: Terrorism, torture, genocide,* Cambridge: Cambridge University Press

Class Acts 2007, *The Invisibility of Upper Class Privilege,* Boston: Women's Theological Centre

Connell, R. 1995, *Masculinities,* St Leonards: Allen & Unwin

Crowe, J. 2011, 'Men and feminism: Some challenges and a partial response', *Social Alternatives,* vol. 30, no. 1, pp. 49–53

Curry-Stevens, A. 2007, 'New forms of transformative education: Pedagogy for the privileged', *Journal of Transformative Education,* vol. 5, no. 1, pp. 33–58

Flood, M. 2009, 'Let's Stop Violence Before it Starts: Using primary prevention strategies to engage men, mobilise communities and change the world.' Notes of a one-day workshop. New Zealand, 28 September to 2 October

Johnson, A. 2006, *Privilege, Power and Difference,* New York: McGraw-Hill,

Katz, J. 2006, *The Macho Paradox: Why some men hurt women and how all men can help,* Naperville: Sourcebooks

Lensmire, T., McManimon, S., Tierney, J., Nichols, M., Casey, Z., Lensmire, A. & David, B. 2013, 'McIntosh as synecdoche: How teacher education's focus on white privilege undermines anti-racism', *Harvard Educational Review,* vol. 83, no. 3, pp. 410–31

Leonardo, Z. 2004, 'The color of supremacy: Beyond the discourse of white privilege', *Educational Philosophy and Theory,* vol. 36, no. 2, pp. 137–52

Levine-Rasky, C. 2010, 'Framing whiteness: Working through the tensions in introducing whiteness to educators', *Race, Ethnicity and Education,* vol. 3, no. 3, pp. 271–92

Logue, J. 2005, 'Deconstructing privilege: A contrapuntal approach', *Philosophy of Education,* pp. 371–9

Manglitz, E. 2003, 'Challenging white privilege in adult education: A critical review of the literature', *Adult Education Quarterly,* vol. 53, no. 2, pp. 119–34

May-Machunda, P. 2005, 'Exploring the invisible knapsack of able-bodied privilege', unpublished paper, Moorhead: Minnesota State University

Mayo, C. 2004, 'Certain privilege: Rethinking white agency', *Philosophy of Education,* pp. 308–16

McIntosh, P. 1998, 'White privilege: Unpacking the invisible knapsack' in M. McGodrick (ed.), *Re-Visioning Family Therapy: Race, culture and gender in clinical practice,* New York: Guilford Press, pp. 147–52

Payson, J. 2009, 'Moral dilemmas and collective responsibilities', *Essays in Philosophy,* vol. 10, no. 2, pp. 1–23

Pease, B. 2006, 'Encouraging critical reflections on privilege in social work and the human services', *Practice Reflexions,* vol. 1, no. 1, pp. 15–26

—— 2008, 'Engaging men in men's violence prevention: Exploring the tensions, dilemmas and possibilities', Australian Domestic and Family Violence Clearinghouse Issues Paper 17, Sydney.

—— 2010, *Undoing Privilege: Unearned advantage in a divided world,* London: Zed Books

—— 2012, 'The politics of gendered emotions: Disrupting men's emotional investments in privilege', *Australian Journal of Social Issues,* vol. 47, no. 1, pp. 125–42

—— 2014a, 'Transforming privileged subjectivities: Towards a pedagogy of the oppressor' in M. Pallotta-Chiarolli & B. Pease (eds), *The Politics of Recognition and Social Justice: Transforming subjectivities and new forms of resistance,* Routledge, New York, pp. 159–72

—— 2014b, 'Theorising men's violence prevention policies: Limitations and possibilities of interventions in a patriarchal state' in N. Henry and A. Powell (eds), *Preventing Sexual Violence: Interdisciplinary approaches to overcoming a rape culture,* New York: Palgrave Macmillan, pp. 22–40

—— 2015a 'Injuries and privileges in: Being a white working-class academic man' in D. Mitchell,

J. Wilson & V. Archer (eds), *Bread and Roses: Voices of Australian Academics from the Working Class,* Sense Publishers, Rotterdam, pp. 85–93

—— 2015b 'Disengaging men from patriarchy: Rethinking the man question in masculinity studies' in M. Flood and R. Howsen (eds), *Engaging Men in Building Gender Equality,* Cambridge Scholars' Press, Cambridge, pp. 55–70

Probyn, F. 2004, 'Playing chicken at the intersection: The white critic of whiteness', *Borderlands,* vol. 3, no. 2, pp. 1–11

Schacht, S. 2003, 'Teaching about being an oppressor' in M. Kimmel and A. Ferber (eds), *Privilege: A reader,* Westview Press, Boulder, pp. 161–71

Smith, A. 2013, 'Unsettling the privilege of self-reflexivity' in F. Twine and B. Gardner (eds), *Geographies of Privilege,* Hoboken: Taylor and Francis, pp. 263–79

Smith, D. 1989, *The Everyday World as Problematic,* Holiston: Northeastern

Stoltenberg, J. 1989, *Refusing to be a Man,* New York: Meridian

Trepagnier, B. 2006, *Silent Racism: How well-meaning white people perpetuate the racist divide,* Boulder: Paradigm

Young, I. 2011, *Responsibility for Justice,* New York: Oxford University Press

7

Social work, class and the structural violence of poverty

Norah Hosken

Introduction

This chapter invites social workers to use a poverty-aware and class cognisant (PACC) approach to doing critical social work. Although written from the perspective of one who has an Anglo-Celtic background in a colonised country, I have aimed to make this relevant for readers from other contexts. I present a view of poverty and class that considers inequalities, and their associated social problems, to be an inherent part of how societies are organised by neoliberal ideology, social relations and practices. Following an introduction to some of the key concepts, assumptions and core principles that underpin a poverty-aware and class cognisant approach, a case study is provided to illustrate potential applications for social work.

I argue that, in neoliberal societies, advantage and disadvantage are allocated in unequal ways that structurally abuse those people and populations who are furthest from the 'mythical norm' (Lorde 1999). Explanations are provided for how these three key concepts—neoliberalism, the mythical norm, and the structural violence of poverty that causes structural abuse—are understood in this chapter.

A neoliberal society is based on a belief in free-market capitalism that involves privatisation, deregulation, and primacy of the individual's rights and of economic growth. The fundamental role of government is to create and maintain the economic, political and cultural framework to facilitate these priorities (Thorsen & Lie 2006; Khan 2015). The cultural framework is where the values of individualism, competition, merit, consumerism and materialism are embedded in how people think about, and treat, themselves and others. Mythical norms are constructed and enacted that normalise the class-based, 'economic pyramid' (Cudd & Holmstrom 2011: 193) hierarchy that is required for neoliberal societies to function. Lorde describes a mythical norm as a socially constructed 'stereotype that is perpetuated by society, against which everyone else is measured' (Lorde 1999: 362) that creates a hierarchy under which others fall.

Class-based structural violence

The class-based hierarchy enables neoliberalism to function and, of particular concern to social work, is achieved through the use of violence. Allen (2001: 47–8) uses the theory of 'structural violence' (Soest 1997; Galtung 1969) to expand the traditional definition of violence from its focus on individual criminal acts against people or property. Structural violence recognises the capacity of people and institutions through 'action and inaction' to inflict harms such as 'discrimination, economic inequality and social injustice' on victims even when not in a direct relationship with them (Allen 2001: 47). These harms include those that are socially approved, and those that are avoidable, that breach human rights or prevent people's access to basic human needs through:

> (1) omission, failing to provide assistance to people in need, (2) as a result of repression, or a violation of civil, political, economic and/or social rights, or through (3) alienation, or severely limiting people's emotional, cultural, or intellectual growth (Allen 2001: 47–8).

In their everyday work, the majority of social workers are witness to, and participants in, the class-based nature of the structural violence of poverty (Ho 2007). Those individuals, families, groups and communities furthest from their society's 'mythical norm' are systematically subjected to the highest rates and impacts of the structural abuse of poverty (Hosken 2013). The majority of the clients of social workers are poor (Sheedy 2012); they disproportionately comprise the people and groups who Marx called the 'reserve army of labour' and the 'relative surplus population' (Marx 1976) sections of the working class. These sub-sections of the working class are predominantly those whose material and social locations such as class, gender, race, dis/ability, age, sexual orientation, religion and geography combine to make them less useful or productive in the paid labour market. Conversely, where the material and social positioning of these groups can make them very useful to the free market, as their need to be part of the waged labour system to survive forces them to accept low wages and poor working conditions (Khan 2015).

Neoliberalism, the 'capitalist fear' and relations of inequality

While comprising many facets, neoliberal theory emphasises individualism and management of the self (Rose 1990). This involves the belief that competition-based market mechanisms are the most efficient and effective allocator of goods and services (including welfare) for people, who are considered to be self-interested, rational and profit-seeking individuals (Hutchinson & Mellor 2004).

Neoliberal theory, and associated practices, foster relationships of inequality through invoking in people the capitalist fear of becoming one of the many 'losers' needed to create the fewer 'winners'. When people experience relationships to employment that are precarious (Standing 2011) and there is institutionalised insecurity (Neilson 2015), the capitalist fear becomes a binding influence with some shared features across workers at low, middle and high wage levels.

In tandem with the capitalist fear is the use of capitalist enticement and entrapment into the neoliberal dream of becoming a winner; that it might just be possible, despite the odds, to become one of the 'haves', instead of remaining a 'have not', or a 'have not enough'. The combination of fear and enticement creates a dominating cultural hold over people (Gramsci 1971). This involves a coercive effect, even on those people and groups who are the worst affected by the values, norms, and practices of dominant economic and political systems. People are coerced into not seeing a society as being organised by people, institutions and practices that promote neoliberalism; they are coerced to accept the 'invisible hand of the market' (Smith 1776 in Olsen 2007) as natural and common sense, and as the only way that a society can be organised to survive.

Relations of class, survival and poverty

Competition to survive is an important component of neoliberalism's logical and cultural framework. This is more clearly evident when neoliberalism is understood as a development from the capitalist system, 'based on commodity production for profitable exchange in which the majority of people are obliged to take part as waged labour if they want to survive' (Hutchinson & Mellor 2004: 7). The conventional

Marxist understanding of the class structure of the capitalist mode of production is seen as producing conflict between two key classes: the ruling class who own the means of production and the working class who must sell their labour power, where these class relations are inherently exploitative, as the ruling class must extract surplus value from workers. These class-based inequalities are normalised and reproduced through time (Ferguson 2011).

Socialist feminism

Socialist feminists advocate the importance of recognising class-based inequalities and fostering class-based resistances to structural violence. They also advocate the potential strengths of class-based, solidarity informed, transformations of unequal relations, organisations and societies. Socialist feminists extend traditional Marxism with understandings of class as always shaped on the lines of gender, race (Acker 2006a), able-bodiedness, heterosexuality and ageism. While acknowledging academic and practitioner debates surrounding socialist feminism, this chapter is based on an acceptance of a socialist feminist view of capitalism and the state, a view that is updated by scholars such as Acker (2006a) and Abramovitz (2006). There are important debates about the degree of benefit or disadvantage of capitalism for women. I agree with Holmstrom's (Cudd & Holmstrom 2011) analysis and conclusion that overall, despite capitalism having created positive opportunities for some women, there are systemic constraints on the lives of women under capitalism. As Holmstrom argues, 'women do not tend to be the winners in the brutally competitive system which is capitalism; indeed they are among the poorest and most vulnerable people on earth' (Cudd & Holstrom 2011: 138).

In exploring how class is always shaped by gender and race, I follow Acker's (2006a) approach and adopt socialist feminism to 'understand women's subordination in a coherent and systematic way that integrates class and sex, as well as other aspects of identity . . . with the aim of using this analysis to help liberate women' (Holmstrom 2003: 38), men and children to achieve a society where the social concerns take precedence over the economic ones (Khan 2015a).

Acker broadens the Marxist definition of the economy which focused on waged labour to provide a gendered theory of class expanded to consist of 'the practices and relations that provide differential control over and access to the means of provisioning' (Acker 2006a: 170) and survival. Classism is understood to be the entrenched oppression of those who must sell their waged labour (or be prepared to do so, as are people who are subject to unemployment) to survive, and those who care for them, by those who have control over the means of production (Acker 2006a; Strier 2009: 240). I suggest Acker's understanding of the economy (that brings in the personal relations and labour performed, mainly by women, in the home or community) and class (as always based on gender and race) is particularly relevant for social workers and social work service users as they interact across areas of care and control.

An analysis of power based on Acker's understanding of 'class as relations always in process' (Acker 2006b: 68) addresses both the structural relations of inequality and domination that underpins subordination and allows for the emancipatory potential of agency by social workers and social work service users, within the making of class.

Social welfare feminism

Traditional conceptions of class have not always included welfare service users, many of whom rely on state-provided income support, on church, family or community support, or, who are without any support. This group of people, in their diversity, have denied access in common, or perceived lack of current value, to the paid labour market. Social welfare feminism brings those who are not in the paid labour market clearly into view (Abramovitz 2006). Thus, it focuses on how the classed relationships between 'neoliberal paternalism' (Soss et al. 2011) and welfare reform (Abramovitz 2006), such as the Australian 'end of the era of entitlement' (Hockey 2012) and compulsory income management (Mendes et al. 2013), are always shaped by gender, race, able-bodiedness and ageism, as they disproportionately impact those furthest from the mythical norm.

Social-welfare feminism makes the link that the inequities generated by the capitalist-market system underpin much social work practice (Abramovitz 2006). Welfare reform involving class and poverty governance does not aim to end class inequality, poverty, homelessness, imprisonment of the poor and the ill, systemic gendered and racialised violence, or child abuse. Rather, it invokes the capitalist fear to bind and manage those who are distanced by varying degrees from the mythical norm.

The key example of the practice of capitalist fear that is highlighted in this chapter is the dual nature of the structural violence of poverty serving to both 'discipline the poor' (Soss et al. 2011) and instil fear, and a precarious sense of superiority of those who, but for a paid job, could also become poor. This structural violence is used against the working class, and it includes the 'reserve army of labor' and the 'relative surplus population' to maximise compliance with prevailing norms, and forces this group to accept the least attractive jobs with the lowest wages servicing the 'low road of capitalism' (Soss et al. 2011: 15).

The delivery and impacts of this violence, including systemic denigration, dehumanisation and patronising contempt (Khan 2015) serve as ongoing reminders to those who have paid jobs of the fate accorded to those not involved in the 'free market' cycle of accumulation, production and consumption. Using the work of Acker (2006a), Smith (2005) and Abramovitz (2006) enables gender, race and social-welfare feminism to be analysed in the context of social work and the class-based structural violence of poverty.

In relation to class, Acker (2006a) alerts us to the fact that while gender and race discrimination are no longer legally legitimated in developed capitalist societies, this is not true in the case of class. Class-based exploitation and structural violence are accepted and normalised in a socioeconomic system that requires these bases for the process of capital accumulation (Acker 2006a). This is particularly relevant for social workers who often work on behalf of the state to discipline the poor (Soss et al. 2011).

Using the methods of institutional ethnography to challenge class-based structural violence

The primary causes of the poverty and inequalities produced by class-based structural violence lie in the ideas, decisions and practices of people and groups of people, in positions of power such as corporate, organisational and political leadership (entrenched across time in institutions and associated documents such as laws, policies and newspapers). Those in positons of power, and those that believe in or benefit most from the neoliberal stage of capitalism, are able to justify and normalise inequalities by using their ownership of, access to, the mechanisms of economic, political and cultural decision making and communication, such as the press. These primary causes of povery and inequality are not in the people and communities who bear the brunt of the actions or inactions of those who seek to maintain class-based power. However, social workers are often, unthinkingly, complicit in structured class-based inequalities when they consider oppression and domination as actions that are only caused by powerful others that are separate from their own actions (Campbell 2003).

Institutional ethnography (Smith 2006) offers a critical feminist sociology and practice that can provide social workers with an orientation and methods to evaluate their work to reveal how, and when, they may take up oppressive or ruling concepts and activate them (see also Chapter 12). Once social workers who seek to create changes towards social justice become aware of their participation in ruling relations, they are then better informed to work to resist and change.

Neoliberalist practices that embed mythical norms are key organisers of how the work of social workers happens within organisations; for example, who are considered to be 'good' workers and 'good' clients. Senior managers of educational and human-service organisations in Western countries often place high value on compliant, low-risk behaviour and can use codes of conduct, performance appraisals, promotional policies, supervision, workload allocations and discretionary leave provisions to discipline those workers who may question or transgress from stated policy and practice (Beddoe 2010; Trounson 2012). Social workers who are compliant, who complete cases, files and tasks in a timely way, and enact organisational policy without question are usually highly valued in neoliberal organisations. Similarly, clients who are compliant, who abide by their care or case plans and attend interviews on time, are often rewarded by being allocated scarce resources, or at least, not punished by being, for example, reported to child protection, social security or housing authorities, or by being refused access to needed resources (Soss et al. 2011). Working in solidarity with others for change is a motivating and protective factor for critical social workers and service users who challenge compliance.

Towards poverty-aware and class-cognisant (PACC) practice

The PACC approach draws on socialist feminism (Acker 2006a), Smith's (2005) feminist sociology and method of institutional ethnography, postcolonial and transnational feminisms (Mohanty 2014), anti-colonial theory (Moreton-Robinson 2004), Strier's 'class-competent social work' model, incorporates Thompson's (2006) personal, cultural and structural 'PCS analysis' and uses critical social work process-orientations (see Chapter 4). My concerns with 'class-competent social work' (Strier 2009: 240–1) are similar to those regarding cultural competence. Invitations to competence, where people are encouraged to aspire towards particular skills sets, can affirm ingrained, often unexamined, classist attitudes that people from dominant class groups have the ability, and right, to learn and become competent in another's class experiences (Hosken 2013).

Strier (2009) and Langhout et al. (2007: 150) provide useful categorisations of types of classism that are adapted here to include Allen's (2001) work on poverty as class-based structural violence, and to correlate with a modified version of Thompson's (2006) 'PCS' analysis:

- Structural level: classism is a component and practice of neoliberalism that normalises class-based structural violence against those individuals, families, groups and communities who are distanced by varying degrees from the mythical norm. This class-based structural violence includes unequal access by people to quality employment, education, housing, health, legal assistance, childcare, community infrastructure and welfare opportunities.

- Cultural/societal/organisational level: classism occurs because of common values and patterns of thought and behaviour, consensus about what is right or 'normal' in organisational and professional discourses, structures, policies, and practices that affect people in different ways based on their class background. People internalise social values and norms through ongoing socialisation and, additionally for social workers, they absorb these values via the inculcation of normative standards, values and processes set by professional bodies that regulate and represent the social work profession. Middle-classed normative standards are those by which others are judged. Workers need to reflect on where they, and service users, get the messages about who is a 'good' worker, a 'good' person, a 'good' child/mother/father/family/community. Workers can critically question whose voice or view is privileged in policies and practices, and are able to set the norms that others are judged against.

- Personal level: interpersonal and internalised classism occurs at the individual/family/ group/community level of thoughts, feelings, attitudes and actions. This includes how social workers interact with each other, and with service users, and the need for social workers to guard against their own complicities and prejudices. Social workers can engage in critical self-awareness and mutual consciousness-raising (see Chapter 4) to become aware of their own class biases and assumptions, those class-based assumptions of other workers in the organisation, and those that underpin policy and practice. By doing so, they can become aware how these may impact same-class and cross-class, worker–client relationships and assessments (Strier 2009: 241). Internalised class biases can affect workers' and service users' self-concept and self-esteem, as well as how they treat, and are treated by, others.

PACC practice draws from the feminist principle of 'the personal is political' to locate the origins of personal experiences, such as women's experience of domestic violence, in political structures, and also encourages practitioners to enact the political change that they seek in their relationships, and actions (Healy 2005: 177). From a PACC approach, this would involve social workers (privately, professionally, publicly and collectively) locating the cause of poverty and unemployment in terms of inequality arising from the capitalist logic of market-based competition, accumulation and growth. Radical egalitarianism (Healy 2005: 177) is another feminist principle that influences PACC practice. It recognises that the knowledge of both workers and service users are needed to understand situations, reduce power inequalities and foster collaborative working partnerships.

Applying the PACC approach and principles to a case study

A case study of 'Vesna, Ms Smith and Mr Jones' follows, which is then used to illustrate potential applications of the key principles of the PACC approach.

Case study: Vesna, Ms Smith and Mr Jones

Vesna is a social worker in a non-government child and family support welfare service. She has been allocated a 'case', Ms Jane Smith and Mr Alan Jones, who were referred to her agency by the state child protection service. Vesna's team leader tells you that this case has been initially assessed as short-term and has limited funding.

The referral states that the child protection service investigated a concern where the eldest child, George, had presented at school with bruising across his back and buttocks from being hit with a belt by his stepfather, Alan. George is the eldest of Jane's four children. Alan is the biological father of the younger two children. The four children missed 40 per cent of school days last term. Alan has been unemployed for three years since the factory where he worked closed down. Jane has a casual job as a night cleaner, but the company has not offered her many shifts lately. The referral states the children's non-attendance at school was due to Jane being inebriated and unable to take them to school. The child protection service was satisfied that George is not currently at risk as Alan agreed to cease using physical discipline, but required Jane and Alan to attend your agency to consolidate the use of non-physical means of discipline, and for Jane to undergo counselling for alcohol abuse.

At your first meeting, Jane tells you that her defacto partner, who is unable to attend the appointment, is a good father. Jane says she feels overwhelmed and exhausted, and has been diagnosed with depression by her local doctor. Jane is worried that they do not have enough money to pay the electricity bill and that she has nothing left to take to the pawn shop to get money for food to put

---

in the kids' school lunches. Jane did not think the child protection workers understood anything about having to live on government benefits.

In detail, Vesna's use of a PACC approach and principles in preparation, and in the first meetings with Jane, may involve the following steps.

Practice principle: Examine the regulatory texts for how they organise normality

Once Vesna is allocated the case and prepares to see the family, she reflects on her immediate frustration that the team leader's rating of this family did not offer the highest level of resourcing available in the family support policy. Reading the referral, Vesna identifies processes of individualisation, where issues are presented as the family's own making, and therefore constructed as being able to be unmade by them. Vesna reflects on her own habit of drinking three glasses of wine most nights, her good wage that provides independence, and sees that the relations of class and poverty permeate her organisation, and child protection, and seem present in every issue that is identified in the referral. The child protection service seem to overly pinpoint the cause and solutions for the identified problems within the family itself. Vesna commences a file and looks at the policy and assessment tool that she is required to use. The language of the policy and tool is paternalistic and individualising in its emphasis on the need for families to self-manage.

Vesna follows the principle to listen ethically and work with people to help them access resources and negotiate problematic situations (Wood & Tully 2013)

At the first meeting, Vesna aims to build trust through using relevant critical social work process-orientations (see Chapter 4) such as deep, respectful and ethical listening, stillness, a culturally friendly attitude using mutual respect inquiry and clear contracting that includes transparency of roles and purposes. Vesna is transparent about the referral from child protection services, and organisational agendas and priorities. She explores with Jane what her views, understandings, experiences and priorities are. If the priorities relate to alleviation of immediate hardship, Vesna can offer food vouchers, advocacy, technical expertise, use of discretion, role authority, strong referrals, among other resources.

Vesna follows the principle to learn from the location and views of those most affected

In exploring these human rights priorities (see Chapter 5), Vesna can learn from, and with, Jane as she shares knowledge of her and her family's history in terms of their subjection to structural violence. Vesna may find her own knowledge building about the relations and practices of class and poverty and her insight into her own organisational practices and those of other agencies that are involved with the family, becomes clearer.

Follow the principle to explore regulatory ideologies, policies and practices for how their organisation of normality might impact the worker and the service user

Discussing the work to alleviate these hardships—obtaining social and economic human rights such as the right to adequate food, income, health care, education, electricity, housing and transport—can reduce individual feelings of blame and inadequacy. The causes of unemployment and poverty are located in the failures of the representatives of the political and economic systems to provide for and protect these and other human rights.

Vesna follows the principle inspired by critical psychology to witness, explore and alleviate the psychic effects of structural violence

Through ethical listening and mutual consciousness raising (see Chapter 4) Vesna would learn about Jane's experiences of living with the structural violence of poverty, among other areas of her life. If Jane has internalised society's messages of blame for her experiences of structural abuse, Vesna can use feminist principles of the 'personal is political', and the feminist-inspired critical social work ideas of 'validation, witnessing, deconstruction' and 'critical questioning' to explore replacing individual inadequacy messages with structural explanations of class and poverty. If Jane shared that she felt stigmatised, patronised or angered by the doctor and child protection services applying the individualising labels of 'depressed' and 'addict', Vesna might discuss the insidious impacts of the structural violence of poverty on individuals, families and communities and countries (Allen 2001; Ho 2007). Vesna would draw on dialogical praxis (see Chapter 4) and take the time, genuine care and interest to explore with Jane how others' experiences and ideas about the structural violence of poverty may resonate (or not) with the particularities of Jane's life. Vesna would benefit from, and be informed by, this deepened understanding the next time she worked with Jane, and with other service users and colleagues.

Vesna follows the principle of working individually and collectively to lobby managers, organisations and funders to change the discourses and institutional work processes

If Vesna also had experience of other service users who were upset by the lack of care, or framing their social issues as medical ones, she could use 'universalising' to share this information in a broad, non-identifying way, with Jane. Vesna could ask Jane if she thought it might be useful for Vesna to raise this issue at her staff team meeting. A networking meeting could then be organised with local health workers to raise awareness of the existence and impacts of structural poverty abuse on individuals, families and communities. Vesna could provide an open invitation to Jane to be part of this education of local service providers if and when she felt she had time. Vesna could investigate funding opportunities so that Jane is paid appropriate remuneration for the work.

Jane may identify that some of the child protection workers did not treat her with dignity or respect, holding her individually responsible as a mother for her family's situation in a community that is devastated by unemployment following factory closures and retrenchments. Vesna and Jane may decide to work together, and with others, to lodge a complaint, review or appeal or lobby for the child protection service to improve their training of, and resources for, workers so they are more transparent, poverty and class-cognisant and effective. They could work together on a combination of these initiatives.

Vesna follows the principle to join with others outside the organisation to strengthen the collective voices demanding change

This networking meeting with local health workers and discussion with other service users could lead to the establishment of a community-based action group that lobbies for increased education of local service providers, increased resources for those who are not able to get meaningful paid work in the region. Vesna would work collaboratively with Jane to explore her response to this circumstance and to investigate other means to improve individual, family and community access to adequate human rights and wellbeing. Critical social workers are aware of how social workers' and service users' opportunities to control or change things are significantly constrained within the relations of structural inequality (Ho 2007). Social workers need to collaborate with service users and engage in solidarity with others to create sustained efforts towards transformative change.

Vesna follows the principle to require no more of those subject to the structural violence of poverty than is required of yourself and others

Literature on critical addiction studies (Granfield & Reinarman 2014b) provides a structural understanding of addiction that identifies the processes of becoming dependant on alcohol, drugs, other substances and activities, and the strategies for continuance, management or change, as strategies that are not solely contained within individuals. They are greatly affected by the locations of people, families, groups and communities within the larger social structure. The cause of the apparent growth of addiction in free-market societies is not a massive epidemic of individual pathology, of neuro-chemical imbalances, but rather 'primarily a political, social, and economic problem' where political action is needed to create greater 'psychosocial integration' rather than the 'dislocation and addiction' spread in freer markets (Alexander 2014: 118).

Dislocation, using Alexander's concept, refers to the near-universal dislocation that is inherent in free market societies' insistence on individualism, accumulation and competition that creates the impossibility of psychosocial integration where people can flourish as individuals and as members of their culture (Alexander 2014: 107 8). The mass dislocation affects those with class privilege as well as those subject to poverty. However, the opportunities to hide, contain and manage are different.

The intersection of poverty, class and gender shaped the likelihood of the sorts of addictive behaviours (onset and trajectories) able to be taken up by and maintained by Jane, and the differential consequences of them (Granfield & Reinarman 2014a: 16). For example, in contrast to Jane, a woman with access to a high income but with an alcohol addiction is unlikely to come under the surveillance of child protection as she would have options to: own her own home in a gated community with little scrutiny of her daily living; purchase private child care; board her children at private schools; organise chauffeurs to drive her children; employ a live-in nanny to feed, bath, clothe, emotionally and educationally enrich the children; and take regular holidays. All of these things could occur while she is able to continue her dependence on alcohol. In the unlikely event that child protection services, or any other authority, investigated any aspect of her, or her family's behaviours, private lawyers could be employed to deal with such matters.

Jane may agree that child protection's identification of her alcohol use interfering with her ability get the children to school is a problem. It may be useful to explore increased material and emotional resourcing to the family to reduce the negative impacts of Jane's alcohol use so there are less child protection issues or other negative consequences. Changing alcohol-use patterns can be a long-term project, with varying results. Possible replacements for negative addictive behaviours, or replacements in peak negative times, could be investigated such as providing gym or yoga memberships that are facilitated by childcare and transport. Emotional and practical support could be provided such as: inhouse help with the children at key stress periods; respite care, before/after-school childcare and transport services; linking up with 'foster grand-parents' or 'big brother/sister' programs. In the short term, provision of taxi vouchers may enable increased school attendance and alleviate significant stress.

Vesna follows the principle of using transparency

Jane acknowledged that her defacto partner did use physical discipline against George, but believes he provides 'good enough' emotional and physical care for the children. Vesna would be transparent in her communications with Jane that the use of physical force was against the law, and that children are now recognised under state and international laws as having legal and human rights to physical safety and wellbeing. Vesna would explain part of the referral requires that Vesna is to discuss with Alan his ongoing willingness and ability to adopt non-physical means of discipline, and that the use of physical discipline would re-involve child protection services and risk separation of the family. Jane may ask that Vesna discuss this in a clear and respectful way with her defacto partner, Alan.

Conclusion

This chapter has outlined a poverty-aware and class-cognisant (PACC) approach to assist social workers to work humanely and proactively with people, families and communities who are subject to class-based structural violence. A PACC approach also requires social workers to consider their complicities, and to work with others to reveal and challenge classism in the policies of their workplaces. Social workers can join with others who seek a more equal society (Ferguson 2008), those who are also dissatisfied and disillusioned with the increasing inequalities and structural violence under capitalism. There are possibilities for social workers to commit to action for social justice that links to the achievement of feminist and anti-capitalist agendas for transformative change.

References

Abramovitz, M. 2006, 'Welfare reform in the United States: Gender, race and class matter', *Critical Social Policy,* vol. 26, no. 2, pp. 336–64

Acker, J. 2006a, *Class Questions: Feminist answers*, Lanham: Rowman & Littlefield, Inc.

Acker, J. 2006b, 'Inequality regimes gender, class, and race in organizations', *Gender & Society,* vol. 20, no. 4, pp. 441–64

Alexander, B.K. 2014, 'The roots of addiction in free market society' in R. Granfield & C. Reinarman (eds), *Expanding Addiction: Critical essays,* New York: Routledge

Allen, J. 2001, 'Poverty as a form of violence', *Journal of Human Behavior in the Social Environment,* vol. 4, no. 2–3, pp. 45–59

Beddoe, L. 2010, 'Surveillance or reflection: Professional supervision in "the risk society"', *British Journal of Social Work,* vol. 40, no. 4, pp. 1279–96

Campbell, M. 2003, 'Dorothy Smith and knowing the world we live in', *Journal of Sociology and Social Welfare,* vol. 30, no. 1, pp. 3–23

Cudd, A. & Holmstrom, N. 2011, *Capitalism, For and Against: A feminist debate,* Cambridge: Cambridge University Press

Ferguson, I. 2008, *Reclaiming Social Work: Challenging neo-liberalism and promoting social justice,* London: Sage Publications

—— 2011, 'Why class (still) matters' in M. Lavalette (ed.), *Radical Social Work Today: Social work at the crossroads,* Bristol: Policy Press

Galtung, J. 1969, 'Violence, poverty and peace research', *Journal of Peace Research,* vol. 6, no. 3, pp. 167–91

Gramsci, A. 1971, *Selections from the Prison Notebook,* London: Lawrence & Wishart

Granfield, R. & Reinarman, C. 2014a, 'Addiction is not just a brain disease: Critical studies of addiction' in R. Granfield & C. Reinarman (eds), *Expanding Addiction: Critical essays,* New York: Routledge

—— (eds) 2014b, *Expanding Addiction: Critical essays,* New York: Routledge

Healy, K. 2005, *Social Work Theories in Context: Creating frameworks for practice,* Basingstoke: Palgrave

Ho, K. 2007, 'Structural violence as a human rights violation', *Essex Human Rights Review,* vol. 4, no. 2, pp. 1–17

Hockey, J. 2012, 'The end of the age of entitlement ', <www.joehockey.com/media/speeches/details. aspx?s=90>, accessed 20 August 2014

Holmstrom, N. 2003, 'The socialist feminist project', *Monthly Review New York,* vol. 54, no. 10, pp. 38–48

Hosken, N. 2013, 'Social work supervision and discrimination', *Advances in Social Work and Welfare Education,* vol. 15, no. 1, pp. 91–103

Hutchinson, F. & Mellor, M. 2004, 'Capitalist malestream monestised markets versus social provisioning: Proposals for the socialisation of the economy', paper presented at ASE World Congress, Albertville, France

Khan, M.A. 2015, 'Putting "good society" ahead of growth and/or "development": Overcoming neo-liberalism's growth trap and its costly consequences', *Sustainable Development,* vol. 23, no. 2, pp. 65–73

Langhout, R.D., Rosselli, F. & Feinstein, J. 2007, 'Assessing classism in academic settings', *The Review of Higher Education,* vol. 30, no. 2, pp. 145–84

Lorde, A. 1999, 'Age, race, class, and sex: Women redefining difference' in A. Kesselman, L. McNair & N. Schniedewind (eds), *Women: Images and realities, a multicultural anthology,* Mountain View: Mayfield, pp. 361–6

Marx, K. 1976, *Capital, volume 1,* Harmondsworth: Penguin

Mendes, P., Waugh, J. & Flynn, C. A. 2013, 'The place-based income management trial in Shepparton: A best practice model for evaluation', *Social Inclusion and Social Policy Research Unit,* Department of Social Work, Melbourne: Monash University

Mohanty, C.T. 2014, '"Under western eyes" revisited: Feminist solidarity through anticapitalist struggles', *Signs,* vol. 40, no. 1, pp. 499–535

Moreton-Robinson, A. (ed.) 2004, *Whitening Race: Essays in social and cultural criticism,* Canberra: Aboriginal Studies Press

Neilson, D. 2015, 'Class, precarity, and anxiety under neoliberal global capitalism: From denial to resistance', *Theory & Psychology,* vol. 25, no. 2, pp. 239–56

Olsen, J. 2007, 'Social work's professional and social justice projects: Discourses in conflict', *Journal of Progressive Human Services* vol. 18, no. 1, pp. 45–69

Rose, N. 1990, *Governing the Soul: The shaping of the private self*, Florence: Taylor & Frances/Routledge

Sheedy, M. 2012, *Core Themes in Social Work: Power, poverty, politics and values*, Berkshire: McGraw-Hill

Smith, D.E. 2005, *Institutional Ethnography: A sociology for people*, Lanham: AltaMira Press

—— (ed.) 2006, *Institutional Ethnography as Practice*, Lanham: Rowman & Littlefield Pub Inc.

Soss, J., Fording, R.C. & Schram, S. 2011, *Disciplining the Poor: Neoliberal paternalism and the persistent power of race*, Chicago: University of Chicago Press

Standing, G. 2011, *The Precariat: The new dangerous class*, London: Bloomsbury Publishing

Strier, R. 2009, 'Class-competent social work: A preliminary definition', *International Journal of Social Welfare,* vol. 18, no. 3, pp. 237–42

Thompson, N. 2006, *Anti-Discriminatory Practice*, 4th edn, London: Palgrave Macmillan

Thorsen, D. & Lie, A. 2006, 'What is neoliberalism', <http://folk.uio.no/daget/What%20is%20Neo-Liberalism%20FINAL.pdf>, accessed 5 August 2015

Trounson, A. 2012, 'Academics at RMIT rebel over niceness policy', *The Australian,* <http://theaustralian.com.au/higher-education/academics-at-rmit-rebel-over-niceness-policy/story-e6frgcjx-1226307739111>, accessed 18 June 2014

Van Soest, D. 1997, *The Global Crisis of Violence,* Washington: NASW Press

Wood, G.G. & Tully, C.T. 2013, *The Structural Approach to Direct Practice in Social Work: A social constructionist perspective*, New York: Columbia University Press

Part III

Developing critical practices within the organisational context of social work

8

Beyond the dominant approach to mental health practice

Noel Renouf

Introduction

Good critical social work practice has proved to be very challenging in the mental health field. This chapter will focus on social work practice within specialised mental health services, which are actually concerned less with mental health than with mental disorder and control (Vassilev & Pilgrim 2007). Much of the challenge relates to the pervasiveness of medical discourses that frame the way that mental distress is assessed and the treatment response. Mental health services rely substantially on coercive power, especially around involuntary treatment, with pervasive attention to the management of 'risk'.

This chapter outlines an approach to mental-health social work practice that focuses on the circumstances of people affected by mental distress and disturbance, and is based on establishing respectful relationships with consumers and their families to support change. 'In Australia, the term "consumer" is used to describe those people who use, have used or, when help has been sought, have been refused use of mental health services' (Olsen & Epstein 2012: 279). Of the core principles of critical social-work practice outlined by Allan (2009), working alongside people who experience oppression and marginalisation is the most fundamental principle in the mental health field. Work of this kind requires an awareness of power relationships, and challenges assumptions and beliefs that are taken for granted and dominate the mental health field. Social work practice that is fundamentally committed to a partnership with consumers and their families goes beyond the dominant mental health discourse, even while it takes place within the mental health system. This chapter describes how this works in practice, paying particular attention to some areas of strategic importance: recovery-based practice, working with involuntary treatment, and forming alliances for promoting social justice and system change.

Working beyond the dominant discourse

The mental health system is dominated by the discourse of psychiatry which combines with organisational imperatives to regulate and constrain the type of 'services' that are provided. In so doing, this combination determines the way that we are led to think about mental distress and disturbance. This has been aptly described as the 'bureau-medicalisation' of mental health care (Nathan & Webber 2010). However, the field is contested and there are contending and overlapping discourses of lesser prominence: human rights, the consumer and carer movements, social perspectives, and the new discourse of recovery.

In the public mental health service in Trieste, Italy, one of the espoused principles of practice is to put each person's mental illness 'into parenthesis' or brackets. The point is to move the centre of attention away from the diagnosis to focus instead on each person's 'human reality' (Norcio et al. 2001). The person (not the illness) is at the centre of things. A similar principle is contained within the emphasis given by the consumer and family carer movements to the 'lived experience' of mental illness (Bland, Renouf & Tullgren 2015). Social workers need to learn about and value the lived experience of the people they work with. This is the starting point for critical mental-health social work practice. Engaging with the particular lived experiences of consumers and families is more important than the 'treatment' of 'illness'.

Consumers and their families all have different understandings of mental health, and some fit more easily than others into the dominant medical paradigm. Diagnoses are sometimes very liberating, serving to make sense of painful and perplexing experiences. Yet it is possible to accept the reality of distress and disturbance without necessarily agreeing with the way that mental illness is constructed and understood by psychiatry and mental health services. Rather, an agnostic view about the classification and causes of mental illness and, in practice, a 'not-knowing' position allows much more openness to the expressed experiences of consumers. Attention can then be paid to the experience itself and the 'illness' is in parentheses.

In conducting mental health assessments, for example, an assumption that the problem lies primarily within the individual tends to skew the focus more towards the form of the distress than to its content and context, leading us to note the presence of symptoms (delusions, depressive thoughts and so on). What we look for profoundly affects what we see. Unless we listen properly and try to understand the meaning of such experiences in the lives of consumers, they may experience the assessment quite literally as a systematic process of not being listened to.

Practice example: careful use of language

Because the medical discourse is carried through language, social workers in the field should watch their own language very carefully. One strategy is to regard the language of diagnosis and treatment almost as a 'foreign' language; one that needs to be learned in order to function well in the system, but not the language to use at 'home', doing social work. An expert grasp of the language can allow us to help consumers make sense of what is occurring, and help us to amplify the voice of consumers within the system to maximise the way it can be acted upon. This applies to the language of psychiatry and expert knowledge about the mental health system; assessment processes and criteria for example. Such are the pressures on the system that social workers often find themselves in the position of supporting consumers to gain access to mental health treatment and care.

Our language will always be 'person-first' such as a 'person with a diagnosis of schizophrenia' rather than 'schizophrenic', to put it very simply. People experiencing distress and disturbance are people first in the sense that there are many other things going on in their life aside from mental illness. Great care needs to be taken to ensure that our language reflects the fact that it is the person, not the illness, that we work with.

> The language of diagnosis and 'helping' powerfully constructs identity. In everyday practice, such language is 'used to formulate the "case history", which is elaborated in reports, referral documents and multitudinous files you construct about us, usually without our knowledge or contribution. Such cascading descriptions can become the dominant stories told about us, entrapping us in our problem-satuated lives and future prospects (Bland, Renouf & Tullgren 2015:37).

Language can be very slippery, of course. It is striking to witness the re-badging of Australian mental health services as being recovery-focused with little (if any) fundamental change to their mode of operation.

Being aware of the operations of power can inform how we use language because power imbalances between staff and patients in a mental health system find their way into the language used by staff in small interactions, sometimes by effectively giving orders, sometimes by presuming to 'know', or understand the consumer's experience, sometimes by presuming to use terms of endearment. In little ways like this, the pattern of control in mental health services is expressed in seemingly benign language and reproduced through relationships, which may have a profound impact on the person's ability to regain control over the rest of their life (Melville-Wiseman 2012).

Psychiatry seeks to associate certain inner experiences with illness, and provide treatment accordingly. Part of the weakness of this approach is its inadequate classification systems, which have failed to produce a stable and reliable basis for diagnosis and treatment (Bentall 2014). Further, it is based in an explanatory system that tends to discount the meaning of experience and relies instead on the authority of medical knowledge and action. Critical psychiatrists (such as those associated with 'post-psychiatry') have responded by adopting an approach that seeks to respond to the meaning of specific symptoms of people as they experience them with less reliance on the medical model of classification and diagnosis (Thomas & Bracken 2004). This is the most pertinent and powerful critiques to come from outside the mental health professions.

Practice example: hearing voices

Hearing voices is one aspect of the experience of (some) mental illness, but the voice hearing 'movement' provides an exemplary approach to practice beyond the dominant medical paradigm. Hearing voices is quite common in the general population—'roughly 5% to 15%' of adults (Beavan, Read & Cartwright 2011: 289). Some people cope well with their voices but many mental health consumers find them to be extremely distressing, disruptive and difficult to control, tending to echo and intensify suffering, despair and previous traumatic experiences such as bullying, sexual abuse and loss. Lives are disrupted and constricted, and the most ordinary activities may require ongoing reserves of conscious willpower (Kalhovde, Elstad & Talseth 2013).

An emancipatory movement of and for people who hear voices has developed that is based on the work of Romme and others (Romme & Escher 1989). One of their fundamental insights was to argue that voices should not necessarily be eliminated but instead that the person should be supported in making sense of the voice experiences:

> hearing voices is a meaning-ful experience; its first lesson is that voice-hearing is not a meaning-less symptom of an underlying illness or disease, but a key part of a person's identity (Woods 2013: 264).

In this way, the inner experience of people hearing distressing voices can be linked with and reflect intense difficulties in their interpersonal and intimate relationships as well as reflect their persecuting, marginalising and ostracising experiences in society.

Groups for people who hear voices may be run by voice hearers or facilitated by professionals. Activities typically include sharing the experiences of hearing voices (what they say, what it is like), discussion of explanatory frameworks for hearing voices (where the voices come from), exploring the meaning of voices in the broader context of the person's life history, exploring and sharing practical strategies for acceptance and change (such as dialogue with the voices), setting boundaries to challenge the power of voices, and not taking them literally. Such groups are often also a place to develop distraction and self-soothing strategies, reflect on recovery stories and explore hopes and dreams (Voices Vic 2009).

The important practice principle here is the focus on the experience, and providing real practical support for managing distressing and disruptive aspects of what might be regarded otherwise as simply a 'symptom' for 'treatment'. The person who experiences the 'symptom' becomes an expert by experience.

If critical psychiatry moves the focus away from diagnosis towards the phenomenology of 'symptoms' such as voices, what marks out the approach of critical social work practice in mental health is its focus on the social context and social consequences of mental health problems, and its fundamental concern with social justice. Social work practice in mental health takes place within the context of relationships. We are all social beings and each life is embedded in that of others. Whatever the impact of biology, there is rarely a psychiatric crisis without a wider context. Social workers have always recognised in their work that recovery takes place within relationships and environments. Because of its different focus, mental health social work can operate alongside psychiatry without offering a real challenge. Critical social work practice, however, is based in a social model (both relational and structural) that challenges the dominant medicalisation model.

Relationships with therapeutic potential

There is a lot of talk about partnership principles in the mental health field, but much of it is superficial. Removing the medical-model lens is a necessary but not sufficient step for authentic engagement. Relationships of the right kind are both the foundation for effective helping and are helpful in themselves. A large recent Australian study found that two-thirds of people who are diagnosed with a psychotic illness reported that their illness made it difficult to maintain close relationships; nearly a quarter reported feeling isolated and lonely; one in eight had no friends at all; and the same number had never known someone they could confide in (Sane Australia 2011).

The quality of the relationship will depend on many factors, including the personality and wishes of the consumer, and will require the willingness and capacity of each social worker to draw upon their own personal attributes and risk emotional vulnerability. Therapies need to be capable of acknowledging and responding sensitively to trauma, abuse and neglect where it has occurred. Some therapeutic approaches are more consistent with critical practice than others. Critical practice problematises the structure of the relationship between worker and client. Dialogue is encouraged in preference to the re-statement of a single-minded view of the situation, which tends to focus on the consumer's behaviour and diagnosis (Seikkula & Arnkil 2006).

To use narrative practice as a brief example, many first-person accounts of recovery provide strong examples of narratives that run in opposition to previously dominant 'illness' narratives, which generally relate to something 'inside' the person. In narrative practice, externalising conversations about the influence of experiences associated with mental illness (such as voices, the symptoms of depression, alcohol and drug use, and so on) help to illuminate the person's effect on the problem as much as the problem's effect on the person. Re-authoring conversations aim to build 'full histories of resistance to the problem and of sources of inspiration and meaning' (Hamkins 2005: 9). A narrative approach may support people with symptoms such as voices to construct the story of their experiences; this is a simple, powerful process of formulation by the voice hearer (Place, Foxcroft, & Shaw 2011). Much of the power of narrative approaches comes from their strongly respectful and ethical position, and their concern with the history, culture and context that affects people's lives.

Among psychosocial approaches in the contemporary mental health system, there is a clear preference for Cognitive Behavioural Therapy (CBT), and current policy in Australia is shaping mental health social work accordingly, especially outside the public-sector services. Some consumers express a strong preference for CBT but, so neat is its fit with the dominant diagnosis–treatment medical paradigm, that social workers who use these techniques need to take particular care to be critically reflective. This is necessary to ensure that they work with consumers in a genuinely dialogic manner. Critical reflection of this kind will most likely lead to a change in practice.

The really important thing is an attitude of respectful curiosity about the experiences of the other person, not just what has been happening *to* them, but also their personal responses and emotions, or what is happening *within*. Often, depending on how much consumers choose to share this information, the social worker needs to be able to hear about and to bear intense inner pain and torment. Really respectful relationships of this kind have therapeutic potential if the social worker has the capacity to pay close empathic attention and engage with these feelings in a sustained manner over time. It is not just a matter of doing things with the person; it is about being with them (Waddell 1989). It is hard to illustrate this work simply, but there are some good published accounts of sustained social work practice of this kind, drawing upon psychodynamic principles (Kanter 2000; Keeping 2008). Disinterest or even hostility to the inner world is inconsistent with an approach to critical social work that aims to understand and connect with the real experiences of people with mental illness. This inevitably involves inner disturbance, turmoil and pain. This has been described as a 'human being with' rather than an 'operational doing to' approach (Bailey 2002: 177). We bear witness to these experiences, acknowledging a responsibility to take action in response.

At the same time, the 'meaning' of experiences includes the way in which dimensions of social structure such as class, gender, race and culture, are played out in the lives of both consumers and workers. Social inequality and individual psychology are related 'like a lock and key' (Wilkinson & Pickett 2010: 33). For example, if a consumer is diagnosed with 'depression' following an accident at a poorly paid job, the plain fact that needs acknowledgement is that poverty and unsafe work practices give rise to psychological distress and disturbance. This is part of the meaning and the cause of the 'symptoms'. To act as if it is simply a case of an illness called 'depression' is a powerful denial of this personal and social reality, and obliterates meaning.

Entering into the consumer's own story is a way of cutting across prejudices and avoiding being an organisational 'functionary' (Parton & O'Byrne 2000). It requires tremendous commitment because, in addition to the personal resources required, it will often tend to bring the social worker up against bureaucratic requirements. It may not be humanly possible for the social worker to sustain this level of engagement with the numbers of people on their 'caseload' in many agencies. The welfare of consumers and workers is interrelated and interdependent (Spandler 2013).

'Recovery'

The concept of recovery, which has become a consistent unifying theme in contemporary mental health policies and services, has radical implications and, even as more and more services adopt the rhetoric, the radical implications are becoming clearer. As Slade puts it:

> People with mental illness don't need treatment; they need a life. Treatment may [be] a means, not an end . . . The overarching principle of recovery is that the impoverished expectations, clinical preoccupations, and stigmatising beliefs sometimes held by mental health workers should not preclude everyday ways of addressing common human problems (Slade 2012: 704).

Mental health professionals can neither define nor bring about someone's recovery; the best they can do is to support it. In practice, this will often mean help with dealing with distress and disturbance, but more often than not it means supporting everyday practical solutions to everyday problems related to how much money that people have to live on, work, issues with family and friends, living arrangements and so on.

Recovery is related to a person's place in society. It involves 'simply being let in' (Davidson et al. 2001), but achieving this under existing social conditions is not simple. Essential components identified by Davidson and his colleagues include friendship, feeling like a worthwhile human being through meaningful activity, and hopefulness through an affirmative stance adopted by professionals and others in the person's world. Social factors can be critical in enabling recovery; factors such as empowerment and control over one's life, connectedness (including both interpersonal relationships and social inclusion) and rebuilding positive identities (often within the context of stigma and discrimination). These can be addressed in work with individuals, families and communities (Tew et al. 2012).

Some of the ideas about recovery in common use put so much emphasis on individual meaning and narrative that the social and political connections are ignored or lost. Recovery discourse can be used in a way that individualises people's problems and, if they do not 'recover', this can be seen as yet another individual 'deficiency'. In this way, 'the recovery model, inadvertently perhaps, decontextualises the environment of poverty, deprivation and unemployment, let alone long-term sequelae of a childhood marked by abuse, parental mental health problems and so on' (Webber 2011: 27).

Actually, it is a struggle for both consumers and workers to 'get into a recovery position' but it can be facilitated, in part, precisely through the kind of democratic dialogical relationship described above (Cameron & McGowan 2012). There are implications, of course, for the power relationship between mental health workers and consumers. From the point of view of social work practice, it means being both willing and able to treat the encounter as an essentially human relationship, 'relinquishing the omnipotent, but a delusional belief that recovery is something which can be prescribed according to the dominant yet misconceived theoretical presuppositions of a particular discipline or mind set' (Cameron & McGowan 2012: 28).

Working with involuntary consumers

Almost all mental-health social work involves actual or potential use of statutory authority. Critical social work practice cannot evade the question of how that authority is exercised. It is no solution to try to leave all of the exercise of authority to other members of the mental health team. As Weinstein (2013) has argued, 'just because statutory powers can be used carelessly or callously does not mean that authority should not be used when people are at risk'.

Voluntary or involuntary status is not the absolute concept in the context of mental-health service systems, nor does it fundamentally determine the quality of the working relationship. So pervasive is the use of statutory power that its shadow casts over all work in the public mental health system. In practice, the issues of safety and risk, as they affect the consumer and those who are close to them (children, partners, parents, etc.) are often complex, and the best decisions require careful thought and moral courage. Writing in the 'critical best practice' tradition, Ferguson (2008) has advanced the concept of 'good authority', which involves a knowledgeable and sensitive use of self on the part of the worker, and a deep and continual awareness of their role and responsibilities. This is combined with the skill to be clear, honest and direct (but not punitively blunt) about why difficult questions need to be asked and difficult decisions may need to be made. This is exactly the kind of authority that can be exercised best in the context of the kind of relationship described in this chapter. Its focus is on the politics of the situation (including interpersonal politics) rather than normalising judgement.

Critical social work practice applies a strong human-rights perspective to work with involuntary consumers. This requires detailed knowledge of mental health, guardianship and other relevant legislation, clarity about exactly what the law allows and requires, the knowledge and experience to know how much discretion may be allowed, and the determination to ensure that the legal limits of the mandate are not exceeded.

Practice example: involuntary treatment

Almost all mental health legislation asserts the principle of least restriction. While there may be no choice about the fact of involuntary treatment, what is the least restrictive setting for the treatment: hospital or community? Specifically, what creative arrangements may be made to make community treatment a realistic option (respite from an aversive living situation, for example, or short-term arrangements for additional support from others such as family members or clinical staff)?

If treatment will be in hospital, what is the best possible way to get to the hospital? It will often be possible here to ensure that choice is available and respected. There can be all the difference in the world between being driven by a family member or friend, going by ambulance, or being brought in by police.

We tend to assume that our role is to 'manage' risk by seeking to minimise or even eliminate it; an impossible idea, but one so pervasive that it might be considered 'the new clinical model' for mental health services (Holmes 2013). Yet this approach tends to draw attention away from the positive benefits of considered risk-taking for clients and their families (Ramon 2005). Risk avoidance in the absence of risk-taking is not an effective strategy for human change. The capacity and right to take risks reflects an empowered position and is an essential element of recovery. So risk is not just something to be avoided. Rather, what is required is a thoughtful approach to risk-taking, with the right balance of risks and protective factors. This will look different for different people in different situations.

Mental-health social workers will be called upon to make assessments of risk. A 'positive' risk assessment will focus on the benefits, advantages and opportunities of a particular course of action as well as addressing the areas of risk, concern and potential harm. The aim is to do what is necessary to minimise harm while working towards the best likelihood of positive outcomes. It is important that we actively ask about the effects of what we do, conscious that 'well-meaning' actions will often have disempowering consequences. In these and other situations, we aim to position ourselves as accountable allies with consumers, rather than experts acting on or even regulating them.

Alliances for change

The development of effective consumer and carer activism and advocacy has been one of the most significant changes in the mental health field. A decade ago, Beresford and Croft (2004: 53) argued that 'social work is unlikely to develop a more emancipatory role, unless social work practitioners . . . develop much closer links and alliances with service users and their organisations and movements'. This is the most important challenge for the profession in a complex service system, but one that mental health social workers as a group have not been able to meet. The most effective recent Australian campaign by social workers concerned access to health care rebates (Mendes et al. 2012) had an overwhelming element of self-interest and weak alliances with consumers.

So strong is the relationship between social inequality and psychological distress and disorder, that almost any action that reduces inequality will have a positive effect on mental health. This chapter has focused on work within the mental health system where the *breadth* of the domain of mental health social work, if combined with a genuine *depth* of engagement with the real-world concerns of consumers and their families, forms the basis for genuine alliances. There are many pressing priorities, including the quality of mental health services themselves, which are regarded by many consumers as an environment for discrimination and re-traumatisation. Violence towards women in psychiatric inpatient wards is a specific example. There are other strategic opportunities for advancing the human rights of people with a mental illness, including reducing the reliance on physical and chemical restraints, strengthening 'advance directives' which are drawn up when a person is legally competent to say what their preferences for support and treatment are at times of mental disturbance (Topp & Thomas 2008), and challenging the reliance on involuntary treatment as a mainstay of the mental health system. This is something that has been achieved in Trieste, for example, where the 'illness' is in parentheses.

Conclusion

Although challenging, critical practice is by far the most satisfying approach to mental health social work. It is engaged and principled, and it requires skill, persistence and courage. Critical practice engages with the mental health system itself and develops detailed knowledge and skill in its language, policies and procedures, and therapeutic approaches, without accepting or cooperating with its premises and assumptions. Instead, the approach described in this chapter seeks to use a social model to achieve genuine and therapeutic partnerships with consumers and their families in a manner that does not reproduce the dominant operation of power relationships in the mental health system.

References

Allan, J. 2009, 'Theorising new developments in critical social work' in J. Allan, L. Briskman & B. Pease (eds), *Critical Social Work: Theories and practices for a socially just world*, 2nd edn, St Leonards: Allen & Unwin, pp. 30–44

Bailey, D. 2002, 'Mental health' in R. Adams, L. Dominelli & M. Payne (eds), *Critical Practice in Social Work*, Houndmills: Palgrave Macmillan, pp. 169–80

Beavan, V., Read, J. & Cartwright, C. 2011, 'The prevalence of voice-hearers in the general population: a literature review', *Journal of Mental Health*, vol. 20, no. 3, pp. 281–92

Bentall, R. P. 2014, 'The search for elusive structure: A promiscuous realist case for researching specific psychotic experiences such as hallucinations', *Schizophrenia Bulletin*, vol. 40, no. 4, pp. S198–S201

Beresford, P. & Croft, S. 2004, 'Service users and practitioners reunited: The key component for social work reform', *British Journal of Social Work*, vol. 34, no. 1, pp. 53–68

Bland, R., Renouf, N. & Tullgren, A. 2015, *Social Work Practice in Mental Health: An introduction*, St Leonards: Allen & Unwin

Cameron, D. & McGowan, P. 2012, 'The mental health social worker as a transitional participant: Actively listening to "voices" and getting into the recovery position', *Journal of Social Work Practice*, vol. 27, no. 1, pp. 21–32

Davidson, L., Stayner, D.A., Nickou, C., Styron, T.H., Rowe, M. & Chinman, M.L. 2001, '"Simply to be let in": Inclusion as a basis for recovery', *Psychiatric Rehabilitation Journal*, vol. 24, no. 4, pp. 375–88

Ferguson, H. 2008, 'The theory and practice of critical best practice in social work' in K. Jones, B. Cooper and H. Ferguson (eds), *Best Practice in Social Work: Critical perspectives*, Houndmills: Palgrave Macmillan, pp. 15–37

Hamkins, S. 2005, 'Introducing narrative psychiatry: Narrative approaches to initial psychiatry consultations', International Journal of Narrative Therapy and Community Work, vol. 1, no. 1, pp 5–17

Holmes, A. 2013, 'Is risk assessment the new clinical model in public mental health?', *Australasian Psychiatry*, vol. 21, no. 6, pp. 541–4

Kalhovde, A.M., Elstad, I. & Talseth, A.G. 2013, '"Understanding the experiences of hearing voices and sounds others do not hear', *Qualitative Health Research*, vol. 23, no. 11, pp. 1470–80

Kanter, J. 2000, 'Beyond psychotherapy: Therapeutic relationships in community care', *Smith College Studies in Social Work*, vol. 70, no. 3, pp. 397–426

Keeping, C. 2008, 'Emotional engagement in social work: Best practice and relationships in mental health' in K. Jones, B. Cooper & H. Ferguson (eds), in *Best Practice in Social Work: Critical perspectives*, Houndmills: Palgrave Macmillan, pp. 71–87

Mass, A and Arcuri, L., 1996, 'Language and Stereotyping' in N. Macrae, C. Stangor & M. Hewstone (eds), *Stereotypes and Stereotyping* New York: Guilford, p. 193

Melville-Wiseman, J. 2012, 'Taking relationships into account in mental health services' in G. Koubel & H. Bungay (eds), *Rights, Risks and Responsibilities: Interprofessional working in health and social care*, London: Palgrave Macmillan, pp. 123–41

Mendes, P., Allen-Kelly, K., Charikar, K., Incerti, K. & McCurdy, S. 2012, *Social Workers and Social Action: A Report for the Lyra Taylor Fund on the AASW campaign to restore Medicare rebates for Accredited Mental Health Social Workers*

Nathan, J. & Webber, M. 2010, 'Mental health social work and the bureau-medicalisation of mental health care: Identity in a changing world', *Journal of Social Work Practice*, vol. 24, no. 1, pp. 15–28

Norcio, B., Baldi, C., Dell'Acqua, G. & Marsili, M. 2001, 'The Trieste mental health services: History, context, principles', paper presented to International conference and workshops, Auckland and Hamilton, New Zealand

Olsen, A. & Epstein, M. 2012, 'The consumer of mental health services' in G. Meadows, J. Farhall, E. Fossey, M. Grigg, F. McDermott & B. Singh (eds), *Mental Health in Australia: Collaborative community practice*, Melbourne: Oxford University Press, pp. 279–81

Parton, N. & O'Byrne, P. 2000, 'What do we mean by constructive social work?', *Critical Social Work*, vol. 1, no. 2

Place, C., Foxcroft, R. & Shaw, J., 2011, 'Telling stories and hearing voices: Narrative work with voice hearers in acute care', *Journal of Psychiatric and Mental Health Nursing*, vol. 18, no. 9, pp 837–842

Ramon, S. 2005, 'Approaches to risk in mental health' in J. Tew & Jessica Kingsley (eds), *Social Perspectives in Mental Health: Developing social models to understand and work with mental distress*, London, pp. 184–99

Romme, M. & Escher, A. 1989, 'Hearing voices', *Schizophrenia Bulletin*, vol. 15, no. 2, pp. 209–16

Sane Australia. 2011, *People Living with Psychotic Illness: A Sane response*, Melbourne: Sane Australia

Seikkula, J. & Arnkil, T.E. 2006, *Dialogical Meetings in Social Networks*, London: Karnac

Slade, M. 2012, 'Everyday solutions for everyday problems: How mental health systems can support recovery', *Psychiatric Services*, vol. 63, no. 7, pp. 702–4

Spandler, H. 2013, 'Letting madness breathe? Critical challenges facing mental health social work today' in J. Weinstein (ed.), *Mental Health*, Bristol: Policy Press

Tew, J., Ramon, S., Slade, M., Bird, V., Melton, J. & Le Boutillier, C. 2012, 'Social factors and recovery from mental health difficulties: A review of the evidence', *British Journal of Social Work*, vol. 42, no. 3, pp. 443–60

Thomas, P. & Bracken, P. 2004, 'Critical psychiatry in practice', *Advances in Psychiatric Treatment*, vol. 10, no. 5, pp. 361–70

Topp, V. & Thomas, M. 2008, 'Advance directives for mental health', *New Paradigm*, pp. 51–5

Vassilev, I. & Pilgrim, D. 2007, 'Risk, trust and the myth of mental health services', *Journal of Mental Health*, vol. 16, no. 3, pp. 347–57

Voices Vic. 2009, *About Hearing Voices Groups: Information pack for managers and clinicians*, Melbourne: Prahran Mission

Waddell, M. 1989, 'Living in two worlds: Psychodynamic theory and social work practice', *Free Associations*, no. 15, pp. 11–35

Webber, M. 2011, *Evidence-Based Policy and Practice in Mental Health Social Work*, 2nd edn, Exeter: Learning Matters

Weinstein, J. (ed.) 2013, *Mental Health*, Bristol: Policy Press

Wilkinson, R. & Pickett, K. 2010, *The Spirit Level: Why equality is better for everyone*, London: Penguin

Woods, A. 2013, 'The voice-hearer', *Journal of Mental Health*, vol. 22, no. 3, pp. 263–70

9

Embedding critical social work in child protection practice

Robyn Miller

Introduction

Social workers in child protection and family services work can have a potent effect when promoting the human rights of family members. Power is implicit and explicit in the statutory child protection role and the ethical, wise use of that authority has initiated a rights-based practice approach and whole-of-system reform in Victoria over the past decade. This chapter focuses on the critical social work principles that have contributed to reform at an overall policy level, and the frontline practice at a more detailed level, in Victoria. I argue that the 'doing' of critical social work in a statutory context is essential when considering the structural disadvantage and complexity of child abuse and neglect.

The Victorian reforms have challenged the earlier polarised position of child protection being child-focused and forensic, and family services being parent-focused and supportive. The social exclusion and structural inequality experienced by many families in the child protection system requires both a child-focused and a family-centred approach. Practitioners need to have emotional intelligence, intellectual rigour, and systemic support to critically reflect on their practice. The reforms promoted a joined-up system in local areas, with a shared-partnership and strength-based practice. This has been a deliberate strategy, in contrast to the 'bureaucratisation' of child protection. As I discuss the 'doing' of critical social work from my perspective as a practitioner who has provided practice leadership within child protection in Victoria for the past eight years, I am aware of the limitations and inherent bias. However, I remain passionate and committed to the importance of critical social work's contribution to both policy and practice in this challenging, yet most rewarding field of practice.

Does critical theory fit in a statutory context?

Allan (2009: 4) gives a powerful reminder that 'it should be stated at the outset that the term "critical theory" does not designate a unified theoretical perspective. It is a term that embraces a variety of different theoretical positions'.

The Canadian work of Donna Baines' (2007) 'anti-oppressive practices' and Bob Mullaly's (2007) 'new structural social work' are influenced by postmodern ideas and provide useful conceptualisations for statutory practitioners. Turbett stresses that the use of authority in a statutory child protection setting aligns with radical social work practice 'if one believes that child protection, and, indeed, social work as a whole, has a positive function'(Turbett 2014: 79). Turbett highlights the need for practitioners' open acknowledgement of the differences in power inherent in statutory work, and the need for practitioners to display openness, honesty and reliability in their interactions with families. Turbett situates relationship building, which is central to Victoria's case practice model, within a radical social work perspective, noting that a practitioner who blames the client for their circumstance may find it difficult to build a good working relationship with that client and in doing so, compromise their ability to best serve the client's interests.

June Allan's position that critical social work is key in addressing issues of social justice and equality (Allan 2009: 40), is one that inspires me and fits the contemporary statutory context in Victoria. Her list of core principles that provide a common ground for different approaches to critical social work are relevant to the Best Interests Case Practice Model that has been used in Victoria since 2008 (see Chapter 1).

Allan also draws on the work of Yeatman (1998) and Healy (2001) to remind us that we should not overlook the sometimes invisible, effective forms of activist work that can be found among government bureaucrats (Allan 2009: 43). This activist work has been evident within the Department of Human Services (DHS) bureaucracy; to develop and implement innovative policy that is informed by current research in order to effectively guide practice. Baines (2007) also notes that, to increase possibilities for social justice, managerial and supervisory positions need to be taken up by critical social workers. I would add that in Victoria, the critical social work values and expertise shown by key leaders within government and non-government settings, who persisted to effect social change, were intrinsic to the incremental success of the system-wide reforms (KPMG 2011; DHS 2013). These remain a work in progress in this state.

The reforms in Victoria have shifted the practice culture towards a different model. This new model is one that both engages families (which wasn't being achieved well before) and partners with other services. This practice shift fits with Allan's (2009) core principle of working alongside oppressed and marginalised populations. Prevention and the need to intervene earlier is prioritised. This is in contrast to previous approaches which involved regular risk assessment of children and monitoring of the perceived risk, through a procedural, task-focussed approach. This shift is towards a practice orientation that is influenced by neuroscience's evidence about the impact of neglect and cumulative harm on the child's voice and experience. Stability for children and their development are prioritised as key considerations under the legislation and practice model, across program silos and sectors, rather than the previously narrow focus on immediate safety.

The historical context

The social construction, causes and meaning of child maltreatment and professional views regarding the most appropriate interventions, have historically been underpinned by the notions of blame and anxiety. The pendulum has swung in different directions over time from blaming children, to blaming parents, social workers or the system (Scott & Swain 2002). Earlier theories were influenced by psychodynamic psychotherapists who conceptualised child abuse as being primarily a disorder of the parent–child attachment that had roots in the parent's early childhood experience. Of note, by the 1970s, Gil (1970) and Gelles (1973) strongly critiqued the parental psychopathology model and developed a structural model that prioritised the significance of social circumstances, such as poverty, unemployment, racism, violence and marginalisation impacting on children and families involved with statutory services.

Robin Clark (1988; 1997; 1998), a preeminent social worker and leader in child protection, highlighted in her work the structural inequalities and over-representation of poor families. Clark critiqued the policy settings of the day and was a strong advocate for a refocusing of services in Victoria to better meet the needs of vulnerable families: 'Large numbers of unsubstantiated reports preoccupy the child protection staff and divert attention from those children most in need. The Child Protection

Service is being asked to respond to an increasing number of families and children, where a short-term investigative service, is not the answer' (Clark 1988: 219).

Thorpe (1994) also critiqued the Australian child protection culture, which had a disproportionate number of Aboriginal and Torres Strait Islander families and single parents who became the focus of the child protection system. Reflecting on the lack of partnership, Armytage, Boffa and Armitage (1998) who were then employed within the DHS, identified the alienation of non-government support agencies and other services by earlier child protection practices that claimed the expert position. They were instrumental in developing earlier partnership approaches and also the well-regarded Victorian Risk Assessment Framework (VRF), which has subsequently been integrated into the Best Interests Case Practice Model (BICPM) (Miller 2012). The lack of analysis of the policy framework and possible alternatives has also received comment from experts in child protection. For example, Dorothy Scott elegantly summarised the dilemma commenting in *The Australian* newspaper that: 'It is not the people working in child protection who are at fault; it is the policy framework in which they operate that is fatally flawed. Rarely is this examined. Instead, more money is poured into bigger child protection systems and more inappropriate referrals flood in' (Scott 2007).

Scott (2009) critiqued the overloading of child protection services, noting that in Australia, only one in five notifications is substantiated or believed to be child abuse and neglect. She strongly advocates a public health approach, requiring an understanding of the underlying social determinants of child abuse and neglect, just as we would with any other public health issue.

Unless proactive strategies are identified to support practice, a more rigid and bureaucratic system can become the reactive response to managing increased demand on the ground. The outcome of such rigidity can be unnecessary statutory intervention in the lives of families who may already be marginalised. For example, Mansell et al. (2011), and Higgins and Katz (2008) have reported the damaging impact of such unwarranted intervention.

Vulnerable children and young people need creative, flexible, dynamic and skilled social work practice. Munro (2010) from the UK has also written about the media's influence on the mistakes made by statutory child protection systems and the increase in regulatory and risk-averse responses which lower the threshold for statutory intervention.

In order to foster creative, flexible and dynamic practice culture, practitioners need to be supported to think critically and to enact social-justice values that underpin our profession. Establishing this culture requires strong leaders within the policy and bureaucratic domains as well as in operational practice.

'Doing' critical social work at a system-wide level

The *Children, Youth and Families Act 2005* (enacted in 2007) articulated a set of Best Interests Principles for the Children's Court, child protection and family services, to place the best interests of children as paramount while aiming to provide the widest possible assistance to the family. For the first time, the legislation focused on the *development* of children and cumulative harm, and the rights of Aboriginal families were specified. The willingness of government- and non-government-sector leaders to engage with the legacy of colonisation and the ongoing over-representation of Aboriginal children, in both the child protection and youth justice services as a rights issue, was significant.

Child FIRST and Integrated Family Services is a major element within the Child and Family Service system reforms in Victoria. After a statewide consultation, evaluation and critical reflection at multiple levels, this strategy focused on radically redesigning the service system to intervene earlier to prevent harm, and to divert families from child protection. Building on the evidence from earlier successful pilots, it was significant to note that from 2002 to 2007 the funding to family service agencies in Victoria almost trebled, which increased their capacity to provide a service for longer where needed and possible, given the demand. Community-based child protection practitioners are now co-located with the Child FIRST sites around the state in local areas, improving collaborative practice, and alliances have been established in each sub-region.

Instead of separate agencies and silos between family services and child protection services, agreement was reached that a lead agency would provide a visible point of contact and coordinate intake processes, joint professional training and reflective practice sessions. It was agreed that more vulnerable families would be prioritised and require outreach services. Muriel Bamblett from Victorian Aboriginal Child Care Agency (VACCA), through her powerful presentations and ongoing dialogue, also challenged the commitment of government and non-government agencies to 'walk' more of the cultural competence 'talk'. The first Commissioner for Aboriginal Children and Young People, Andrew Jackomos, was appointed in Victoria in 2013, and the continuing attention on cultural planning and outcomes for Aboriginal children in care remain sharply in focus.

Victorian services use the BICPM that has been collaboratively developed and endorsed across sectors. The model symbolises the increased partnerships and integration of services and creates a shared language and commitment to systemic, relationship-based practice.

Figure 1: Best Interests Case Practice Model (BICPM)

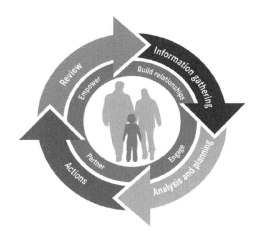

Source: Miller (2012: 5:)

The essence of the BICPM is simple: the child and family are at the centre and the process of what we do as practitioners, and how we do it effectively, is symbolised in a circular and dynamic way. Practice is not a linear process where we tick boxes on computers. The BICPM acknowledges the structural inequalities inherent in the work with vulnerable families and of the interpersonal skills required to be effective. There is a BICPM summary guide, one-page practice tools, and a series of ten specialist practice resources, many of which have been co-authored by colleagues from the Australian Institute of Family Studies and are used by other jurisdictions. These resources are freely available online.

The BICPM positions practice as iterative, interactive, and a practice that requires practitioners to be intelligently responsive to emerging information. The model acknowledges forensically astute practice in which risk is skilfully assessed. As noted by Dumbrill, failing to take an 'investigative and policing' approach when necessary and, on occasion, to remove a child from their home, will 'ultimately fail the children they serve, and failing to protect a child who was relying on a social worker to protect them from harm has to be considered oppressive' (Dumbrill 2011: 53). However, Victoria continues to have the lowest rate of children in care compared to other states, and effort is made to keep children within their family wherever possible.

While there is an inevitable difference in power that is at its most explicit in statutory child protection, if this is respectfully transparent and the practitioner's engagement is skilful, the partnership with families and young people towards safety is generally possible. Research that has looked at the factors that lead to change in families where children have been at risk, consistently highlights the significance of the quality of relationships between children, families and practitioners (Department of Health, UK, 1995; McKeown 2000; De Boer & Coady 2007; Brandon et al. 2008; Furlong 2013; Trotter 2013).

The BICPM has consistently embedded the critical importance of culturally safe practice and the healing power of connection to culture. The lens of culture is not conceptualised as an 'add-on'. Instead, it is the lens through which everything else should be understood. This does not mean that practice in regions is necessarily immediately improved by such a document. As Fixsen et al. noted, 'it is clear that paperwork in file cabinets plus manuals on shelves do not equal putting innovations into practice with benefits to consumers' (Fixsen et al. 2005: 6). Regular cross-sector training opportunities based on BICPM, the development of practice tools and the continued focus on practitioners receiving personal supervision are some of the efforts being made to promote the understanding and use of the model in practice. These training opportunities have been well received.

Judy Atkinson, from the contextual perspective of Aboriginal experiences of violence and healing from trauma, writes powerfully of the transgenerational transmission of trauma that results from colonisation and genocide: 'These create chronic endemic crisis. Government interventions may increase the trauma' (Atkinson 2002: 83). The BICPM stresses that practitioners remain committed to not repeating the oppression of the past and understand the impact of the dispossession of Aboriginal lands and language, and the cruel impact of having their children taken away. At the same time, there is a clear message from Aboriginal leaders such as Muriel Bamblett, that the expectations around safety should not be seen as less of a right for Aboriginal children today, and that there should not be higher thresholds for intervention where the pendulum swings the other way, and children are harmed through a lack of response from professionals. This is an ongoing conversation in Victoria.

Systemic changes and improvement

Practice that privileges building good working relationships with families requires a stable workforce that develops the experience and knowledge of new practitioners. This was an ongoing issue prior, during and following the development of the BICPM. The rate of frontline practitioners leaving the profession in the years prior to 2009 was around 26 per cent per annum, which was clearly unsustainable. This contributed to broad concerns about the performance and competence of the program. However, over the past six years, through very purposeful actions that demonstrate support for practitioners, the exit rate of frontline practitioners has reduced markedly to a healthier 12–15 per cent.

Concurrent strategies that promote good practice and a learning culture have made a difference, despite a 14 per cent increase in demand on services from new reports each year. The new operating model in child protection, which was introduced in 2012, created structures to enable improved practice. It has established specialist senior practitioner positions in every team, strengthened supervision and regular reflective practice sessions, and increased support of new practitioners with more experienced practitioners who work with the most challenging situations.

Significantly, DHS has also funded postgraduate training in child and family practice, provided by a consortia of universities. Over 300 professionals in child protection and family services have enrolled in this training in the past five years.

Leadership support and training has been a feature of the reforms, as it is one of the key ways to enable good outcomes with families. The modelling, the way we talk about families, and the attitudes towards other professionals permeate the work culture, and are prevalent in formal supervision and meetings. The team culture is more powerful than any training, and the way social justice is enacted within a statutory context is very much influenced by it. Supervisors' attitudes and conceptualisations powerfully shape less experienced practitioners.

All of these professional development actions have had a coherent focus on critical reflection, which stems from earlier work and literature on reflective practice. Are we walking our talk or is it just rhetoric and jargon? The difference between what we say we do (espoused theory) and what we actually end up doing in action (theory in use) is central to Argyris and Schon's work: the theory which actually governs his [sic] actions is his [sic] theory-in-use, which may or may not be compatible with his [sic] espoused theory; furthermore, the individual may or may not be aware of the incompatibility (Argyris & Schon 1974: 7).

The ways in which individuals can be made aware of these discrepancies in their own professional situation was the subsequent creation of what Schon (1983) went on to name 'reflective practice'.

However, as Furlong observed, while the directors of agencies and those who set the development of agencies are in a unique position to influence the attitude and skill set of employees, 'this is not a 'monkey-see-monkey-do' exercise, staff are not robots and may kick back against unwelcome change' (Furlong 2013: 209). Of note, evaluations have found that practitioners across sectors have had a positive response to the BICPM, despite the practical implementation and demand problems, because it provides a shared language and understanding, and it aligns with the social justice values that inspired many people to work in the field. It aspires to integrate evidence from research and critical reflection at every phase of practice.

An independent evaluation undertaken by KPMG (2011) made an overarching finding that outcomes of the reforms 'are extremely positive' and suggest that the intent of the reforms is being met. KPMG note: 'This suggests that the quality of case work is improving, as is the relationship with community-based services (such as Child FIRST and Integrated Family Services) so as to sustain change for families' (KPMG 2011: 8. Of key significance is the consistency between the KPMG data with compelling data from the *Child and Family Services Outcome Study* (DHS 2012), which independently found that practice has become more child- and family-focused, and informed by research evidence. Results from focus groups undertaken in 2012 with those working at a range of levels in child protection and family services further corroborated these findings (Miller 2014).

Empowerment in practice

Early engagement with families and where appropriate, facilitating family meetings where problems are shared and outcomes negotiated is one practice representing 'empowerment'; providing the process is one of genuine participation which is transparent and respectful in negotiating the power inequality between the practitioner and the family.

Practitioners need to understand the parent's perspective while keeping the child's needs front and centre. Dumbrill describes engagement as being the 'process of a worker's establishing an agreement with a parent to work together towards a shared purpose' (Dumbrill 2011: 54). Further, an 'alliance' is described as 'the interpersonal bond through which worker and parent work toward that purpose' (Dumbrill 2011: 54)

The empowerment of children through hearing their voices and acting to keep them safe is a key part of the statutory role, as is the building of an alliance with parents; some who may have been victimised by an oppressive partner or have been groomed by a sex offender. Supporting victims of family violence to seek intervention orders, for example, can be seen as an empowerment intervention and clearly the notion of social justice is closely aligned to such practices. Helping families to 'get on with their lives' with full respect to their human rights is central to this concept.

White and Epstein (1989) and McCashen (2005), from a strengths-based perspective, see empowerment as an expansion of choices, a 're-authoring' of one's life; the concept of taking responsibility and agency to reclaim one's life in an enhanced way. While disempowerment and disconnection are core experiences of trauma, reconnection and empowerment occur when people choose and are supported to reclaim and make sense of their stories (Herman 1992: 133). Understanding of the power of stories underpins the strengths-based theoretical models of change that focus on strength, knowledge and resilience rather than predominantly on problems or deficits (McCashen 2005); the BICPM has drawn on these approaches.

However, I will never forget the powerful lesson given by a father in a very troubled family, when I was working as a family therapist trainee. In a session one day, using the narrative approach I clumsily referred to his pain as 'his story'. He looked up at me, with a distressed look and said, 'Love, that's no story; it's my bloody *life*'. Jargon, even if used with good intention, can alienate people and minimise deeply painful experiences, which is the antithesis of skilful critical social work in action.

Case study: Sally

I recently joined a residential carer and a child-protection case manager with Sally (a pseudonym), who was a profoundly sad adolescent who had attempted suicide. She had been sexually abused as a preschooler by her stepfather and, as is the norm, had kept it a secret. Her primary school years were uneventful and she only came to the attention of services at the age of thirteen when she began running away. At the age of fourteen she was in a secure unit where I first met her as she showed us her recent self-harm; the fresh cuts were evidence that she 'just wants to die'. In these situations, providing immediate support and remaining curious about *what has happened to her rather* than quickly assuming *what is wrong with her* can powerfully influence a different care team response and future planning. A trauma-informed approach means working with her to unpack what she is feeling, and how this is normal given the circumstances that underlie her distress. Central to this approach, which is supported by recent advances in neuroscience (Perry 2001), is the hope that can be offered to the person and that with the right therapeutic care things can be different. Sally felt enraged and so hurt by her mother's rejection, but Sally ached for connection. It was very reassuring to help her to know that she was not 'weird' and that her feeling overwhelmed is a 'normal' response to the trauma she has experienced. Cutting was a strategy to manage unbearable emotional pain, and intrusive feelings and thoughts that she could not stop.

Understanding her trauma helped others remain effectively engaged with her and reframed the unhelpful view that she was

---

'attention seeking' or 'sabotaging the placement'. For Sally, it was the relationships with her carers and her child protection practitioner that made the immediate difference and gave her some reassurance that she was not on her own. Sally loved animals and some creative casework set up work experience at the local vet surgery (which later became a part-time job). She was unwilling initially to go to formal counselling, but the skilled and compassionate engagement by her practitioner eventually helped her to see the point in going back to school. These conversations often took place in the car as they were doing other practical things.

None of this would have been as effective if her child-protection practitioner had not also built an alliance with her mother who was initially still living with the offender. Gradually she engaged and was helped to understand that her daughter was not 'attention seeking,' and that the earlier sexual abuse that she had suffered was 'not a lie' and was deeply disturbing. Sally's mother was trapped in an overwhelmed state herself, as her partner had been the perpetrator, and Sally had only recently disclosed this information when she was already in trouble for shoplifting, and had started using drugs and alcohol. Her mother had struggled to believe her as Sally retracted her initial disclosure and then was angry, distant and rude to her. Sally's mother was deeply confused and regularly heard her 'nice, middle-class' partner saying: 'Would I do that? Your daughter is off the rails! No wonder she's in resi; she needs help!' Sally later reflected that her child-protection practitioner 'hanging in there' with her mother enabled her to separate from the offending step-father and was the turning point in her recovery.

Care team meetings with Sally and her mother involving mental health and other services sometimes got stuck, and respectful dispute-resolution skills were critically important. However, Sally has now returned to live with her mother and she is still attending school with the aim of becoming a lawyer. She has met with police and is getting ready to make a sworn statement to assist the criminal investigation.

These complexities underline the acute need for facilitation and partnerships that can deliver what the young person needs rather than maintaining territorial service boundaries. Practitioners all over the state are required to respectfully deal with conflict and difference, remain creative, assertive and 'think outside the square'. Listening to everyone in the room (including those cynical and critical of child protection services), remaining curious, while managing the practical issues of time, urgency, placement issues, waiting lists for assessments or adult treatment, and legalities are daily challenges.

Conclusion

Fiona McColl strongly challenged the lack of critical reflection in child protection systems in Australia as contributing to the retention problems of experienced frontline practitioners and noted that other community services are becoming 'increasingly risk aversive and proscriptive' (McColl 2009: 128). Mindful of this analysis, a consistent theme throughout the BICPM publications is that a culture of critical reflection is crucial so that professionals: can be astute to the possibilities for change; *think* about what they are observing; reflect on *how they are feeling* about the dilemmas; experience support; have robust debate; integrate relevant theory and research; draw on the practice wisdom of their colleagues and not become stuck and biased in their views (Miller 2010: 116–119).

I witness the critical social work principles as articulated by Allan (2009) being worked on the ground by good practitioners who are committed to ongoing critical reflection in action, and about our actions. These skills are vital in being able to think about complexity and multiple versions of truth, judgements and possibilities for change; never more important than when children have been hurt, and we have the chance to make a difference.

References

Allan, J. 2009, 'Theorising new developments in critical social work' in J. Allan, L. Briskman & B. Pease (eds), *Critical Social Work: Theories and practices for a socially just world*, 2nd edn, St Leonards: Allen & Unwin, pp. 30–44

Argyris, C. & Schon, D.A 1974, *Organisational learning II: Theory, method and practice*, Reading: Addison Wesley

Armytage, P., Boffa, J. & Armitage, E. 1998, 'Professional practice frameworks: Linking prevention, support and protection', paper presented at the Twelfth International ISPCAN Congress on Child Abuse and Neglect, 'Protecting Children: Innovation and Inspiration', Auckland, New Zealand, 6–9 September

Atkinson, J. 2002, *Trauma trails: Recreating song lines—the transgenerational effects of trauma in Aboriginal Australia*, Melbourne: Spinifex Press

Baines, D. (ed.) 2007, *Doing Anti-Oppressive Practice: Building transformative politicized social work*,

Halifax: Fernwood Publishing

Brandon, M., Howe, D., Belderson, P., Black, J., Dodsworth, J., Gardner, R. & Warren, C. 2008, *Analysing Child Deaths and Serious Injury Through Abuse and Neglect: What can we learn? A biennial analysis of serious case reviews 2003–2005*. London: Department for Children, Schools and Families

Clark, R. 1988, *Whose Children? A review of the Substitute Care Branch*. Canberra: Department of Education and Community Services

—— 1997, *A Review of Intensive Out-of-Home Care Support Services*. Sydney: Department of Community Services, NSW

—— 1998, *A Framework for Development of Intensive Out-of Home-Care Support Services for NSW Department of Community Services research report*, Sydney: Deakin Human Services

De Boer, C. & Coady, N. 2007, 'Good helping relationships in child welfare: Learning from stories of success', *Child and Family Social Work*, vol. 12, pp. 32–2

Department of Health (UK) 1995, *The Challenge of Partnership in Child Protection: Practice guide*, London: HMSO

Department of Human Services 2012, *The Child and Family Services Outcomes Survey*, prepared by Queensland University of Technology and the Social Research Centre. Melbourne: Department of Human Services, Victorian government

—— 2013, *The Child and Family Services Outcomes Survey*, prepared by Queensland University of Technology and the Social Research Centre. Melbourne: Department of Human Services, Victorian government

DHS *see* Department of Human Services

Dumbrill, G. 2011, 'Doing Anti-Oppressive Child Protection Casework' in D. Baines (ed.), *Doing Anti Oppressive Practice*, Fernwood Publishing: Halifax, pp. 52–63

Fixsen, D.L., Naoom, S.F., Blase, K.A., Friedman, R.M. & Wallace, F. 2005, *Implementation Research: A synthesis of the literature*, Tampa, Florida: The University of South Florida, The National Implementation Research Network

Furlong, M. 2013, *Building the Client's Relational Base: A multidisciplinary handbook*, Bristol: Policy Press

Gelles, R. 1973, 'Child Abuse as Psychopathology: A socio-logical critique and reformulation, *American Journal of Orthopsychiatry*, vol. 43, pp. 611–21

Gil, D.G. 1970, *Violence Against Children: Physical child abuse in the United States*, Cambridge: Harvard University Press

Healy, K. 2001, 'Reinventing critical social work: Challenges from practice, context and postmodernism,' *Critical Social Work*, vol. 2, no. 1, pp. 1–17

Herman, J. 1992, *Trauma and recovery: The aftermath of violence*, New York: Basic Books

Higgins, D.J. & Katz, I. 2008, 'Enhancing service systems for protecting children,' *Family Matters*, vol. 80, pp. 43–50

KPMG 2011, *Evaluation of child and family services reform, evaluation summary report*, Melbourne: Department of Human Services, Victoria

Mansell, J., Ota, R., Erasmus, R., & Marks, K. 2011, 'Reframing child protection: A response to a constant crisis of confidence in child protection', *Children and Youth Services Review*, vol. 33, pp. 2076–86

McCashen, W. 2005, *The Strengths Approach: A strengths based resource for sharing power and creating change*, Bendigo: St Luke's Innovative Resources

McColl, F. 2009, 'Where have all the social workers gone? Critical reflection and child protection', *Advances in Social Work and Welfare Education*, vol. 11, no. 1, pp. 127–30

McKeown, K. 2000, *Supporting Families: A guide to what works in family support services for vulnerable families,* unpublished report, Dublin: Department of Health and Children

Miller, R. 2010, 'Practice Reflection: The knowledge and skills that child protection practitioners need today', *Advances in Social Work & Welfare Education*, vol. 11, no. 2. pp. 116–19

—— 2012, *Best Interests Case Practice Model: Summary guide, State* Government of Victoria, www.dhs. vic.gov.au<www.dhs.vic.gov.au>, accessed 27 October 2014

—— 2014, *Walking the Same Talk*, internal unpublished presentation, Melbourne: Department of Human Services

Mullaly, B. 2007, *The New Structural Social Work*, 3rd edn, Don Mills: Oxford University Press

Munro, E. 2010, 'Conflating risks: Implications for accurate risk prediction in child welfare services', *Health, Risk and Society*, vol. 12, no. 2, pp. 119–130

Perry, B.D. 2001, 'The Neurodevelopmental Impact of Violence in Childhood' in D. Schetky & E.P. Benedek (eds), *Textbook of Child and Adolescent Forensic Psychiatry*, Washington: American Psychiatric Press

Schon, D.A. 1983, *The Reflective Practitioner: How professionals think in action*, New York: Basic Books,

Scott, D. 2009, *Seminar Report: A public health approach to child protection.* Adelaide: Centre for Learning in Child Protection

Scott, D. & Swain, S. 2002, *Confronting Cruelty: Historical perspectives on child protection in Australia,* Melbourne: Melbourne University Press

Scott, D. 2007, 'Children let down by the rules', *The Australian* Newspaper, 14th November

Steiner, G. 1976, *The Children's Cause*, Washington: The Brookings Institute

Thorpe, D. 1994, *Evaluating Child Protection,* Buckingham: Open University Press

Trotter, C. 2013, *Collaborative family work: A practical guide to working with families in the human services*, St Leonards: Allen and Unwin

Turbett, C. 2014, *Doing Radical Social Work*, Houndmills: Palgrave Macmillan

White, M. & Epston, D. 1989, *Literate Means to Therapeutic Ends*, Adelaide: Dulwich Centre Publications

Yeatman, A. 1998, *Activism* and the *Policy Process*, St Leonards: Allen & Unwin

10

Critical social work in Centrelink: an oxymoron or an opportunity?

Peter Humphries

Introduction

A few years ago, while participating as a panel member at a public seminar with a focus on 'welfare reform' (and at that time working with Centrelink), I mentioned that social workers had been active participants in Australia's income-support agency, the Department of Social Security, and then Centrelink, for over 60 years. This prompted a question about how social workers had survived in such a bureaucratic and potentially hostile environment. The questioner asked whether I thought the longevity of the social work service was a result of them being either very clever or very compliant. My response was that they had been 'cleverly compliant'. This off-the-cuff comment encapsulates the challenges of social work practice in Centrelink (which is now a part of the Commonwealth Department of Human Services). As public servants, social workers in Centrelink have to recognise the right of an elected government to set policy directions and have their policies implemented by the public service. As Briggs notes the *Public Service Act 1999* 'requires public servants to be responsive to the Government of the day' and 'this means that the public service acts non-politically and professionally in support of the Government of the day' (Briggs 2007: 501). So this is where the 'compliance' comes in, as it does for any social workers directly employed by government. 'Clever compliance' involves the interpretation of policies and guidelines in the 'interests of the client', and this is where the opportunities for critical social work practice in Centrelink emerge. Carey and Foster explore similar territory when they talk about 'deviant social work', which for them is about providing 'tangible support to vulnerable people' and being able to largely evade 'managerial or policy-led forms of location, surveillance and control' (Carey & Foster 2011: 576).

Fook comments that 'critical social work practice is primarily concerned with practising in ways which further a society without domination, exploitation and oppression' (Fook 2012: 18). Healy echoes this, stating that critical social work is 'concerned with the analysis and transformation of power relations at every level of social work practice' (2005: 172). Allan observes that there are many different ways of understanding critical social work, while identifying what she considers to be five inherent 'core principles' (Allan 2009: 40; see also Chapter 1).

Allan considers there are many challenges for critical social work that emerge from these principles, not the least of which is 'how to realistically promote social change in a neoliberal context with its stringent managerial controls and account-abilities' (Allan 2009: 42). It is difficult to see Centrelink in the context of this debate as anything other than a 'neoliberal' organisation that undoubtedly displays 'strin-gent managerial controls and accountabilities'. For this reason, I have often been confronted by the view that social workers in Centrelink have essentially 'sold out' their social work values in exchange for secure well-paid employment as 'agents of the state'. This may be true of some social workers working in Centrelink, but in my view it is an unfair assessment of the majority who are in there doing all that is possible to support vulnerable people and act as advocates for a fairer approach to social policy. So yes, critical social work practice in Centrelink has its challenges but, in my view, it is possible.

Ife makes a strong argument that community-based social work is 'the most fruitful position from which to develop significant alternatives to the managerial and economic rationalist orthodoxies' (Ife 1997: 75). Ife's view is that the practice context is the key determinant of the possibilities for critical practice and he does not consider it to be possibile in a large government bureaucracy. In this chapter, I explore an alternative view that critical social work practice can also occur in a large government organisation such as Centrelink.

Centrelink in the 'service system'

As noted earlier, social workers have been working in Centrelink, and its predecessor, the Department of Social Security, for nearly 70 years. Centrelink currently employs over 600 social workers (DHS 2011). It was fully integrated into the Commonwealth Department of Human Services in 2011 and its key function remains to provide income-support payments including Newstart Allowance (unemployment benefits), the Disability Support Pension and the Age Pension. Centrelink is a key 'point-of-first-contact' agency in the Australian welfare system and has contact with over six million Australians every year. Most of those who have contact with Centrelink do so because they have to, as they need income support payments, rather than because they want to, but this contact does allow for other support to be offered. As an example, a sixteen-year-old person who is unable to live at home will come to Centrelink to obtain income support, but also brings a range of other possible issues and concerns. It is the extent of this contact with the Australian community that creates possibilities for critical social work practice in Centrelink, acknowledging that there is a strong view that these possibilities have been greatly reduced over the past few years (for example, McDonald & Chenoweth 2009; Hart 2013).

Social work in Centrelink

Centrelink (DHS 2014) describes its social workers as offering 'help during difficult times' by providing confidential counselling, support and information, and that this social work support and information can include:

- short-term counselling and support for difficult personal or family issues
- exploring options
- providing information about, or referring to, government and community support services
- discussing difficulties in meeting activity tests or participation requirements.

The Centrelink pamphlet goes on to state that 'people of all ages can talk to social workers about a range of issues, including domestic and family violence, homelessness, relationship breakdown, loss and bereavement, mental health and addictions' (DHS 2014). The 'priority customer groups' are said to be:

- customers expressing suicidal thoughts or experiencing mental illness
- young people without adequate support
- customers experiencing severe distress, family and domestic violence, homelessness or hardship
- individuals caring for an adult or child with a disability or serious illness.

Much of this contact with Centrelink 'customers' tends to involve crisis intervention. A recent survey of Centrelink social workers found that 48.2 per cent of the 460 social workers who completed the survey reported that their most common contact with Centrelink customers focused on crisis intervention (Humphries & Morgan 2010). The same survey also found that 80.6 per cent of the social workers who responded reported that at least 50 per cent of their work involved 'direct customer contact' (Humphries & Morgan 2010: 4). The 'crisis' nature of the contact is not surprising given that the social workers are in contact with the poorest Australians; that is, those reliant on Government income support payments. Also, social work practice in Centrelink is unquestionably focussed on the frontline of Centrelink's service delivery to its 'customers'.

Welfare reform in Australia

Ife considers that 'another area where this is a tension between mainstream social work and the critical theory approach is in the area of authority and control' (1997: 146). Ife is primarily focused on areas such as child protection and corrections but there are aspects of social work practice in Centrelink where issues regarding authority and control emerge. This can be in the generic work associated with determining the customers' eligibility for income-support payments, but has become more noticeable as the 'welfare reform' agenda initiated by the Howard Government has emerged over the past ten years. In Australia, 'welfare reform' and concerns about 'welfare dependency' have led to stricter conditions being put in place to retain eligibility for particular payments (such as Newstart Allowance for those who are unemployed), with a focus on compelling active job seeking, generally through a government-funded employment services provider. The paternalistic use of authority so often inherent in approaches to welfare reform (Mestan 2014) has, and still does, create difficulties for social workers in Centrelink as they attempt to balance their ethical obligations to work in their clients' 'best interests' and with their responsibilities, as public servants, to implement government policy. Turbett sets out this dilemma well: 'Social work is riven with ambiguities that underlie its position as mediator between state agencies and the desire to control social problems on the one hand, and social workers' trained response to exercise compassion and outcomes that favour the individual service user on the other' (Turbett 2014: 66).

Financial Case Management (FCM)

An example of this issue is the provision introduced during the Howard Government that allowed for any person who received an 'activity tested' income-support payment (that is, one with provision for some employment-orientated activity) who failed to keep an appointment with their employment-services provider on three occasions, with no 'reasonable excuse', would lose their payment for eight weeks. The social workers in Centrelink responded to this policy by drawing together hundreds of case studies that clearly demonstrated the harm that this policy was doing to very vulnerable Australians. While the policy continued, this internal policy feedback did lead to some moderation in the harshness of the policy's application. This was a good example of how well-targeted and accurate feedback on the impact of social policy can influence its application in practice. I want to focus on just one aspect of this policy, which demonstrates how critical practice can be possible even in the most seemingly difficult circumstances.

Eight weeks without any income support would create serious difficulties for most people, some of whom would be particularly vulnerable as they had dependent children or some form of disability. To avoid putting these people at further risk, Financial Case Management (FCM) was introduced. FCM enables 'exceptionally vulnerable' people to receive some assistance during this eight-week non-payment period. Initially, this assistance was to be provided on a contract basis, through case managers working for non-government welfare organisations. These case managers were authorised to provide non-cash assistance for 'essential' items up to the value of the person's usual income support payment (for example, food vouchers, medication and school clothes) for this eight-week period. There were many parts of Australia where social workers in Centrelink were also required to provide this service due to a lack of non-government organisations (NGOs) that were willing or able to take on these contracts. Many of these NGOs were opposed to the broader policy, believing it to be too harsh and hence were not prepared to be involved. Many social workers in Centrelink also had moral and ethical concerns regarding this and other welfare-reform policies and had mixed feelings, to say the least, about engaging in this work. Hart (2013) conducted in-depth interviews with ten experienced social workers in Centrelink, which highlighted their concerns regarding the implementation of welfare reform/work first policies.

There was an active debate in the Centrelink Social Work Service around the ethics of social workers undertaking the FCM work. One group of social workers decided to approach the Australian Association of Social Workers (AASW) with a complaint that they were being asked to undertake 'unethical practice'. My view at the time (from a 'decision-making' position in Centrelink), was that it would have been unethical for social workers in Centrelink not to deliver FCM, as this would have further disadvantaged an already vulnerable group. FCM did, in part, moderate some of the harsher aspects of this policy and it was a case of providing as much as possible given the situation. It is also important to note that some of the FCM services provided by NGOs at that time were both authoritarian and overly directive. The challenge was to provide FCM in a manner that allowed the person as much dignity as possible within the parameters of the policy. FCM provided the opportunity for a Centrelink social worker to have regular supportive contact with a person who otherwise would have been without income for eight weeks and to ensure that they continued to receive a form of income support. To do this work ethically did require a critical approach to practice as questions of power, oppression and social justice had to be considered. The FCM work also provided the opportunity for many case studies of those affected to be included in the policy review process. At this time, there were few genuine opportunities to influence the 'what' of welfare reform policy, but the experience of providing FCM services did allow for some influence on the 'how' these policies were implemented. Are we looking at critical social work practice or at these social workers being merely co-opted as participants in an oppressive and discriminatory policy? I think this question well illustrates the contradictions inherent in this work. I want to briefly explore another couple of areas where social workers in Centrelink have been active before I discuss the concept of 'front-line autonomy' as a vehicle for critical practice, in even the most potentially difficult practice contexts.

Responding to homelessness

Centrelink has always been a key agency in responding to homelessness and this continues to be an important focus for the social work service. The only homelessness prevention program directly funded by the Commonwealth Government, the HOME Advice Program, was partly developed by social workers in Centrelink (in partnership with the CEO of a Victorian-based homelessness agency). The HOME Advice Program continues, with a site in each state and territory, and focuses on assisting families at risk of becoming homeless to not lose their accommodation. The program at each site is staffed by a Centrelink social worker in partnership with workers from a local NGO. (Of note is that the program has been fully evaluated twice, and shown to be a cost-effective response to preventing homelessness, but has not expanded beyond the initial eight sites in the twelve years it has operated).

A strong focus on homelessness and homelessness prevention in the early years of the Rudd Government, from its election in late 2007, created the opportunity for social workers in Centrelink to further expand Centrelink's role in this area. The Rudd Government's 'white paper' on homelessness described Centrelink as a key 'first to know agency that was well placed to identify people at risk of homelessness and to refer them to appropriate services' (PM&C 2008: 35). Also included was the development of a 'homelessness indicator' to be placed on the Centrelink 'system' to identify any 'customers' who were homeless or at risk of becoming homeless, additional support for young people applying for youth allowance on the basis they were unable to live at home, and putting in place a team of ninety Centrelink community engagement officers whose explicit focus was to provide outreach services to those who were homeless (and those at risk of becoming homeless). These were all initiatives of the social work service in Centrelink and demonstrate a concerted attempt to look at the issues surrounding homelessness beyond the provision of income support to 'eligible' customers. The homelessness indicator, for example, provided valuable information about who was homeless in Australia and, just as importantly, raised the awareness of Centrelink's frontline staff around Australia to the need to identify and support those who were homeless or at risk of becoming homeless.

These initiatives were supported by social workers in Centrelink through the provision of regular 'homelessness awareness' training for all Centrelink staff. In my view, the social workers were able to broaden the response to homelessness, well beyond their own efforts in providing crisis intervention and support services, to a more broadly based organisational response that influenced the service delivery system as well as government policy.

Place-Based Services Program

My final example of potentially critical practice in Centrelink is the Place-Based Services Program (PBSP) which was developed in 2008 and 2009. Social workers again provided a strong underlying 'practice framework' and direction in implementing the actual service delivery to Centrelink customers. The social workers in Centrelink had long argued that each community has different characteristics and hence needed a different and better-targeted service response from Centrelink. They also consistently promoted the idea that Centrelink provided the opportunity to connect with, and support, marginalised and disadvantaged Australians who had no other contact with the broader 'service system'. The then Commonwealth Government's social inclusion agenda, which was based on the premise that a socially inclusive society is one in which all Australians feel valued and have the opportunity to participate fully in the life of our society (PM&C 2009), provided the impetus to establish the PBSP, particularly as the role of 'place' factors in the creation and maintenance of disadvantage was overtly acknowledged. Tony Vinson's study highlighting what he termed areas of 'concentrated disadvantage' (Vinson 2007: xi) also influenced the Government's support for the PBSP and all of the sites initially chosen for the program were identified as being 'disadvantaged' in Vinson's study. The challenge here, from a critical social work point of view, was to maintain a focus on the structural and economic issues inherent in these areas, and not to see those who lived in these locations as being in some way inadequate.

The first three PBSP sites were the Peachey Belt in the northern suburbs of Adelaide, Logan in the southern suburbs of Brisbane and Morwell, a regional town in Eastern Victoria. The focus of work for each site was established through a participative workshop involving the local Centrelink social workers and a representative group of other frontline staff (and I was fortunate enough to facilitate these workshops). Peachey Belt decided to provide better-targeted and more intensive support to disadvantaged sole parents, young people and Aboriginal people; Logan decided to focus on people experiencing domestic and family violence, young people leaving care and people with 'unmet' mental health needs (a full account of the development of the Logan project can be found in Hall et al. 2012); while Morwell decided to provide additional assistance to 'very long-term' unemployed men aged between 35 and 55 years. Without question, these workshops would have been more effective had they also included some representation from Centrelink 'customers', but even the level of local decision-making that was included was hard fought for at the time.

Four additional PBSP sites were subsequently established. They were Broadmeadows in Melbourne and Fairfield in Sydney, which both focused on increasing the 'social and economic participation' of young refugees; Cooma in NSW that focused on assisting young carers; and in Darwin where the initiative aimed to provide further assistance to itinerant and homeless people (most of whom were Aboriginal people). An evaluation of the PBSP by Darcy et al. concluded that these initiatives 'demonstrated the effectiveness of holistic approaches and a more collaborative approach to service provision in improving the wellbeing of participants' and 'this approach contrasts with the traditional approach of applying rule-based compliance rather than addressing problems in partnership with the individual' (Darcy et al. 2009: 83). They went on to conclude that 'the effectiveness of the interventions in assisting individuals who have been very difficult to reach in the past was clear' (Darcy et al. 2009: 83). The evaluators documented a range of what they termed 'social inclusion outcomes' including better connections for 'customers' to key services such as mental health and domestic violence services, decreased social isolation, increased engagement in education and to some extent, increased engagement in employment (Darcy et al. 2009: 61).

The achievement of the PBSP, with social workers in active leadership roles, was to demonstrate that flexibility and individualised responses, along with more equal and respectful relationships with other services in the community, could make a difference to the lives of the most marginalised and disadvantaged Australians. There was a further expansion of this approach under the previous Labor Government but the various trials ended in June 2014, following the election of the Coalition Government the year before. What is important though, is that this more activist and respectful approach to service delivery has been demonstrated to be effective, it and can be reintroduced when the political will is there. It is also important not to forget the positive impact this work had on the frontline staff who had the opportunity to work in a more relationship-based and less process-orientated way with Centrelink's clients. As the PBSP evaluators noted, program participants 'were overwhelmingly positive about having their perspectives heard and most responded by taking steps to improve their circumstances' (Darcy et al. 2009: 83). This is indicative of a critical approach to practice, in that questions of power in the worker–client relationships were actively considered, and more equal and participatory approaches were utilised in this work. The achievement was to create the 'room' to work in this way within a very large and procedurally driven organisation and to demonstrate that, given some support and additional resources, people living in some of the most disadvantaged and stigmatised parts of Australia could improve their circumstances.

Critical practice in Centrelink?

By describing the role of social workers in implementing FCM, developing Centrelink's response to homelessness and in the development and implementation of the PBSP, I have attempted to demonstrate that critical practice can, with thought and effort, happen in a large, regulated government bureaucracy such as Centrelink. This does not mean that all social workers in Centrelink think about the 'core principles' of critical social work identified by Allan (2009) that were discussed earlier. While many bring a well-developed awareness of the nature of power and inequality in our society, and the capacity to critically reflect on their practice, there are others who merely succumb to the 'invitation' to follow the rules and who define their practice in purely procedural terms. For me, the difference between these two groups is their capacity to utilise the level of frontline autonomy that can be found within social work practice in Centrelink.

The use of frontline autonomy

White observes that 'a growing number of writers have presented social workers as having turned into unreflective people-processors by waves of managerialism over the last thirty years' (White 2009: 129). Jones (2001) argues strongly that this has created a new working environment within state social work. He describes a new type of highly regulated and much more mundane and routine-based relationship with clients, which many of the social workers whom he interviewed believe could not even be described as social work. The argument that frontline discretion has been greatly reduced by ever-increasing managerialism has been made by a number of writers (for example, Ife 1997; Ellis et al. 1999; McDonald & Marston 2006). Evans and Harris, however, offer a strong argument that the 'death of discretion' in social work is 'greatly exaggerated' (Evans & Harris 2004: 871), and while we may debate the extent of the discretion that exists in social work practice, the key point is that it does still exist. This point is made most strongly in Lipsky's seminal text, *Street-level Bureaucracy* and the progressive 'potential' inherent in his work has only recently been restated by Turbett (2014). Lipsky's central argument is that no matter what the rules are, when implemented, they are always 'interpreted' by the frontline worker (the street-level bureaucrat) when interfacing with the organisation's clients (Lipsky 1980). This is where the opportunities for critical practice exist, even in the most apparently regulated of service delivery organisations. There are undoubtedly some social workers in Centrelink who have become 'unreflective people processors' and utilise very little of their 'discretion' in their practice but I do also agree with White (2009) that the continuing existence of professional discretion offers 'spaces for resistance' (White 2009: 130).

The examples I have provided illustrate how positive change can emerge through the creative use of the discretion that social workers can utilise in their practice. It is also important to note that these examples were all informed and influenced by the frontline experience of social workers in Centrelink.

Conclusion

Centrelink provides a powerful, and at times difficult and ambiguous, practice context for social workers. It is a large government bureaucracy that is highly managerialised and with a responsibility to implement the policies of the 'government of the day'. The challenges for social workers are acknowledged by both McDonald and Chenoweth (2009) and Hart (2013), who are the only external researchers to have explored the experience of social workers in Centrelink. McDonald and Chenoweth, in the context of discussing the inherent challenges of social work practice in Centrelink, comment that 'nevertheless we have demonstrated that social workers can and do exercise agency in experiencing institutional change and in shaping outcomes' (McDonald & Chenoweth 2009: 158). Similarly, Hart comments that existing accounts of social workers within state welfare institutions have 'conceptualised social workers as mostly passive and resigned recipients of the discourses of change ... resulting in either active or passive compliance with contested organisational practices, or withdrawal from regulated public services' (Hart 2013: 207). Hart then adds that 'the conclusion reached by this thesis in the case study organisation Centrelink, demonstrated active processes of reflection and engagement that drew upon various elements of self-identity' (Hart 2013: 207). Both of these key studies do not underestimate the challenges facing state-employed social workers, but both acknowledge that social workers, on the 'inside', can contribute to progressive social change through utilising a critical approach to their practice.

Fook observes that 'there seems to be an assumption that practice is determined by context and therefore it is not possible to counter the influence of context'. (Fook 2012: 184) Fook goes on to challenge this idea by suggesting that:

> reframing our practice as contextual therefore means we reframe our practice as working with environments, rather than working despite environments. We see ourselves as part of a context, ourselves responsible for aspects of this context. In this way we see possibilities for change, for creating microclimates within broader contexts (Fook 2012: 185).

This does not mean that context does not matter, but Fook suggests that we aim to influence the context rather than just trying to work around the context when difficulties arise. The practice examples that I have discussed have equally focused on influencing the broader practice context as on providing more effective intervention and support to the organisation's clients.

Bringing a critical perspective to bear in a neoliberal organisation such as Centrelink is always going to have its challenges. Perhaps it would have been better to call this chapter 'Towards Critical Social Work in Centrelink'. However, I do believe that these examples can be understood as seeing possibilities for change in Centrelink and creating opportunities where some change can occur. Critical practice involves seeing the possibilities for change, rather than continuing to argue that change is not possible.

Opportunities for critical practice exist within Centrelink from the way in which a social worker engages and supports a young person applying for Youth Allowance, to influencing governments to implement more active approaches to prevent homelessness. It all matters; it can all make a difference.

References

Allan, J. 2009, 'Theorising new developments in critical social work practice' in J. Allan, L. Briskman & B. Pease (eds), *Critical Social Work: Theories and practices for a just world,* 2nd edn, St Leonards: Allen & Unwin, pp. 30–44

Briggs, L. 2007, 'Public Service secretaries and their independence from political influence: The view of the Public Service Commissioner', *Australian Journal of Public Administration*, vol. 66, no. 4, pp. 501–6

Carey, M. & Foster, M. 2011, 'Introducing deviant social work: Contextualising the limits of radical social work whilst understanding (fragmented) resistance within the social work labour process', *British Journal of Social Work*, vol. 41, pp. 576–93

Darcy, M., Gwyther, G., Perry, J., Wood, J. & Richardson, R. 2009, *Centrelink Placed Based Services Evaluation*, Sydney: University of Western Sydney

Department of Families, Housing, Community Services and Indigenous Affairs 2008, *The Road Home: A National Approach to Reducing Homelessness,* Canberra: Australian Government Publishing Service

Department of Human Services 2011, *Centrelink Annual Report, 2010–11,* Canberra: Australian Government Publishing Services

—— (Centrelink) 2014, *Social Work Services,* Canberra: Australian Government Publishing Service

DHS *see* Department of Human Services

Department of Prime Minister and Cabinet 2009, *A Stronger, Fairer Australia*, Canberra: Australian Government Publishing Service

Ellis, K., Davis, A. & Rummery, K. 1999, 'Needs assessment, street level bureaucracy and the new community care', *Social Policy and Administration*, vol. 33, no. 3, pp. 262–80

Evans, T. & Harris, J. 2004, 'Street-level bureaucracy, social work and the (exaggerated) death of discretion', *British Journal of Social Work*, vol. 34, pp. 871–95

Fook, J. 2012, *Social Work: A critical approach to practice*, London: Sage Publications

Hall, G., Boddy, J., Chenoweth, L. & Davie, K. 2012, 'Mutual benefits: Developing relational service approaches within Centrelink', *Australian Social Work*, vol. 65, no. 1, pp. 87–103

Hart, D. 2013, *Processes of Social Work Engagement with the Reforming State in Australia: The case of Centrelink*, PhD thesis, Sydney: University of Sydney

Healy, K. 2005, *Social Work Theories in Context: Creating frameworks for practice*, London: Sage Publications

Humphries, P. & Morgan, G. 2010, Centrelink Social Work Mental Health Survey, unpublished survey, Canberra: Department of Human Services (Centrelink)

Ife, J. 1997, *Rethinking Social Work: Towards critical practice*, Melbourne: Longman

Jones, C. 2001, 'Voices from the front line: State social workers and New Labour', *British Journal of Social Work*, vol. 31, pp. 547–62

Lipsky, M. 1980, *Street-level Bureaucracy: The dilemmas of individuals in public service,* New York: Russell Sage Foundation

McDonald, C. & Chenoweth, L. 2009, '(Re)shaping social work: An Australian case study', *British Journal of Social Work*, vol. 39, pp. 144–60

McDonald, C. & Marston, G. 2006, 'Room to move? Professional discretion at the frontline of welfare-to-work', *Australian Journal of Social Issues*, vol. 41, pp. 171–82

Mestan, K. 2014, 'Paternalism in Australian welfare policy', *Australian Journal of Social Issues,* vol. 49, no. 1, pp. 3–22

PM&C *see* Department of Prime Minister & Cabinet

Turbett, C. 2014, *Doing Radical Social Work*, Houndmills: Palgrave Macmillan

Vinson, T. 2007, *Dropping off the Edge: The distribution of disadvantage in Australia*, Melbourne and Canberra: Jesuit Social Services/Catholic Social Services

White, V. 2009, 'Quiet challenges? Professional practice in modernised social work' in J. Harris & V. White (eds), *Modernising Social Work,* Policy Press, Bristol, pp. 129–144

11

Building relationships and effecting change: critical social work practice in prison settings

Sophie Goldingay

Introduction

Social work has a stated concern 'to alleviate social suffering and improve the quality of people's lives' (van Heugten 2001: 14). It was my first choice of profession as it aligns with my belief in the innate worth of every human being. I have spent much time observing how oppressive power relations caused by differences in race, sexuality, gender and class diminish choices, create suffering and generally impair the quality of life for those who are on the receiving end of social work practice. When I trained to be a social worker in the mid-1990s, I learnt a number of theories, which I hoped would serve me well in the world of practice to enact these quality-of-life goals. Over time, I realised that the theories, devised in contexts other than those I was working in, did not take into account the complexity, contradictions and 'messiness' of frontline social work. I was not aware of post-structural theory or critical post-structural theory while I was involved in practice in the prison setting so this chapter is written in hindsight.

Some of the strategies which proved successful in shifting oppressive power relations and improving the quality of life for prisoners and their families could be theorised as being consistent with a critical post-structural approach (Fook 2012) due to a focus on changing oppressive dominant discourses, working to moving beyond polarised identity positionings (for example, compliant/manipulative) and creating possibilities for new identities for prisoners, custodial staff and me. In this chapter I integrate theory and practice in such a way that it may be helpful to others who are interested in working in this or a similar field. It discusses a recurring practice scenario that I encountered while I worked as a prison social worker/social work team leader for the six years leading up to 2003. While the scenario is drawn from real life, some aspects of it have been combined or removed to ensure it is not possible to identify any prisoner or staff member.

Critical social work in criminal justice settings: what really happens

Principles that are common to critical social work include a 'commitment to social justice and equality . . . to working alongside oppressed and marginalised populations . . . [and] an orientation towards emancipatory personal and social change' (Allan 2009, pp. 40–1). Extensive research has demonstrated that the majority of women prisoners are from disadvantaged backgrounds (Carlen & Worral 2004; Chesney-Lind & Pasko 2004; Gaarder & Belknap 2004). Further, researchers have identified a high prevalence of mental health problems, self-harm, trauma and substance abuse among women prisoners (Morash, Bynum & Koons 1998). It has been cited that 81 per cent of women prisoners have been victim to physical or sexual abuse or both at some point in their lifetime (Ambrose, Simkins & Levic as cited in Chesney-Lind & Irwin 2008: 168). Clearly, this is a particularly marginalised population.

Nevertheless, goals of social justice and equality become more complex in an institution that is already set up to deliver its unique form of 'justice' to a population that is seen as inferior, bad and unworthy by the very nature of their status as prisoner. For example, prisoners are constructed by many people in society as 'oppressors'; they have created victims as a result of their criminal activity, whether it is against a person or property. I do not agree with this construction due to structural disadvantages experienced by women who are identified as criminals. Tax payers expect a number of outcomes from the delivery of public penal services, including that the person will be punished (retributive function) and that the imprisonment will be so unpleasant that the person avoids future offending (deterrent function). With these functions of prisons being made clear by government policy and the media, a social worker may wonder where they might fit in with the purposes of day-to-day prison life. This was certainly my experience, particularly in the early months of my employment there.

There is another, less populist, goal of imprisonment, which is rehabilitation. This has the potential to align more with the goal of social work improving people's quality of life and alleviating suffering, than the other two goals of retribution and deterrance. While rehabilitation is not the answer to the problem of crime because offending is generally caused by structural disadvantages that impact on a person's life choices (not a fault in prisoner psychology), rehabilition was a discourse that staff and management within the institution understood. A key to a postmodern critical approach to social work is working within dominant discourses to transform and create new ones, which may shift oppressive power relations (Fook 2012). For the remainder of this chapter I describe how I worked to transform the oppressive power relations through a process of analysing those power relations and questioning 'taken-for-granted and dominant assumptions and beliefs' (Allan 2009: 41) while working within the dominant discourse of rehabilitation within the prison setting.

In order to do work to change oppressive power dynamics, I had to learn to analyse how power was operating at any given moment. Theorising how power is operating is central when considering how life is experienced by both prisoners and staff who are working in the prison setting, where 'prison is the only place where power is exercised in its naked state, in its most excessive form, and where it is justified as a moral force' (Foucault 1979: 210). While the exercise of oppressive power is sanctioned by government, power operates in multiple and complex ways, and is influenced by prevailing ways of constructing events and practices through language. It is used within the media, within staff members and prisoners' families and friends, in management meetings and in everyday conversations in the lunch-room, the corridor and the prison control room.

Allan (2009) gives an account of one of the key tensions in how to address inequitable power relations in critical social work. She notes that while both modernist and postmodern social work are influenced by a concern for the impact of social structures on people's life opportunities and experiences, critical postmodern social work allows for consideration of how power relations are played out both at micro and macro levels, not just at the government level (Allan 2009).

Post-structuralism is related to postmodernism (Fook 2012) and is an approach, which explores the role of language in social life and its influence on power relations, truth claims, and identity (Burr 2003; Fook 2012). Critical post-structuralists adopt a stance that seeks to foreground the perspectives of those who are marginalised, with the view of alleviating oppressive power relations, which cause suffering and impair quality of life (Fook 2012).

My practice experience in mental health and criminal-justice social work settings means I can recognise the existence of multiple, context-dependent truths about the cause of (and hence multiple and context-dependent ways of addressing) oppressive social dynamics and power relations. Examples of this will be explained in more depth in the vignettes. In brief, however, this means that each setting will have its own unique power relations. This will be due to the unique combination of person-alities, authority lines, context-related problems to solve and dominant ways of constructing identities and events through language in that setting. In being open to multiple and context-dependent causes, one then becomes open to multiple and creative solutions which would not otherwise be considered. This possibility is one full of promise, especially in an institutional setting, despite the fact that such solu-tions are likely to take a lot of time, effort and careful planning.

While I was not aware of critical post-structural thinking during my time at the prison, I was acutely aware that those who had power in the institution were able to define what discourse or version of events and identities was 'true'. As demon-strated in the vignettes below, there were some established ways of talking about prisoners, drug addiction, prisoners as mothers and the institution's role, and this way of talking was oppressive to prisoners and limiting for staff, and the overall culture and function of the institution.

To analyse what was happening, I draw on an adapted version of Fook's (2012) critically deconstructive process, whereby I name the discourses operating, how my beliefs fit with these discourses, what perspectives were missing and devalued, and how these discourses and related practices reinforced power relations, thus constructed the various actors in the vignette. I will problematise assumptions that were embedded in my initial account of what happened, explore where these assumptions may have originated, and discuss how I developed alternative ways of constructing my own role and that of others through exercising power via discursive practices. I do this by presenting a vignette in two parts, with analysis and discussion in-between.

Vignette: part 1

I would like to introduce you to a typical Monday morning working as a social worker for the women's division of the public prison service. Imagine it is 9 a.m. and you drive through the gates, past the razor wire, and through the time-locked electronic doors with paint peeling off them. You go into the control room (like a nursing station for officers and set up in a panopticon style) where you issue yourself your key set and chat to the female officer who is stationed in the control room. Another female officer arrives and they bemoan the latest exploit by a prisoner whom they label 'manipulative' due to her attempts to request visits with her children through various officers. They outline their perceptions of the prisoner's moral failings, the number of times she has received a prison sentence, her entrenched drug use, her 'obvious' lack of real care for her children. They snigger about how the current caregiver of the children is likely to try to smuggle drugs into the prison via the children's nappies while they are wearing them. They shrug their shoulders and declare their prediction that these children are already lined up to be the next generation of prisoners.

Your heart sinks as you realise you will have to think carefully about how (or if) you will advocate for this prisoner when you receive the inevitable request for help from her. Her request 'chit' is probably waiting for you in your pigeonhole. You walk down the corridor to your office and hear the rattle of keys, the echo of metal doors slamming, the buzz of the radio intercoms, and the voices of prisoners and staff. The corridor is bleak and as you enter your office you are reminded that there is an element of neglect or lack of value in your role since you are greeted with dated, tatty carpet and a rather damp odour. You see the large pile of prisoners' requests to see you in your pigeonhole. Mondays are always busy following what is the usual chaotic weekend for the prisoners. A partner has taken up with another woman, housing has been lost, pets have been abandoned, children have got into trouble, become ill or had an accident, phone calls have reawakened intense grief or family conflict, or a family member has been victimised or died. You feel the burden of being the only social worker for a group of over 100 highly vulnerable, traumatised and marginalised women based in an institution that is set up to contain and punish them.

In the first of my five years working as a prison social worker I wondered how long I could last. I certainly could not imagine I would be there for over five years. I was acutely aware that, at best, in those early months, I was positioned as 'naive' if I spoke out directly in conversation with officers about my views about the well-being and quality of life of prisoners and their children. When I tried to advocate for prisoners to management I was constructed as not only being irrelevant to the core business of the institution, but as undermining its purpose as well.

The custodial staff were positioned as 'judge, jury and executioner' every day. There was an expectation that they enlist punitive discursive practices and use these to justify a restrictive, limiting and punishing regime. I identified the discourses as 'women prisoners as sneaky, manipulative and dishonest', and 'women who are addicted to drugs are thoughtless, selfish and irresponsible'. From these discourses came others which include that 'women prisoners are dangerous or damaging to their children', that 'these mothers do not care about their children and only want to see them to get drugs', that 'their children would be better off without them', and even that 'their children already possessed a degree of criminality that is inevitable due to the actions of their mothers'. From this, the implication is that there is no point in striving to help them as they are already on an unstoppable path to criminality and hence worthlessness.

I did not agree with these constructions of the value of relationships between prisoner mothers and their children because several things are missing from these accounts. For example, the perspectives of the prisoners and children in relation to the impact of the prison sentence on them are not included. Nor is the value of ongoing contact and regular visits, or the positive benefits to prison staff in relation to prisoner behaviour should regular visits be facilitated.

Those custodial officers who did not join in with these discourses tended to be marginalised in the workplace, and they were discussed in disparaging terms as being a 'softie' or 'naive'. The discourse of prisoners being victim to oppressive life circumstances was never used, nor was the rehabilitative function of the prison service considered in discourse at this point. Thus, there was a dichotomy of 'soft' versus 'effective' approaches where effective was defined as restricting and punishing prisoners and 'soft' was defined as undermining the goals of the institution and possibly putting its role at risk.

Vignette: part 2

I would like to invite you back into the prison now, where you have looked through your large pile of chits and seen the request from the prisoner who was discussed by the custodial staff in the control room earlier. You know this prisoner as she has been inside before. You double-check the client card that you have made for her when you saw her last, which details hers and her children's personal situation. She has three children between the ages of three and twelve, and battled a drug addiction since she was a teenager. She has a history of being physically and sexually abused as a child and an adult. You recall the prisoner's expression of grief from being separated from her children during her last sentence and her remorse about how her drug addiction significantly interfered with her ability to parent them. The children have all had behavioural problems and issues at school, and the child protection services have been involved a number of times. You visualise the grief and disruption the children will be experiencing with the loss of their main caregiver yet again, moving house, being separated from each other, either living in foster care, or with extended family members who are barely managing themselves.

You have a gut feeling that even though this family has multiple and complex problems, supporting the ongoing relationship between the mother and her children is important for the wellbeing of all of them both now and in the future. Armed with this view, and seeing that the initial request for a visit has been denied, you make an appointment to talk to the unit manager to advocate for the prisoner, and you feel confident, anticipating a positive outcome. You are therefore unprepared for the response, which is: 'Well, she should have thought about that before she came here! No I will not approve her visits. Last time we did that, her family tried to bring drugs in the kid's nappies!! No! It would be a security risk.'

You leave the manager's office crestfallen and wonder what move you can make next. You also mull over the fact that alleviating suffering and promoting wellbeing for the prisoner and her children are not the highest priority for this senior officer and others like her. They are charged with the role of upholding the security of the institution, and promoting the retribution and deterrence function of the prison. Should they be seen to step outside this, they risk undermining their own credibility within the institution.

One of the assumptions that is embedded in my account above is that social workers are the only group who are concerned about improving the culture of the prison and the situation for these women; setting up a 'me against the institution' mindset, which was unlikely to be helpful. This assumption comes partly from the way I interpreted people's talk as a reflection of their set views and unable to be changed, as opposed to the way they had learnt to talk in order to have a place among their colleagues. It took me some time to move beyond this. In the next section of this chapter, I will discuss some of the practices that I began to trial in my struggle to improve the quality of prisoner's lives within the prison.

I would like to note that while the following practices may have had some influence in this particular setting at this time with these particular people, it is not the only way to practice critical post-structural social work. In fact, Fook (2012) emphasises that it is important to be flexible enough to adjust one's practice to the setting and not try to impose knowledge from outside. She draws attention to the inductive process needed to practice critical social work, which needs to be suitable for the specific context. This process requires a social worker to watch and gather empirical evidence of the dynamics of the context and their impact on those people involved. From this, contexts can be analysed through a process of deconstruction; that is, resisting discourses that cause oppressive power dynamics through naming them, challenging them by considering alternative or missing perspectives, and then constructing alternative discourses that enable the situation to be seen and acted on in new and non-oppositional ways (Fook 2012).

As mentioned earlier, I entered the social work profession with core values of the intrinsic worth of all people, irrespective of their circumstances, history, or social location. Alongside these values, and through personal experience, I have adopted the habit of striving to see issues, events and practices from numerous perspectives. My belief in the intrinsic worth of all people extends to my attitudes towards my colleagues as well as those I am employed to 'help'. While I did not agree with many views held by my colleagues in the prison service, I was committed to working as a team and acknowledging their experience as custodial staff.

One of the first tasks I prioritised was to understand the dynamics of a prison and how it was experienced by those involved, since I saw myself as a 'context' worker rather than one who was only there to work directly with prisoners. I read work such as Goffman's (1961) *Asylums* and Zimbardo, Maslach and Haney's (1999) Stanford Prison Experiment. Such reading led me to conclude that the way prisoners *and* staff may talk and act in prison settings has little to do with any in-built personality or personal deficiency. Rather, I theorised at the time that it is the power relations created by the authoritarian structure of the prison and its perceived purpose, which may encourage staff to talk and behave in ways that dehumanise, demean and denigrate prisoners in their care. I acknowledge, however, that while staff may have been co-opted by the oppressive environment and its discourse, staff still have some degree of agency or choice in their beliefs and actions.

This knowledge enabled me to move beyond polarising constructions of officers (for example, at times custodial staff were constructed as callous or lazy) which I had overheard others in my field use, which served to alienate allied health and welfare staff and custodial staff from each other. I stopped blaming the custodial prison staff for their apparent callous and punitive practices and I focused on building positive relationships with them. I volunteered for the dragon-boat racing team and ensured I always came to practice and competed at events. I joined them for Friday night drinks. I began to really value their professionalism and commitment to their role as custodial officers even though I did not necessarily agree with how it was carried out or the premises that it was based on. While the oppressive dimension of prisons needs to be acknowledged, through many informal conversations it occurred to me that we did actually have a shared goal, and that was the organisation's goal to 'reduce reoffending'. The differences between custodial staff and myself lay in regimes of truth or interpretations about how this could or should be achieved and why. While I was concerned for the wider forces in society that defined these women as criminals, other prison staff were focused on the psychological factors that led women to offend.

At the same time this was happening, I was fortunate to be in a senior social work role and was invited to attend ongoing meetings with a senior manager who was involved in developing policy. I do think that he was open to taking my views seriously because I had established a positive reputation as one who worked closely with custodial staff, respected them in their role and therefore was respected in my role. I had also kept abreast of some global advances in ways of conceptualising the reduction in reoffending, which at this time was the Risk Needs Responsivity framework (Andrews & Bonta 1998). This framework conceptualises the causes of criminal behaviour in terms of 'criminogenic needs' and these include poor family relationships, unstable housing, and lack of employment, among other more psychological issues such as poor impulse control and substance addiction.

While there have since been important critiques of this model (for example, Ward & Stewart 2003; Hannah-Moffat 2005), at the time the framework offered some promise to transform the regime of everyday life within the prison walls into one where prisoners and staff could adopt less restricted and more empowered identities. At the time it seemed that working to transform the discourse from within might offer some opportunities to move towards more emancipatory possibilities at the micro level.

I began to speak with this senior manager about how all staff shared the goals of reducing reoffending and how each of the professional groups contributed to this outcome. While custodial staff controlled prisoners' behaviour and prevented crime from occurring by their efforts to contain prisoners, professions like social work reduced reoffending by supporting positive relationships between prisoners and their children/families and attending to reintegrative needs to help them fit back into society. These reintegrative needs included advocacy and community development, which addressed the impact of the more structural causes of crime such as income inequality and its associated issues. We discussed the potential for all the staff's involvement in supporting prisoners to address their 'criminogenic' needs, not just social work and psychology. I shared with him some research I had located from overseas about the positive correspondence between maintaining mother–child relationships and female prisoner motivation for rehabilitation (for example, Clarke 1995), and how this may reduce prison misconduct and the incidence of mental health problems.

A development occurred when the manager agreed for me to present this information to a unit management meeting. How was I to respond to this invitation from a critical social work approach? One possibility was to refuse to participate on the basis that the criminogenic model has its potential, through its location of deviance in the individual woman, to further oppress. On the other hand, I was being given the opportunity to reframe (even to a minor extent) elements of the model that might result in greater freedom and support for the women in prison. As I was witness to the daily pain and suffering experienced by both women and children as a result of the punitive and restrictive environment, I chose the latter option.

As a result of discussions at the management level, where the prison leadership was endorsing this new way of conceptualising what we all as a team were working towards, I noticed positive changes in the responses to prisoner requests for visits with family. I received fewer request chits for help from prisoners for social work advocacy, as prison management were now more likely to approve requests straight-away. There were fewer discussions by custodial staff about requests being a threat to security.

While there were times when the previous discourse of prisoners not 'deserving' visits were used, these were replaced by the less oppressive discourse that family visits were a part of their rehabilitative plan and as such matched the goals of the institution to reduce reoffending. I was delighted when I was no longer the only one drawing on this discourse. My role was to continue to support this way of thinking and talking about family visits through relevant discussions in a respectful way with custodial staff and our focus on shared goals as a team.

In reflecting on these events, I can see that the team of various staff roles were able to move beyond the dichotomies that kept the old punitive discourses alive. This had occurred through creating a new discourse, which included attending to prisoners' wellbeing and their connectedness with family as one pathway to reha-bilitation. For example, prior to my presentation at the management meeting and the shift in practices that followed, there was a binary between custodial and welfare staff which kept us polarised in our roles, one to control and punish (custodial) and one to protect, care and support (social work and other allied health professions). By aligning all staff to a clear aim of reducing reoffending, we were able to focus on what united us, not what set us apart from each other.

While some may note that this process replaced one form of disciplinary prac-tice with another, it is important to remember that we are all disciplined in every field but the impact is felt in how this plays out on a day-to-day basis. Foucault (1984: 343) said that 'my point is not that everything is bad, but that everything is dangerous'. My interpretation of this is similar to that of Fook (2002: 16), in that ideas are not good or bad in themselves; it depends on how they are enacted. In the case of the prison, the enactment of rehabilitation as a disciplinary practice was less oppressive for both prisoners and workers than the enactment of retribution and deterrence as disciplinary practices.

I observed prevailing discourses moved away from discourses of blame and as a result I noticed fewer oppressive interactions between prisoners and custodial staff. Not all the custodial staff agreed with this new way of thinking and talking about their role in relation to prisoners but over time, more staff did see it that way. From a critical post-structural perspective, custodial staff were able to legitimately adopt an expanded and more flexible identity, so that their roles were less oppressive for both them and for those they were charged to contain. Prisoner perspectives and experiences were now also taken into account in decisions that affected them, which constituted a small step towards emancipatory social change, while acknowledging that as long as the model remains the dominant discourse, women will continue to be oppressed. However, I had been able to carve out an effective and valued social work role, thereby expanding the possibilities for my own and my social work colleague's identity in the prison setting as well.

Conclusion

This chapter conveys my own experience as a social worker in a prison setting while I struggled to find a meaningful and relevant role as a critical social worker. Prison is an institution that is already established to inflict pain and take power away from its inmates, so the traditional critical social work goals of social justice, equality and emancipation may struggle for relevance. Social workers may at times feel frustrated and even despair if they are expecting that direct advocacy with managers at the unit level will achieve social work's goals of alleviating suffering and improving the quality of life for prisoners and their families. This can be especially so if workers do not work closely with custodial staff in a respectful way or if social workers adopt adversarial ways that pit them against management or the institution's goals.

Nevertheless, the goals of social work practice to reduce suffering and improve quality of life through emancipatory social change can be achieved in an institutional setting through analysing power relations and questioning dominant assumptions, especially our own assumptions as workers. In particular, carefully observing the localised practices of power, including discursive practices, enables social workers to develop a plan that can improve the overall culture of an institution over time. Such a plan may involve identifying where staff are polarised, what discourses are leading to oppressive uses of power, and where marginalised or silenced discourses may have the potential for being foregrounded in new ways.

A key learning from these vignettes is that power can be exercised in creative ways by taking control of what discourse is dominant; or in other words, what version of events, accounts, or causes of problems (and hence the solutions) are seen as 'true'. There are multiple ways of doing this. I chose to do it in this prison setting through building respectful relationships with staff at all levels and different disciplines, working hard to acknowledge and respect perspectives that were different to my own. I used the language of alliance to develop shared goals among the team of various staff including myself, as opposed to being adversarial. This was particularly the case when advocating on behalf of prisoners to management. Importantly, I created opportunities to build shared understandings with management, and together we created a new vocabulary and way of talking about prisoners and their family visits which did not polarise staff or blame prisoners. This was just one small achievement in an ongoing struggle for emancipatory social change for those who have been convicted of crime.

References

Allan, J. 2009, 'Theorising new developments in critical social work' in J. Allan, L. Briskman & B. Pease (eds), *Critical Social Work: Theories and practices for a socially just world*, 2nd edn, St Leonards: Allen & Unwin, pp. 30–44

Andrews, D. & Bonta, J. 1998, *The Psychology of Criminal Conduct,* 2nd edn, Cincinnati: Anderson Publishing Co.

Burr, V. 2003, *Social Constructionism,* 2nd edn, London: Routledge

Carlen, P. & Worral, A. 2004, *Analysing Women's Imprisonment*, Devon: Willan

Chesney-Lind, M. & Irwin, K. 2008, *Beyond Bad Girls: Gender, violence and hype*, New York: Routledge

—— & Morash, M. 2013, 'Transformative feminist criminology: A critical re-thinking of a discipline', *Critical Criminology*, vol. 21, no. 3, pp. 287–330

—— & Pasko, L. 2004, *The Female Offender: Girls, women and crime,* 2nd edn, Thousand Oaks: Sage

Clarke, J. 1995, 'The impact of the prison environment on mothers', *The Prison Journal*, vol. 75, no. 3, pp. 306–29

Fook, J. 2002, *Social Work: Critical theory and practice,* London: Sage

—— 2012, *Social Work: A critical approach to practice*, London: Sage

Foucault, M. 1979, *Discipline and Punish: The birth of the prison,* New York: Vintage Books

—— 1984 'In the interview with Paul Rainbow and Hubert Dreyfus' in P. Rabinow (ed.), *The Foucault Reader*, Harmondsworth: Penguin

Gaarder, E. & Belknap, J. 2004, 'Little women: Girls in adult prison', *Women and Criminal Justice*, vol. 15, no. 2, pp. 51–80

Goffman, E. 1961, *'Asylums': Essays on the social situation of mental patients and other inmates*, London: Penguin

Hannah-Moffat, K. 2005, 'Criminogenic needs and the transformative risk subject: Hybridizations of risk/need in penalty', *Punishment & Society*, vol. 7, no. 1, pp. 29–51

Morash, M., Bynum, T. & Koons, B. 1998, *Women Offenders: Programming needs and promising approaches*, National Institute of Justice Research in Brief, Washington DC: National Institute of Justice,

van Heugten, K. 2001, 'Social work: its role and task' in M. Connolly (ed.), *New Zealand Social Work: Contexts and practice*, Oxford University Press, Melbourne, pp. 3–17

Ward, T. & Stewart, C. 2003, 'Criminogenic needs and human needs: A theoretical model', *Psychology,*

Crime & Law, vol. 9, no. 2, pp. 125–43

Zimbardo, P., Maslach, C. & Haney, C. 1999, 'Reflections on the Stanford prison experiment: Genesis, transformations, consequences' in T. Blast (ed.), *Obedience to Authority: Current perspectives on the Milgram paradigm*, Mahwah: Lawrence Erlbaum

12

Professional practice standards and critical practices: addressing the tensions in social work field education settings

Norah Hosken, Lesley Ervin and Jody Laughton

Introduction

This chapter considers the constraints and possibilities for university staff and agency-based field educators to enable social work students to practise critical social work while on placement. While recognising the differences in power, students are placed in a unique position to respectfully introduce and model critical social work views and practices to their placement field educators and teams. We authors are members of a university social-work field education team (the team) who draw on our collective experience to write this chapter. This experience includes teaching of field education units and placement integration seminars, organising social work placements and providing liaison visits to students and their field educators during placements. The examination of constraints and possibilities for critical social work practice occurs in an Australian context. We hope that readers from other locations may find the discussions and suggested critical responses relevant when these concern the normalisations of the ideas and practices of neoliberalism as they relate to social work field education.

The team identify a major constraint on critical social work practice as the influence of neoliberal values and associated implementations that affect funding, accreditation, management, policies and service provision of universities and human service organisations. We explore the possibilities for creating environments that foster greater opportunity for students to practise and model critical social work with a focus on working in solidarity and using suggested critical social principles and process orientations within locally developed frameworks for change. It is suggested that 'listening ethically' (see Chapter 4) informs people's capacity to think and see critically to reveal the policies, or their components, that constrain the practice of critical social work for social justice. Policies are contained in a variety of texts that organise much of the work and behaviours of social work academics, field educators and students in education and human service organisations.

A case study frames the chapter, describing the efforts we have made to enact critical social work practice. The case study introduces and illustrates suggested critical social work practice principles, drawing on many critical social work process orientations (see Chapter 4), and located within the Framework for Critical Social Work Action (FCSWA) that we have developed. The principles and framework could be nuanced for different situations, including students' practice of critical social work on placement. Central to FCSWA is the experience of the authors that the value of the day-to-day use of critical social work is increased when listening ethically to those who are most affected by policies and practices, and when forming part of collective efforts. This collectivity involves working in solidarity and purpose with others, towards the longer-term goals of transforming practice, organisations and societies towards social justice.

Practice principle: draw on experience and critical theories for one's own work and working with others

In early 2014, when we as an author team planned the content for this chapter, we as the *team*, were concerned at the lack of opportunities for social work students to practise critical social work on placements. Over the following twenty months, using a process inspired by feminist participatory action research, we endeavoured to improve our own understanding and enactment of critical social work within our educational setting as a form of praxis aimed at social change. This was a parallel process that would guide our efforts for improved structure and support for social work students' opportunities to be prepared for, learn and do critical social work on placements. The dual process of using the writing of the chapter to inform the way we align the ideas, texts, teaching and practices of social work field education more strongly to critical social work are referred to as the *'project'*. Students and practitioners may find similar ways to use this parallel project process within teams and organisations to increase motivation, resources and collaborative critical reflectivity towards social-justice-oriented change.

Practice principle: develop shared understandings of theory to increase practice

The opportunity to discuss and develop shared understanding of the theoretical base of critical social work directly influenced the *team's* practice of critical social work during the *project,* an outline of which follows. The team arrived at a shared understanding of critical social work to include a range of social work practice approaches that were primarily informed by critical theories as supplemented by postmodern insights (Allan et al. 2009; Pease 2013). A theory is critical 'to the extent that it seeks social transformation as forms of justice and emancipation' (Gray & Webb 2013: 77). A major impetus for the development of critical social work was professional's dissatisfaction with perceived limitations of the dominance of traditional social work that involved 'taken-for-granted professional assumptions of the time, which gave prominence to individualist explanations of social problems' (Healy 1993: 4). These individualist explanations primarily focused on the individual in a casework model, which were often underpinned by psychological theories that recognised the causes of clients' problems as mainly located within them, and the aim was to promote the clients' adjustment. The *team* had observed many instances of our own policy-shaped practice in the university setting, and of social work in placement agencies, that aligned with this individualistic model of understanding and responding to the problems of those using services. In contrast, while critical social work comprises different approaches, there is a common view of the problems that social workers and service users experience being primarily caused by hardships entrenched in economic, social, political and cultural stratifications (Weiss-Gal et al. 2014), and the goal is to support service users while working individually, and with others, to change these inequalities. This understanding of critical social work acknowledges the inter-relationships between interpersonal, institutional and macro or structural levels of critical practice. Explanation of the *team's* use and localisation of these core principles of critical social work to the *project* follow.

Practice principle: listen ethically and learn from the location and views of those who are most affected

We adopted the feminist perspective embedded in Dorothy Smith's (2005) institutional ethnography as has been applied in social work contexts (for example, de Montigny 1995; Brown 2006; Hosken 2013). Using this method, inquiries into how organisations and practices are structured to create their outcomes commence from the partial views from the locations and experiences of those most affected, often the least powerful and least privileged, in particular situations (Smith 2005). In terms of positioning, inquiries into how social justice and critical social-work practices are constructed or are absent from these views aims to 'create the vision, and ability, to challenge [unjust and] discriminatory policies and practices as they are normalised and inflect at individual, supervisory, organisational and societal levels' (Hosken 2013: 91). Social work students on placement have discussed, expressed numerous concerns and posed many questions to us; some of these points are referred to in this chapter, and served to orient the *project*.

Practice principle: examine the regulatory texts for how they organise normality

Texts can standardise and exert control

The examination of the texts regulating placements commenced from the views and experiences of those most affected, field education staff and the many students who expressed concern and stress while navigating their roles in their unpaid placements. In particular, we were interested in how the regulatory documents governing field placements might support, or inhibit, the ability of field education staff, and placement students, to do critical social work. Smith's concept of the 'text-reader conversation' (Smith 2005: 105) alerted us to how texts that regulated student placements may 'exert significant control' (2005: 108) in activating certain actions in the daily work of educators, practitioners and students. One key purpose of a regulatory text, such as a code of ethics, is to standardise and control how people reading the text then act. Regulatory texts often embed dominant discourses and majority culture expectations as norms (Hosken 2013). The term, discourse, as used here, refers to a: 'systematic way of knowing something that is grounded in expert knowledge and that circulates widely in society through language, including most importantly language vested in texts . . . [and] appears almost as common sense' (Mykhalovskiy 2002: 39).

Identifying the regulatory texts

The day-to-day work of the field education team included developing the curriculum and teaching of academic units that related to field placement; editing the field placement manual and associated documents; telephone, video-conferencing, email and face-to-face conversations with students and staff to organise and manage field placements; and providing liaison visits for first- and final-year social work students on placement.

We observed and identified the key documents that organised our own work in these areas, finding: university staff members' position descriptions, workload agreements, complaints procedures, assessment policies, audit regimes, performance appraisals and the field education budget; the *Australian Social Work Education and Accreditation Standards* (AASW 2012c) [the *ASWEAS*] that set out required principles, standards, graduate attributes and core content for accredited social work courses in Australia; ASWEAS *Guideline 1.5: Guidance on reaccreditation reviews* (AASW 2012a); ASWEAS *Guideline 1.2: Guidance on field education programs* (AASW 2012b); the *Practice Standards* (AASW 2013b) [the *Standards*]; the *Code of Ethics* (AASW 2010), [the *Code*] and *Ethics and Practice Guideline—Ethics and Field Education* (AASW 2013a). Even when the subject of debates and tensions regarding value of their content the authors noted that these AASW documents remained instrumental in organising the work of social work staff in the field education team and the agencies that provide placements, and the students who were undertaking placements.

Dominant discourses that organise normality

The *team* identified how government-led, neoliberal-informed values and business management practices were a major influence that shaped our work. Examples of neoliberal values infiltrating the thinking and behaviours of *team* members included:

- *team* discussions during the *project* meetings of our own experiences and feelings of individualised inadequacy, accountability and responsibility, for our performances in demonstrating compliance with university and professional body regulations governing placements;
- how the construction of students and services users as purchasers of a product or service invoked risk management, rather than holistic, responses to issues;
- the *team's* exposure to regular emails from management that promoted competitive funding and staffing processes and 'successful' individual staff who self-managed within expected behaviours and ideals as contained within strategic plans, accreditation processes and corporate brands.

The *team's* experience appeared consistent with others in the way that staff organisation of student placements takes place in Australian universities have been subject to government-led corporatisation, 'transformed into a business by mobilising processes, discourses, and practices of marketisation, managerialism and privatisation' (Blackmore 2014: 285). The authors observed first-hand that students undertake placements in the human services sector which has been the 'proving ground for NPM [New Public Management]-inspired market-focused service provision' (Butcher & Dalton 2014: 142). The *team* talked with workers in organisations that had traditionally taken students on placement who were not able to do so due to staff retrenchments and funding instability.

Regulation of mythical norms

The requirement that universities delivering professional social work programs must meet accreditation, and re-accreditation, standards as set by the Australian Association of Social Workers (AASW) was a major influence on how the *team* understood and organised our work. One example of the significant disciplinary control of the AASW regulatory texts was the additional work activated from field education staff, and students, as they aimed to comply with the ASWEAS Guideline 1.2.3 that placement students can have no leave of any kind included in their completion of a minimum of 1000 hours in at least two field education subjects (AASW 2012b: 3).

We found that the ASWEAS Guidance on field education programs (Guideline 1.2.3) produced disproportionate negative impacts on those students who were furthest from the 'mythical norm' of the social work student (Hosken 2013: 96) on placement being 'young, Anglo, unencumbered, and financially supported by parents'. A mythical norm is a socially constructed 'stereotype . . . perpetuated by society, against which everyone else is measured' (Lorde 199: 362), forming a hierarchy under which others fall. For example, we found that students from a range of non-Anglo-Celtic cultural backgrounds experienced greater disadvantage under the 'no leave of any kind' rule than students closest to the mythical norm placement student. Those students from a minority-culture background explained to the authors that absences from placement were needed due to cultural requirements associated with birth, bereavement or mourning, or participation in decision-making forums within interdependant family and community structures. Some of these students talked about the additional burdens on students from minority-culture backgrounds that arise when Anglo-Celtic cultural norms (reflected in regulations) conflicted with their own cultural requirements. In other situations, experiences of racial micro-aggressions and racism (Szoke 2012) combined with poverty (Brough et al. 2015) to create extra physical, emotional and financial work, and stress, when undertaking placement. A number of these students expressed emotional distress to us where feelings of personal and cultural inadequacy were invoked by having to request permission for absences from their placements and then request to extend placements to cover those absences. In conversations with these students, some authors actively drew on their under-standing of critical social work developed in the *project* to define problems in ideologies, policy and practices first, rather than in individuals. Some of the critical social-work process orientations (see Chapter 4) were used by authors including witnessing, ethical listening, mutual consciousness-raising, acknowl-edging, validating, resisting, universalising, individualising, and critical reframing of experiences. A number of students reported to the authors that their feelings of inadequacy lessened after these discussions, particularly in relation to exploring possible deficiencies in policies that were not culturally inclusive. These and other conversations with students about the adverse impacts on them of policy and regulations were a major impetus in our developing a localised FCSWA to critique and challenge aspects of university, and AASW policy and practice.

Neoliberal enforcement of individualism

The impacts of the ASWEAS Guideline 1.2.3, as discussed above, appears to both contradict and invite action regarding the AASW's own requirement to eliminate violations of human rights, to 'challenge, and/or report … policies, procedures, practices and service provisions which: are not in the best interests of clients … are in any way oppressive, disempowering or culturally inappropriate …' (AASW 2010: 32). Enforcing individualism and eroding capacities for collectivism, which appears to be one of this guideline's unintended outcomes, is one way that the *ASWEAS* could be said to promote neoliberalism and constrain the potential for critical social work. Similarly, efforts by the AASW to concentrate on the 'professional project' (Olsen 2007) that seeks to elevate the standing of the profession, while understandable on some levels, also dovetail with neoliberal concerns that prioritise self-interest. Not just 'one discourse among many', neoliberalism is identified as a 'strong discourse' that has the goal of individualism through eradication of collectivism at its core (Bourdieu 1998).

Texts that activate discriminatory effects

We discussed how our shared understanding of students as being diverse and often subject to 'poverty as structural violence' (see Chapter 7), influenced our responses to the needs and concerns of placement students. One of these responses was to work in solidarity with a larger group to advocate that the AASW amend the

ASWEAS Guideline 1.2.3 as it appeared to produce unintended, discriminatory effects. The understanding of this guideline producing discriminatory effects is consistent with the Australian Human Rights Commission's view that policies and practices can be discriminatory with, or without, intent being present on behalf of those designing them to be so. The measure is if these practices have 'an unequal effect on the rights and freedoms of the individual or group involved' (HREOC 2000 in Hosken 2013: 95).

Practice principle: critically interrogate the ideologies, policies and practices of employing, funding and regulatory organisations

Our understanding of critical social work appeared, on one level, as compatible with the stated principles and key provisions in the *AASW Code of Ethics*. The AASW statement of the social work profession's responsibilities for social justice is the section of the *Code* most clearly aligned with a critical social work approach: promote justice and social fairness . . . ; advocate for change to social systems and structures that preserve inequalities and injustice; oppose and work to eliminate all violations of human rights . . . ; promote the protection of the natural environment . . . ; and promote community participation (AASW 2010: 13).

The AASW's statement that the social work profession has an 'equal commitment' to working across personal, cultural and political domains to 'support personal and social wellbeing' and to 'achieve human rights and social justice through . . . social and systemic change . . . ' (AASW 2010: 7, clause 1.2) is another example of a stated commitment that appears to balance working to support people with structural change towards creating a more equal society that is consistent with the vision of critical social work.

Dissonance is present, however, within and between, the *Code* and the *Standards*. The assertion that social work is, or should be, underpinned by social justice and human rights principles (AASW 2010: 7) and works to eliminate all violations of human rights can easily contrast with aspects of the *Code* that guide social workers in ethical practice and decision-making. For instance, where tension exists between 'observing the *Code* and complying with legal or organisation requirements' social workers are instructed by the *Code* to 'act in accordance with the law and with organisational directives' (AASW 2010: 14). This contradiction has been mentioned by field educators and students during liaison visits as excusing social workers from the requirement to work to eliminate violations of human rights, to 'challenge, and/or report . . . policies, procedures, practices and service provisions which: are not in the best interests of clients . . . are in any way oppressive, disempowering or cultur-ally inappropriate' (AASW 2010: 32). Moreover, of the eight *Standards*, only one appears to require that social workers, and students on placement, demonstrate that they not only understand, but 'practice', what is required in the standard.

More students means more risk and less placements

Now there are more enrolled students due to deregulation (Koshy 2014), it has intensi-fied existing social work placement shortages across much of Australia. The increased caution arising from government funding cuts across the human services sector alongside output-focused funding contracts have combined to embed management and audit regimes that invoke risk-averse work cultures (Keevers 2010) that are not easily amenable to supporting the learning needs of students. In this environment, human-service sector organisations increasingly seek compliant, 'job-ready' gradu-ates, 'high performing' and 'low-risk' placement students (Cleak & Smith 2012).

From the view of field education team members, it is clear that the organi-sation, progress and experience of student social-work placements in the human service sector are inevitably full of risks. Things can go awry in small and big ways as students navigate their lengthy field placements, which are frequently in organisa-tions experiencing turmoil, with service users subjected to harsher welfare regimes. This is amid the students' own life situations, often involving part-time paid work, financial and time-shortage stresses, and the pressures of caring responsibilities (Brough et al. 2015).

Current assessment of social work student placements

The *Standards* identify requirements and practice expectations for a qualified social worker and are also the basis for students to develop learning goals, and to evaluate students' performance on placements. The 23 specified practice standards are segmented into 8 components of practice and 102 detailed indicators to illustrate the requirements for meeting that standard (AASW 2013a).

The AASW require an assessment of whether students on placement have demonstrated an acceptable level of understanding and enacting of the standards, and that a range of learning activities and methods of assessment should be used to assess the student's level of achievement and whether they have met the perfor-mance outcomes specified (AASW 2012b). The *Standards*, indicators and *ASWEAS* Graduate Attributes use a competence-based approach of measuring a student's performance on placement. These centre on the descriptions of the standards and indicators.

The majority of Australian universities delivering social work programs have additional assessment requirements for placements involving student contributions to university-run integration seminars, portfolios and written reflections to demonstrate critical reflection and an ability to integrate theory and practice. Contributions to student teaching, assessment and passing or failing field placement units are shared between students, field educators and university staff. The responsibility for the final assessment, however, rests with the university.

Our experience indicates some support from workers and students in universities, and human-service sector organisations for the structuring, consistency, clarity and seeming transparency contained in specified standards and outcomes. However, there is also recognition of a philosophical divergence between the use of practice standards, measured by outcomes and competence, and of critically reflective practice that accepts complexity, uncertainty, ambiguity and humility.

Fragmentation and technicism

Social work courses at universities have to meet the requirements of the AASW to gain and maintain accreditation. The regulatory documents of the AASW are, therefore, a dominant influence on how university staff write field education manuals and construct the student placement learning and assessment processes. The AASW definition, purpose, value base, core curriculum, practice expectations, supervision requirements and some guidelines for assessment of student placements for social work are in different places, not necessarily aligned or coherent, across a range of documents including: the *Code* (AASW 2010); the sixteen online Ethics and Practice Guidelines (AASW 2013); the *ASWEAS* (AASW, 2012) as revised in 2014; the *Standards* (AASW, 2013a); specific practice standards for school social workers (AASW 2008) and for mental health social workers (AASW 2008) and *Supervision Standards* (AASW 2014).

The following vignette, drawn from a number of liaison visits carried out by us during the *project*, highlights the interface between regulatory documents and human service organisations, both shaped within neoliberal work values and practices.

Vignette

Running late, I grab my liaison pack with the *Manual*, the *Code* and pop in the student's learning plan. Between the jerks of station stops, reading the student's learning plan, while making notes of points to discuss, I am struck by the realisation that, again, many students are interpreting the learning plan in a 'technicist' manner. Is the learning

---

plan itself inviting this response? Where is the inspiration, the sense of social justice purpose, the requirement for students to learn and practise critical social work among these fragmented standards and endless indicators?

Absorbing this reflection, I prepare to go in to the liaison, intending to create a space for critical social work informed reflection. I imagine meeting the student and field educator in the organisation with the aim to cohere threads of the *Manual*, learning plan, the *Code*, *Standards* and indicators—using artistry to make a holistic and meaningful learning experience out of siloed columns and clauses, decoupled from context. I hear about the most recent restructuring of this agency to accommodate the new programs that reduce the length of time for client involvement. This includes the types of services allowed to be offered.

The student shows and explains the various intake, assessment and planning documents. I see that our learning plan is similar in style, another tick-the-box template form, divorced from what it is meant to represent, familiar in the everyday life of social workers here; our competency-based learning plan with rating scales is perfectly compatible with, and contextualised to, risk-averse, time- and resource-poor, predefined outcome-focused, organisations.

I gently explore with the student and supervisor some changes to the learning plan that could enable the student to undertake tasks to learn and demonstrate competence in *Standard One*, which was seemingly missed: 'works to eliminate all violations of human rights; identifies social systems and structures that preserve inequalities . . . and advocates for change; challenges policies and practices that are oppressive and fail to meet international standards of human rights'. (AASW 2013b:9). The field educator looks at me and says quietly, 'You know of course there is no way that we can actually do these things like challenge policies and practices. If we did, that would become our whole job. I can try to create an understanding with the student of how they might do it, but we can't actually do it.'.

Identifying dissonance

The vignette above points to the dissonance between how prominent the discourse of social justice and human rights is in the definition and core principles of social work adopted by the AASW and many universities' Schools of Social Work, and the lack of this discourse's coherent, holistic and contextualised presence in the university's *Manual* as influenced by the *Practice Standards* and indicators. This disjuncture also occurs between those *Practice Standards* requiring students (and practitioners) to do social justice, human rights, and critical social work and its lack of implementation by many social workers in education and human service organisations. The language used in most of the eight *Practice Standards* only requires that students and social workers demonstrate an 'understanding of' what is defined in the standards. However, Practice Standard One requires social workers, and students on placement, to demonstrate not only understanding but 'practising' what is required in the standard, that social workers:

> uphold their ethical responsibilities and . . . act appropriately when faced with ethical problems, issues and dilemmas . . . practice within a social justice and human rights framework . . . work to eliminate all violations of human rights, identify . . . inequalities . . . and advocate for change, challenge policies and practices that fail to meet . . . standards of human rights (AASW 2012: 9).

The *Standards* and indicators are a fragmenting and technicist influence when experienced by the social work field education team member in the above vignette. The liaison person does what seems possible in a given moment, to use 'spheres of influence' to achieve more critical social work cognisant, 'micro-climates' (Fook 2012: 185) within broader business-like contexts. It appears, though, given the prevalence of NPM in their respective organisational contexts that the university liaison person and the social work supervisor make a private pact to settle for the student just demonstrating an understanding of social justice, human rights and critical social work practice, rather than the student demonstrating they can actually do these things. The liaison person found that individual critically reflective practice was important, but not enough on its own. The team found the ability to achieve small or big changes was increased when working with others to form plans to challenge the embedding of neoliberal values and practices within people, within practices, within texts and within organisations.

Principle: use critical reflection, informed by those most affected, in purposeful solidarity with others

Our experiences of using the competency-based approach are that it invites an uncritical tick-the-box response to learning and assessment (Aronson & Hemingway

2011: 283) against the contextual backdrop of neoliberalism and NPM that impact on social work educators and field education team members at universities, liaison staff, students and field educators in busy organisations. Our conclusions, based on 20 months and comprising some 30 liaison visits, is that learning and assessment processes are needed to complement or replace competency-based methods, enabling 'integrated knowledge', 'highly developed intuition', that provide for combinations of 'critical reflection, practice experience, discipline-specific theories, and empirical research' (Regehr et al. 2011). We agree with Pease that learning and assessment would benefit from a foundation in: 'critical knowledge-informed practice to encompass radical sociological thought, ethnographic qualitative research, tacit knowledge, critically reflective practice, parity of participation and citizen based knowledge' (Pease 2013: 32).

We suggest the assessment process needs to match the values and processes of learning and practice. This could be achieved by the assessment of a student's performance on placement having a greater integration of reflection, holistic approach and critical thinking as part of the assessment culture and practice (Wilson 2011). This would include considering how the university, placement agency and societal context differentially affects the opportunities for students to learn rather than just viewing a student's pass or fail of a placement unit as a function of atomised, individual competence (Bourdieu 1998). The *team* is currently working to trial placement learning and assessment processes that incorporate these understandings.

Practice principle: work in solidarity while recognising differences with others, towards social-justice oriented change

Working in solidarity, in a team, provided much needed inspiration and motivation to sustain us while undertaking this *project*. Involvement in the *project* fostered collective, rather than individualised, responsibilities and responses. This strengthened the ability of the *team* to understand and respond to the complex issues surrounding student placements to be responded to as structural, rather than individual problems. We feel this is a good example of how working in solidarity with others creates opportunities, and a sense of protection, for people to practise critical social work. The collective nature of the *team* work also provided validating occasions to acknowledge each other's work and moments of safe reprieve, to 'let off steam'.

Drawing on this experience, the team member responsible for teaching integration seminars with students on placement further emphasised fostering a sense of solidarity between herself and students, and between the students as a group. Students' own placement experiences, an ongoing case study (see Chapter 4) and critical policy analysis practice were scaffolded across the three placement integration seminars to explore, and support students to practise, critical social work in their placement contexts.

Practice principle: 'good enough' critical social work within a 'Framework for Critical Social Work Action'

Although we were disappointed that our workloads prohibited a full re-think and re-write of the *Manual* and the learning plan it contains, we decided an incremental review was possible and worthwhile. Despite falling short of our initial goals, this 'good enough' progress initiated the development of a 'Framework for Critical Social Work Action' (FCSWA) in the social work field education team that broadened as the *project* developed. The FCSWA provided a longer-term plan and approach that alleviated feelings of inadequacy, the pressures of perfection, and an 'all-or-nothing' mentality.

Practice principle: work alongside marginalised groups to advocate for change

The inclusion of other goals into the FCSWA included applying for seed funding for a number of projects to provide and share learning from: opportunities for student placement that promote critical social work practice; developing the university social-work simulation website to share ways of providing opportunities for the practice of critical social work in student placements; and improving the educational preparation, and support, for critical social work placement practice. Importantly, the FCSWA was broadened to include work and goals that were already underway but that had previously lacked coherent prominence in the plan. In this way, we could honour our witnessing (see Chapter 4) of the students' experience to advocate for changes to those university and regulatory provisions that adversely impact social work students on placements in Australia such as lack of cultural inclusivity in 'no leave of any kind provisions'.

Conclusion

The accumulated learning by the *team* in this *project* includes how regulatory texts, covering those of the professional body representing social work in Australia, and the university social work field education manual plus the learning plan that it contains, are influenced by neoliberal values and practices. The neoliberal discourse embedded in regulatory texts activates certain responses in social work staff and students in the university, and in placement organisations, to constrain the practice of critical social work. Our plan, within our locally developed FCSWA, is to continue to be informed by students to challenge policies and regulations that are not inclusive or social-justice oriented, and to change the *Manual* to invite responses from readers that enable critical social work. This is part of the process of critical social work, to question, to reflect, and to work with others to create change.

References

AASW 2008, *AASW Practice Standards for Mental Health Social Workers*, Canberra: AASW

—— 2010, *The AASW Code of Ethics*, Canberra: AASW

—— 2012a, *Australian Social Work Education and Accreditation Standards (ASWEAS) 2012, Guideline 1.5: Guidance on reaccreditation reviews*, AASW, Canberra

—— 2012b, *Australian Social Work Education and Accreditation Standards (ASWEAS) 2012, Guideline 1.2: Guidance on field education programs*, AASW, Canberra

—— 2012c, *Australian Social Work Education and Accreditation Standards (ASWEAS) 2012 v1.4*, (revised July 2014), AASW, Canberra

AASW 2013a, *Ethics and Practice Guideline—Ethics and Field Education: Important reflections for educators and students*, Canberra: AASW

—— 2013b, *Practice Standards 2013*, Canberra: AASW

—— 2014, *Supervision Standards 2014*, Canberra: AASW

Allan, J., Briskman, L. & Pease, B. (eds) 2009, *Critical Social Work: Theories for a socially just world*, 2nd edn, St Leonards: Allen & Unwin

Aronson, J. & Hemingway, D. 2011, '"Competence" in neoliberal times: Defining the future of social work', *Canadian Social Work Review*, vol. 28, no. 2, pp. 281–85

Australian Association of Social Workers *see* AASW

'Blackmore, J. 2014, '"Still hanging off the edge": An Australian case study of gender, universities, and globalization' in N. Stromquist & K. Monkman (eds), *Globalization and Education: Integration and contestation across cultures*, Lanham: Rowman & Littlefield Pub Inc, pp. 285–303

Bourdieu, P. 1998, 'Utopia of endless exploitation: The essence of neoliberalism', *Le Monde Diplomatique*, <http://mondediplo.com/1998/12/08bourdieu>, accessed 15 August 2015

Brough, M., Correa-Velez, I., Crane, P., Johnstone, E. & Marston, G. 2015, *Balancing the Books: An assessment of financial stress associated with social work and human service student placements*, School of Public Health and Social Work, Brisbane: Queensland University of Technology

Brown, D. 2006, 'Working the system: Re-thinking the institutionally organized role of mothers and the reduction of "risk" in child protection work', *Social Problems,* vol. 53, no. 3, pp. 352–70

Butcher, J. & Dalton, B. 2014, 'Cross-sector partnership and human services in Australian states and territories: Reflections on a mutable relationship', *Policy and Society,* vol. 33, no. 2, pp. 141–53

Cleak, H. & Smith, D. 2012, 'Student satisfaction with models of field placement supervision', *Australian Social Work,* vol. 65, no. 2, pp. 243–58 de Montigny, G. 1995, *Social Working: An ethnography of front-line practice*, Toronto: University of Toronto Press

Fook, J. 2012, *Social Work: A critical approach to practice*, London: SAGE

Healy, B. 1993, 'Elements in the development of an Australian radical social work', *Australian Social Work,* vol. 46, no. 1, pp. 3–8

Hosken, N. 2013, 'Social work supervision and discrimination', *Advances in Social Work and Welfare Education,* vol. 15, no. 1, pp. 91–103

Keevers, L. M. 2010, *Practising Social Justice: Community organisations, what matters and what counts,* PhD thesis, Sydney: University Of Sydney

Koshy, P. 2014, *Student Equity Performance in Australian Higher Education: 2007 to 2012,* Perth: National Centre for Student Equity in Higher Education (NCSEHE)

Mykhalovskiy, E. 2002, 'Understanding the social character of treatment decision making' in M. Bresalier, L. Gillis, C. McClure et al. (eds), *Making Care Visible: Antiretroviral therapy and the health work of people living with HIV/AIDS,* report prepared by the Positive Action Fund, Toronto: Ontario Ministry of Health

Olsen, J. 2007, 'Social work's professional and social justice projects: Discourses in conflict', *Journal of Progressive Human Services,* vol. 18, no. 1, pp. 45–69

Pease, B. 2013, 'A history of critical and radical social work' in M. Gray & S. Webb (eds) *The New Politics of Social Work,* Houndmills: Palgrave Macmillan

Regehr, C., Bogo, M. & Regehr, G. 2011, 'The development of an online practice-based evaluation tool for social work', *Research on Social Work Practice,* vol. 21, no. 4, pp. 469–75

Smith, D.E. 2005, *Institutional Ethnography: A sociology for people,* Lanham: AltaMira Press

Szoke, H. 2012, 'Racism exists in Australia—are we doing enough to address it?', *Faculty of Law at Queensland University of Technology, Public Lecture Series,* Australian Human Rights Commission, <www.humanrights.gov.au/news/speeches/racism-exists-australia-are-we-doing-enough-address-it>, accessed 16 July 2015

Weiss-Gal, I., Levin, L. & Krumer-Nevo, M. 2014, 'Applying critical social work in direct practice with families', *Child & Family Social Work,* vol. 19, no. 1, pp. 55–64

Wilson, G. 2011, 'Evidencing reflective practice in social work education: Theoretical uncertainties and practical challenges', *British Journal of Social Work,* vol. 43, pp. 154–72

Part IV

Doing anti-discriminatory and anti-oppressive practice in social work

13

Anti-oppressive practice with people seeking asylum in Australia: reflections from the field

Sharlene Nipperess and Sherrine Clark

Introduction

In this chapter we reflect on our practice of working with people seeking asylum in Australia over nearly two decades. Over this period, we have experienced several new governments, multiple changes of policy and witnessed a number of critical events that have had a significant and detrimental impact on the lives of asylum seekers in Australia. In this chapter, we define key terms including 'refugee' and 'asylum seeker' and explore the context of practice with asylum seekers in contemporary Australia. This is followed by an overview of anti-oppressive practice in relation to asylum seekers. We then explore anti-oppressive practice with asylum seekers at the personal, cultural and structural levels, using three case studies from our practice. Finally, we outline some principles of anti-oppressive practice with asylum seekers that we have found useful to guide our work.

Seeking asylum in Australia

There is significant confusion around the labels that define who is and who is not a refugee in Australia and other countries (Zetter 2007; McAdam & Chong 2014). Terms such as 'economic migrant', 'economic refugee', 'environmental refugee', 'genuine refugees', 'illegal asylum seekers' and so on abound in political and public discourse and are used pejoratively to restrict access to the protection offered by the United Nations Convention Relating to the Status of Refugees (1951) to which Australia is a signatory. According to the Convention a refugee is a person who:

> As a result of events occurring before 1 January 1951 and owing to a well-founded fear of being persecuted for reasons of race, religion, nationality, membership of a particular social group or political opinion, is outside the country of his [sic] nationality and is unable or, owing to such fear, is unwilling to avail himself [sic] of the protection of that country; or who, not having a nationality and being outside the country of his [sic] former habitual residence as a result of such events, is unable or, owing to such fear, is unwilling to return to it (United Nations High Commissioner for Refugees [UNHCR] 2010: 14).

The 1967 Protocol Relating to the Status of Refugees is the only amendment to the Convention and removed the geographical limit ('events occurring' in Europe) and temporal limit ('before 1 January 1951'). Asylum seekers are people who have fled to another country and have applied under the Convention to be assessed as a refugee. Asylum seekers then are people who have not yet had their refugee status determined. Essentially, refugees and asylum seekers are forced migrants as opposed to voluntary migrants who leave their own country for a range of economic and other reasons. Questions of definition are vexed. In the highly charged political debates that have been experienced in Australia and around the world, the claims of refugees are commonly thrown into doubt; that they are not 'true' refugees according to the UN definition. However, the distinctions are increasingly arbitrary as Papademitriou (cited in Marfleet 2006: 12) notes: 'Both pure refugees and purely economic migrants are ideal constructs rarely found in real life; many among those who routinely meet the refugee definition are clearly fleeing both political oppression and economic dislocation'.

Australia ratified the Convention in 1954 and the Protocol in 1973, which means that Australia has voluntarily agreed to treat 'refugees in accordance with internationally recognised legal and humanitarian standards, and [commits] its willingness to share the global responsibility for protecting refugees' (McAdam & Chong 2014: 11).

In this chapter, we define refugees according to the Convention and contrast the protection that is afforded to people who arrive in Australia on refugee visas with people who claim asylum in Australia. In Australia, the rights and entitlements offered to people seeking asylum and those that have been granted protection under the Convention vary markedly. Anyone has a right to claim refugee status but increasingly access to this fundamental human right is restricted, not only in Australia but across the developed world (Zetter 2007). Although the terms 'refugee' and 'asylum seeker' are to some extent legal constructs existing in national legislation and in the various international human rights instruments, we acknowledge that the risk of using such labels is to reduce a person to a single identity. Although we use the term 'asylum seeker' throughout this chapter we also use the phrase 'people seeking asylum' wherever possible, to emphasise the person, rather than the label or category of asylum seeker. In doing this we acknowledge that people who are seeking asylum in Australia are diverse and hold multiple identities.

The most recent figures from the UNHCR (2014, pp. 6–7) show that as of the end of 2014 there were 13,685,507 refugees, 1,796,310 people seeking asylum (an enormous increase from the previous year of 928,230) and numerous other populations of concern. These include returned refugees, internally displaced peoples and stateless people worldwide. The majority of refugees were located in Africa whereas the largest number of asylum seekers were located in Europe. Traditionally, developing countries host the majority of refugees and in 2012 Pakistan hosted 1,616,500 refugees, by far the highest number of any nation (UNHCR 2013). However, by the end of 2014, Turkey (1,587,374) leaped ahead of Pakistan (1,505,525), which had hosted the most number of refugees for more than ten years (UNHCR 2014).

In 2013, Australia granted 20,019 visas under the Humanitarian Program. Of these, 12,515 were granted under the offshore component of the program (under the Refugee category and the Special Humanitarian (offshore) category) and 7504 visas were granted under the onshore component of the program (Department of Immigration and Border Protection 2013). In 2012–13, the Humanitarian Program was increased to 20,000 places from a relatively stable 13,000 places over the previous ten years. In comparison to many countries throughout the world, Australia's program is relatively small.

Of the 20,019 visas, only 37.5 per cent were granted under the onshore component of the program and people who arrived by boat represented only a proportion of this number. However, despite the small numbers of people arriving by boat, the onshore component of the Humanitarian Program has proven to be the most controversial aspect of Australia's Humanitarian Program (Gibney 2004). The Australian Government treats the refugees who arrive by boat, known in popular discourse as 'boat people', very differently to those who arrive via the offshore resettlement program. This is despite the government having ratified the Convention and Protocol and incorporated these international obligations into domestic immigration legislation (McAdam & Chong 2014). Though most people seeking asylum are granted refugee status according to the Convention, they are treated with suspicion, labelled and stigmatised, and are forced to endure conditions in remote detention centres that have major consequences for their health and wellbeing (Austin et al. 2007; Lusher et al. 2007).

Australia's response to refugees and asylum seekers cannot be understood without also understanding that racism and exclusion have been central to the nation's development and its immigration policy (Hollinsworth 2006; Chappell et al. 2009). However, the year 2001 was a watershed in Australia's response to refugees and asylum seekers. A number of highly controversial events occurred. This included the boarding of the Norwegian ship, the *Tampa*, the children overboard case and the 352 drowning deaths that occurred after the Suspected Illegal Entry Vessel (SIEV) X sank. At the same time, the then Federal Government led by Prime Minister John Howard introduced or further developed a number of contentious policies, including offshore processing, mandatory detention and temporary protection visas, which have all had a significant impact on the wellbeing of people seeking asylum. Public policy and political leadership in relation to these events and policies, was widely criticised by the international community for being punitive and unsympathetic and at times in breach of international law and human rights (Burnside 2007).

The election of the Rudd Labor Government in 2007 seemed to signal a change in refugee and asylum seeker policy and in 2008 the government announced that it would close the detention centres on Nauru, an island nation in the Pacific Ocean, and Manus Island, part of Papua New Guinea, and abolish temporary protection visas. However, since then, successive Labor and Liberal governments have reintroduced offshore processing and temporary protection visas, re-opened the detention centres on Nauru and Manus Island, and introduced new and deeply concerning policies that discourage people from claiming asylum in Australia. Despite the sustained international and national condemnation, repeated polls demonstrate that a great deal of the Australian population supports the government's harsh measures and there are many people that call for even tougher policies (Marr 2011).

Anti-oppressive social work practice with people seeking asylum

Anti-oppressive social work is one of a number of approaches that fits within the overarching tradition of critical social work. Anti-oppressive and anti-discriminative approaches to social work practice came out of the UK and Canada in the 1980s and 1990s. They emerged in response to a critique of earlier class-based approaches and targeted 'the failure of individualistic theories of social work to recognize the impact of discrimination against minority groups in society' (Mendes 2009: 26).

Informed by theories including Marxism, critical social theory (incorporating the Frankfurt School and later iterations), feminism, post-colonialism and post-modernism, social work writers have explored anti-discriminatory and anti-oppressive practice (Dominelli 2002; Thompson 2006; Mullaly 2010; Baines 2011). Although diverse, these practice approaches share a commitment to both understanding the experience of oppression and challenging that oppression across interrelated personal, cultural and structural domains.

Oppression is complex. While the literature has explored oppression in terms of particular oppressed groups (as this chapter does), it is important to recognise that people may experience multiple forms of oppression. Understanding that the different dimensions of oppression intersect and interrelate is vital for the development of anti-oppressive practice. It is also important to note that people may occupy contradictory positions and be both oppressed and privileged at the same time on the basis of different social divisions such as class, gender, race/ethnicity, age, sexuality, religion and so on (Pease 2010).

Many people seeking asylum have experienced significant discrimination and oppression and they are one of the most vulnerable groups in Australian society (Briskman, Latham & Goddard 2008). They have often endured significant physical and psychological trauma in their home country, during their journey to Australia and upon arrival in Australia when they are placed in detention and in the resettlement process (Leach & Mansouri 2004; Austin et al. 2007).

At the same time, it is also important to acknowledge that people who have sought asylum in Australia and in other countries have diverse and complex experiences. Some of these differences relate to the experience of oppression and privilege based on a range of social, cultural, political and geographic identities and experiences. These include class, gender, ethnicity, national origin, language, age, physical appearance, ability, religion, education, sex or gender identity, and sexual orientation or preference. The complexity and diversity of their situation is also evident in their experiences of war, torture and trauma in the home country, their method of escape, their experience of refugee camps and detention centres, the numbers of their family and community members remaining in the home country, who are still displaced and who have resettled in Australia.

It is also crucial in anti-oppressive practice to recognise that refugees and asylum seekers demonstrate resilience, strength, and rich and diverse histories and cultures. As Zetter notes, a stereotypical label such as refugee or asylum seeker 'fails to capture the rich and multilayered "identity" of any one of' (Zetter 2007: 183) the millions of forced migrants that seek refuge all over the world. In Australia, after four years as a permanent resident, refugees can apply for citizenship. Some people embrace and retain their refugee status as an important part of their identity; others reject the label outright. Other refugees remake and reuse the label for their own political, cultural and familial ends.

Anti-oppressive practice with people seeking asylum requires understanding the experience of oppression and privilege and a commitment to personal, cultural and structural change. Anti-oppressive practice with asylum seekers also recognises the vulnerability and the complexity, diversity and strengths of the women, men and children who comprise asylum-seeking communities in Australia. A commitment to reflective and reflexive practice is also an important component of anti-oppressive practice with people seeking asylum. Although there are various understandings of reflectivity and reflexivity in the social work literature (D'Cruz, Gillingham & Melendez 2007), we understand reflectivity to refer to the process of reflecting on our practice and reflexivity as the process of understanding how our values, beliefs, experiences and assumptions—our social location or positioning—impacts on practice and how the practice context impacts on us.

Social work practice with people seeking asylum at the personal level

Upon arrival in Australia, people on refugee visas commence the process of resettlement, which can be experienced very differently depending on a range of factors. In general, refugees need to undertake a number of settlement tasks all within the first few months of arrival (Bowles 2005; Fiske & Briskman 2013). People seeking asylum, on the other hand, have not yet had their claims for refugee status recognised and therefore must go through a process of proving that they should be recognised as a refugee under the Convention. This means that they have considerably less access to rights and entitlements than people who have already had their refugee status recognised. It also means that people seeking asylum experience unique challenges primarily because of their uncertain future.

Social workers have a longstanding history of working with newly arrived refugees in a range of generalist and specialist agencies, although arguably it has not been part of mainstream practice and has largely focused on the personal rather than the political or structural level (McMahon 2002). However, working with asylum seekers has primarily been the domain of the non-government funded sector such as of church-funded services and independent organisations. In late 2010, the release of people from detention meant that many agencies accepted government funding to work with asylum seekers. These agencies provided community detention facilities and administered the asylum seeker assistance scheme and community assistance support program, now known as Status Resolution Support Services. With these relatively recent policy changes, social workers in generalist agencies are increasingly providing a range of services to people seeking asylum to meet their immediate needs as well as to deal with the impact of discrimination and oppression. For example, in relation to health, hospitals and community health centres in some jurisdictions, provide a range of services to asylum seekers.

Seeking asylum in Australia is a complicated and stressful process. This is further compounded by the initial experiences that result in a person seeking asylum in the first place, and reach the point where they apply for protection in Australia. Asylum seekers will often reveal a number of issues that impact on their experience while they await the lengthy refugee determination process. This may include a history of trauma and at times torture, significant health and mental health issues (especially if they have spent time in detention), lack of income, housing, material aid supports and grief and loss as a result of separation from family, friends and culture. People seeking asylum often require support to navigate the complex welfare and legal process which will determine their legitimacy to be recognised as a refugee, as well as other rights and entitlements. Support needs to be provided for a range of different issues including health, housing, immigration, legal, social and recreational, financial, material aid, employment, education and counselling throughout the entire refugee determination process or for as long as the person seeking asylum is able to access the service.

In addition, given the recent shifts in asylum seeker policies (this relates to the structural level), the harsh political rhetoric, media misrepresentation and the general public's attitudes to asylum seekers and their issues (this relates to the cultural level), refugees and asylum seekers often experience internalised oppression at the personal level. Social workers working in the community will often witness the impact of reduction of rights, exclusion and misinformation for asylum seekers on a personal level resulting in low self-esteem, powerlessness, fear, anger, isolation and alienation.

When working with asylum seekers, it is important to be mindful that once a person applies for protection, they are required to tell their story (often repeatedly) and provide proof of their claims for asylum, and as a result this can often be very emotionally challenging. Common experiences in the initial stages of seeking asylum include living with uncertainty, triggering memories of difficult experiences that forced asylum seekers to flee their country, including torture, trauma, and profound grief and loss.

Anti-oppressive practice at the personal level can include providing relevant and up-to-date information supporting opportunities for people seeking asylum to make informed choices, encouraging self-determination, trauma counselling, individual advocacy in relation to immigration issues, individual advocacy to enable access to rights and entitlements, referral to appropriate services, settlement work including facilitating access to housing, language classes, schools, medical treatment and groupwork. Anti-oppressive practice at the personal level also involves connecting the personal experience of discrimination and oppression with social work practice at the cultural and structural levels in order to contribute to social change. For example, a social worker might note that a number of people accessing a service experience discrimination on the same issue. The socal worker could use these experiences to inform a social policy submission to advocate for change at the appropriate governmental level.

Case study: supporting Mary to seek asylum in Australia

Mary is a female student, twenty years of age, who arrived in Australia in 2011 and attended the Asylum Seeker Resource Centre (ASRC) for support. Mary indicated that she did not understand the asylum seeker process; she appeared very distressed, stated that she had no money or accommodation, and that she had been sleeping on the streets for the last three nights. Mary said that she had come to Australia on a student visa. However, after one year, her uncle told her that her father had disappeared; his business had been burned as a result of a fundamentalist political party's actions, and he advised her not to go back home.

In partnership with the social worker, Mary identified her immediate needs. The social worker was able to provide relevant information regarding Mary's options, supported Mary to consider the range of options regarding appropriate services which may be able to assist her, provided advocacy in relation to accessing

---

emergency accommodation for female asylum seekers, provided a referral to the ASRC legal service and attended to her immediate needs by providing a hot meal.

The next day the social worker supported Mary to see a female lawyer who explained the process for seeking asylum. Mary became anxious, distressed and appeared to experience a panic attack during the appointment and the social worker accessed the health team who supported Mary through the incident. Mary, the social worker, and the legal and health teams identified that she required additional support to enable her to tell her story in order to lodge a protection application. The social worker arranged a priority referral to a trauma counsellor who could then support this process.

With all these supports in place, Mary was able to tell her story and apply for protection. Her social worker advocated for Mary to obtain federally funded government support (89 per cent of a Centrelink benefit), and continued to support her throughout the process. While waiting for an outcome from the Department of Immigration and Border Protection (DIBP), the government depart-ment responsible for assessing her application, Mary and her social worker explored her goals and hopes for the future. Mary identi-fied that she was interested in sporting activities and would like to learn how to reduce/manage her panic attacks. The social worker provided information and support to link Mary to relevant services and sporting organisations.

Mary was requested to attend an interview at the DIBP, which concerned her as articulating her story previously had resulted in a panic attack. Mary and her social worker developed a plan of support, ensuring that letters from medical professionals attesting to her medical condition, which may have compromised the hearing, were provided. The social worker and lawyer explained the process so that Mary knew what to expect and to get through the interview safely.

While waiting for a decision from the DIBP, Mary engaged with sporting activities, accessed appointments independently and managed her anxiety. Approximately eighteen months later, Mary was advised that she was granted protection and was linked to settlement services to support her to continue to obtain support and manage her mental health concerns. Over a period of time and

> with the support of the social worker Mary began to engage in the political activities of the organisation; in particular, she participated in campaigns challenging federal asylum seeker policies. Mary is now safe, managing her anxiety, a keen soccer player, studying aged care and working at the ASRC as a volunteer to support other people seeking asylum.

Social work practice with people seeking asylum at the cultural level

Although it is true that many people within the Australian community have resisted the dominant discourses about refugees and asylum seekers, the political rhetoric of being 'tough' on border protection and people smugglers has continued to be popular in the general community. This has contributed to the election or re-election of successive governments in Australia (Gibney 2004; Minns 2005). The difference between refugees and asylum seekers began to be publicly articulated following the arrival of the first Vietnamese people seeking asylum by boat in 1976. Since then there has been a gradual tightening of policies from the introduction of mandatory detention in 1992, through to various incarnations of offshore processing and the implementation of temporary protection visas, which have all had a significant and detrimental impact on the wellbeing of people seeking asylum. Over the same period of time, the public and political debate has become tougher. Labor Prime Minister Bob Hawke in the 1980s introduced into the public vernacular the idea of 'queue jumpers' and other labels followed including the use of terms such as 'illegals', 'not genuine refugees' and 'boat people'. Like most stereotypes, these labels have proven difficult to challenge and have contributed to the discourse on asylum seekers that seeks to demonise those who arrive by boat as opposed to those who arrive via other means (Rowe & O'Brien 2014).

The media have been willing partners in the demonisation of asylum seekers. Research has consistently showed that media reporting has generally been negative in relation to asylum seekers (McKay et al. 2011). Despite the Australian Press Council's guidelines to use more appropriate terms, some sections of the media still insist in using labels such as 'illegals' or 'illegal immigrants' even though it is inaccurate and misleading to do so. Further, it suggests they are criminals, which continues to stigmatise people seeking asylum.

The impact of the political rhetoric, public opinion and negative discourses perpetrated by the media on the wellbeing of asylum seekers has also been demonstrated extensively in the research (Suhnan et al. 2012). In particular, many refugees and asylum seekers experience direct discrimination and oppression at the personal level through verbal and physical violence and significant psychological impacts.

Case study: a community education program to tackle racism

This case study describes the development of a community education program designed to challenge the myths and stereotypes of refugees and asylum seekers evident in political rhetoric, in the media and in public discourses. Using an action research model, built on a cycle of planning, action, evaluation and reflection, the program was developed by a social worker and trialled in a number of community organisations and schools (both primary and secondary) in two federal municipalities, and was auspiced by a metropolitan migrant resource centre.

This program was developed within the context of an anti-discriminatory/anti-oppressive framework. It sought to go beyond the usual 'cultural diversity programs' that focus on cultural sensitivity to one that recognised and was committed to changing the structures that perpetuate racism and oppression in Australia. The developed program explicitly explored racism and its role in the development of Australia generally, including the development of Australian political attitudes and culture, and immigration policy in particular. It included modules exploring invasion, colonisation and the development of Australia's particularly oppressive brand of immigration policy, known as the 'White Australia Policy'. These modules also explored policy shifts from assimilation, to integration and eventually, multiculturalism, and the legacy of racism and its impact on refugee and asylum seeker policy in contemporary times.

The program explicitly challenged the dominant discourses of refugees and asylum seekers by exploring the stereotypes and language that had been promoted through the political rhetoric and in the media. Finally, critical reflection was embedded in the program. In particular, students and practitioners were invited to consider their own social context, which included exploring their own ethnicity, standpoint on racism and privilege, gender, religion and spirituality. Participants were also offered the opportunity to explore

---

their own migration experiences, and their values and assumptions that shape their understanding of colonisation and the experience of Australia's Indigenous peoples, Australia's migration policy and the legislative framework and the experience of seeking asylum in contemporary Australia. Practitioners were invited to consider the implications that arose from this opportunity for critical reflection including the commitment to practising across the personal, cultural and structural levels with the goal of social change.

Social work practice with people seeking asylum at the structural level

Asylum seeker advocacy groups have lobbied hard, especially over the last decade, to challenge the numerous punitive policies that have been introduced or re-introduced in relation to asylum seekers. There are some examples of success including the repeal of temporary protection visas (although this, like many policies, has been reinstated) and the Pacific solution and in more recent times, the removal of the 45-day rule (whereby in coming to Australia an asylum seeker must lodge a protection visa within 45 days, otherwise face a long process without work/study rights and Medicare), and the release of people seeking asylum in detention to the community in 2011. This latter initiative paved the way for many mainstream agencies that had not previously worked with asylum seekers to be funded by the Federal Government to support asylum seekers in the community. Essentially it reduced the harsh impact that mandatory and indefinite detention has had upon asylum seekers' mental health and wellbeing, by providing Bridging visas, which entitled asylum seekers to work and study and access Medicare. Overall, the story of Australia's asylum seeker policy is one of ever-increasing restrictive policies designed to dissuade people of their right to seek asylum in Australia.

The introduction, occasional repeal and re-introduction of oppressive and inhumane policies and practices, have resulted in asylum seekers (especially those arriving by boat) presenting with significant levels of destitution and despair, especially to agencies working with asylum seekers. Cuts to vital services such as the Immigration Advice and Application Assistance Scheme in 2014 mean that people seeking asylum in Australia are unable to access the right to seek legal advice and representation and further add to this disadvantage.

It is therefore important that social workers ensure that they continue to advocate at a systemic level, despite the hostile environment and the challenges of doing so. There are certainly consequences of systemic advocacy. There is a well-founded fear that if concerns are raised in the public domain, organisations may lose their funding. Since the Abbott Liberal Coalition Government was elected, a culture of secrecy has permeated through the asylum seeker sector and government departments, and has resulted in social workers being afraid to speak up for fear of losing their jobs. The current political climate, shrouded in misinformation and secrecy, results in workers in government-funded agencies facing real penalties for informing and educating the community, including their agencies losing funding, as the experience of the Refugee Council of Australia (2014) attests. It is becoming clearer for the asylum seeker sector that independent agencies that do not rely on government funding are in a far stronger position to advocate for asylum seekers. Social workers employed in government-funded services can contribute to social change by providing de-identified information (that is, information that removes any identifying information about the individual or the particular experience) to enable these peak advocacy groups to continue to raise awareness, and advocate for the human rights of refugees and asylum seekers in Australia. The value of independence also indicates the role that the social work academics can have in relation to systemic advocacy and there are a number of important examples of social work academics advocating publicly against the Federal Government's punitive policies and oppression in general (see ACHSSW 2006).

Case study: advocating access to transport concessions

In the state of Victoria in Australia, a variety of policies have been challenged successfully. Change has been initiated through targeted campaigns, lobbying from key groups including the Network of Asylum Seeker Agencies of Victoria (NASAVic) and a series of position papers (ASRC 2009; 2010). The following case study describes a process of policy advocacy in relation to transport concessions that resulted in immediate and significant benefits to asylum seekers.

The ASRC along with other key agencies in Victoria identified that, due to the large number of unjust policies and the lack of welcome provided by much of the Australian community, the many asylum seekers coming to the agency were socially isolated from other community members, had limited ability to access essential services, received high rates of infringement notices and limited capacity to address their needs. The material-aid services of the ASRC identified they could potentially meet the transport needs of asylum seekers if they were able to access transport concessions from the state government. The ASRC and other key agencies lobbied the State Government of Victoria and in May 2010 three key agencies, the ASRC, Red Cross and Hotham/Lentara were able to provide access to transport concessions for asylum seekers. Providing transport tickets at a reduced rate has had a significant impact on the wellbeing of some asylum seekers in Victoria. It has helped to reduce some asylum seekers' social isolation and marginalisation, and enabled them to have access to essential health, welfare and legal services.

In addition to approving transport concessions, the State Government of Victoria, over successive Labor and Liberal governments has increased access for people seeking asylum in Victoria to emergency services such as ambulance and public hospitals, to Vocational Education and Training (VET) courses and to the Housing Establishment Fund (HEF). These initiatives have reduced aspects of the level of inequality for some asylum seekers in Victoria. However, the structural oppression created and experienced in the federal government policies has been significantly different.

Conclusion

A number of practice principles can be identified from our reflections on our practice with people seeking asylum over the past two decades. These include: working at all levels of practice to achieve personal, cultural and structural change for asylum seekers; engaging in ethical self-reflective and reflexive practice; keeping up to date with the rapidly changing policy environment and recognising the implications of this for people seeking asylum in their everyday life; recognising the importance of resilience and persistence; having realistic expectations and maintaining critical hope; and actively monitoring self-care.

While the role of a social worker working with asylum seekers can be uncertain and challenging due to the significant discrimination and oppression that is experienced at the personal, cultural and structural levels, it can also be incredibly rewarding, enlightening and life-changing work. Anti-oppressive practice offers a framework for practice with asylum seekers that is aligned to the profession's ethical commitment to human rights, and strives for social justice and social change.

References

ASRC *see* Asylum Seeker Resource Centre

Asylum Seeker Resource Centre (ASRC) 2009, 'Locked Out: Position paper on homelessness of asylum seekers living in the community', ASRC, <www.asrc.org.au/pdf/locked-out.pdf>, accessed 10 August 2014

—— 2010, 'Destitute and Uncertain: The reality of seeking asylum in Australia', *ASRC*, <www.asrc.org.au/wp-content/uploads/2013/07/asrc-welfare-paper.pdf>, accessed 10 August 2014

Austin, P., Silove, D. & Steel, Z. 2007, 'The impact of immigration detention on the mental health of asylum seekers' in D. Lusher & N. Haslam (eds), *Yearning to Breathe Free: Seeking asylum in Australia*, Sydney: Federation Press, pp. 100–12

Australian Council of Heads of Schools of Social Work (ACHSSW) 2006, *We've Boundless Plains to Share: The first report of the Peoples Inquiry into Detention*, ACHSSW

ACHSSW *see* Australian Council Heads of Schools of Social Work

Baines, D. (ed.) 2011, *Doing Anti-oppressive Practice: Social justice social work*, 2nd edn, Halifax: Fernwood

Briskman, L., Latham, S. & Goddard, C. 2008, Human rights overboard: Seeking asylum in Australia, Melbourne: Scribe Publications

Bowles, R. 2005, 'Social work with refugee survivors of torture and trauma' in M. Alston & J. McKinnon (eds), *Social Work: Fields of practice*, 2nd edn, South Melbourne: Oxford University Press, 249–67

Burnside, J. 2007, *Watching Brief: Reflections on human rights, law and justice*, Carlton North: Scribe Publications

Chappell, L., Chesterman, J. & Hill, L. 2009, *The Politics of Human Rights in Australia*, Melbourne: Cambridge University Press

D'Cruz, H., Gillingham, P. & Melendez, S. 2007, 'Reflexivity, its meanings and relevance for social work: A critical review of the literature', *British Journal of Social Work*, vol. 37, no. 1, pp. 73–90

Department of Immigration and Border Protection (DIBP) 2013, 'Fact Sheet 60—Australia's Refugee and Humanitarian Programme', DIBP, <www.immi.gov.au/media/fact-sheets/60refugee.htm>, accessed 10 August 2014

Dominelli, L. 2002, *Anti-oppressive Social Work Theory and Practice*, Houndmills: Palgrave Macmillan

Fiske, L. & Briskman, L. 2013, 'Working with refugees and asylum seekers' in M. Connolly & L. Harms (eds), *Social Work: Contexts and practice*, 3rd edn, South Melbourne: Oxford University Press, pp. 151–62

Fook, J. & Gardner, F. 2007, *Practising Critical Reflection: A resource handbook*, Maidenhead: Open University Press

Gibney, M. 2004, *The Ethics and Politics of Asylum: Liberal democracy and the response to refugees*, Cambridge: Cambridge University Press

Hollinsworth, D. 2006, *Race and Racism in Australia*, 3rd edn, Katoomba: Social Science Press

Leach, M. & Mansouri, F. 2004, *Lives in Limbo: Voices of refugees under temporary protection*, Sydney: UNSW Press

Lusher, D., Balvin, N., Nethery, A. & Tropea, J. 2007, 'Australia's response to asylum seekers' in D. Lusher & N. Haslam (eds), *Yearning to Breathe Free: Seeking asylum in Australia*, Sydney: Federation Press, pp. 9–20

Marfleet, P. 2006, *Refugees in a Global Era*, Houndmills: Palgrave Macmillan

Marr, D. 2011, *Panic: Terror! Invasion! Disorder! Drugs! Kids! Blacks! Boats!*, Collingwood: Black Inc

McAdam, J. & Chong, F. 2014, *Refugees: Why seeking asylum is legal and Australia's policies are not*, Sydney: UNSW Press

McKay, F., Thomas, S. & Blood, W. 2011, '"Any one of these boat people could be a terrorist for all we know!" Media representations and public perceptions of "boat people" arrivals in Australia', *Journalism*, vol. 12, no. 5, pp. 607–26

McMahon, A. 2002, 'Writing diversity: Ethnicity and race is Australan social work, 1947–1997, *Australian Social Work*, vol. 55, no. 3, pp. 172–183

Mendes, P. 2009, 'Tracing the origins of critical social work practice' in J. Allan, L. Briskman & B. Pease (eds), *Critical Social Work: Theories and practices for a socially just world*, 2nd edn, St Leonards: Allen & Unwin, pp. 17–29

Morley, C., Macfarlane, S. & Ablett, P. 2014, *Engaging with Social Work: A critical introduction*, Melbourne: Cambridge University Press

Mullaly, B. 2010, *Challenging Oppression and Confronting Privilege*, 2nd edn, Don Mills: Oxford University Press

Pease, B. 2010, *Undoing Privilege: Unearned advantage in a divided world*, London: Zed Books

Refugee Council of Australia (RCOA) 2014, 'Government removes Refugee Council's core funding', media release, 30 May, RCOA, <http://refugeecouncil.org.au/n/mr/140530_RCOAfunding.pdf>, accessed 10 August 2014

Rowe, E. & O'Brien, E. 2014, '"Genuine" refugees or illegitimate "boat people": Political constructions of asylum seekers and refugees in the Malaysia Deal debate', *Australian Journal of Social Issues*, vol. 49, no. 2, pp. 171–93

Suhnan, A., Pedersen, A. & Hartley, L. 2012, 'Re-examining prejudice against asylum seekers in Australia: The role of people smugglers, the perception of threat and acceptance of false beliefs', *The Australian Community Psychologist*, vol. 24, no. 2, pp. 79–97

Thompson, N. 2006, *Anti-discriminatory Practice*, 4th edn, Houndmills: Palgrave Macmillan

UNHCR *see* United Nations High Commissioner for Refugees

United Nations High Commissioner for Refugees (UNHCR) 2013, 'The global report 2013', UNHCR, <www.unhcr.org/gr13/index.xml>, accessed 10 August 2014

—— 2014, 'The global report 2014', UNHCR, <www.unhcr.org/gr14/index.xml>, accessed 30 August 2015

Zetter, R. 2007, 'More labels, fewer refugees: Remaking the refugee label in an era of globalization', *Journal of Refugee Studies*, vol. 20, no. 2, pp. 172–92

14

Challenges for Indigenous and non-Indigenous practitioners in the neoliberal context

Stephanie Gilbert

Introduction

There are a number of factors that have changed employment conditions for social workers in modern Australia. Gone are the times when the social worker (whether Aboriginal or not) was seen to be one of a limited group of professionals working in welfare supported by a team of professionals and paraprofessionals, including vocationally educated welfare workers. The modern workplace has workers who have similar job roles but are employed with a degree, vocational qualifications or without a degree but with life or work experience or both. Alongside this major change in the professional circumstances, there has been the devolution of the core work of statutory agencies to non-government agencies. This has occurred in most areas within the social services including employment support services, out-of-home care for children or adolescents, and family support.

This chapter examines the nature of these changing circumstances with particular focus on economic change. In addition, the question of how critical theory might assist social workers to understand and construct social work with both colleagues and clients is examined. The chapter looks closely at the neoliberal construct of workers as ahistorical and what this means for Aboriginal workers, and in particular Aboriginal social workers, who may require some compassionate understanding of the historical injustices that may have occurred to affect them. This examination explores what an Aboriginal worker is perceived to bring to the workplace and what is their expertise, as well as the conditions of the workplace for that worker including whether racism is routinely or randomly practised.

Why take a critical stance?

Briskman, Pease and Allan (2009) advocate that social workers ought to see the situation through the lens of critical theory to actively reflect on their practice. This reflection must consider how dominant ideologies or ways of thinking and societal institutions impact on all people's lives. This reflection can create an impetus for social workers to challenge institutions, whether family, policy or governance, when the worker identifies they are creating or reinforcing structural inequality. This impetus exists even more acutely now at the coalface where the newest social workers operate. The challenge to construct meaning of the organisational dynamics surrounding our work has always existed but has reached a critical level since the world financial crisis of 2008. Briskman et al. encourage social workers to look to their own and their client's lives for the links between experience 'and the material conditions and dominant ideologies in society' (Briskman et al 2009: 5), ultimately with the aim to take action to transform it. This transformation occurs by taking this reflection into their work and challenging the norms operating within organisations, between organisations and their clients and the underlying premises embedded in the funding models that finance our work. As will be discussed later in this chapter this critical stance is crucial for Aboriginal workers as their presence within the services sectors as providers is relatively new and still very much a work in progress. There are necessary considerations everyday of which type of services to provide to Aboriginal people. This consideration must also apply to services provided by Aboriginal people as well. Aboriginal workers need to consider how they operate in both mainstream services as well as when they operate alongside mainstream services from within Aboriginal organisations.

Taking a wider perspective

It is worthwhile to pause and take a global perspective of locally experienced trends. According to Iamamoto (2005), the implementation of the neoliberal agenda is the implementation of a conservative perspective with its focus being oriented to capitalism. This way of constructing the world sees the resulting social inequalities as inevitable. They are seen as a consequence of the behaviour of individuals who are unable to perform effectively within the capitalist mode of operations. These social inequalities are not seen as a collectivistic experience by, for instance, the working class. They are seen as just the isolated issues or difficulties of individuals. This perspective of seeing issues as individually located ignores the structural context and can result in a wider pattern of dismantling universal social rights. These rights may have been the result of accumulated social advocacy or struggles and their loss can be felt very acutely.

Iamamoto (2005) encourages us to note how the response to difficulties or issues can become the site for exceptional measures like philanthropic initiatives and voluntarism. Particularly as it is advocated that earlier responses to broader social issues affecting the communities have led to 'excessive social spending' and hence the 'fiscal crises of the States' (Iamamoto 2005: 143). This leads social commentary away from a broader 'social question' of public, political and national interest. It also leads it away from the notion of a civil society in which societal organisations manifest the interests and will of its citizens (Iamamoto 2005: 143).

Advocating for social protections

The International Labour Organisation's (ILO) research has shown the more we embed social protections into our nations the better that nation's economic life becomes. This is an interesting challenge to the neoliberal project. Iamamoto contends that the result of winding back social protections with the neoliberal policy approach have included 'unemployment, recession, economic denationalisation and an increase in foreign vulnerability' (Iamamoto 2005: 144). As the ILO state, any winding back of social security protections in either developing or developed countries results in increased poverty and social exclusion (ILO June 2014a). In spite of this evidence expounding the negative outcomes of winding back social protections, only 27 per cent of the world's population are comprehensively enjoying their fundamental human right to social security (ILO 2014c: 3).

The ILO contend that effective access to essential health care and basic income security, which then ensures dignity through the life cycle, is the necessary national social protection required for any nation. These should include at least:

- access to essential health care, including maternity care
- basic income security for children

- basic income security for persons of working age who are unable to earn sufficient income, in particular in cases of sickness, unemployment, maternity and disability
- basic income security for older persons (ILOb 2014b: 6).

The ILO advocates that by boosting human capital and productivity nations can reduce poverty and inequality, and support inclusive growth. Nations can then create domestic-based demand, and support and further develop their own economies (ILO 2014c). Unfortunately, since the fiscal crisis in 2008, countries have tended to adopt measures disproportionately affecting poor households such as cutting wages and rationalising services. Hand-in-hand measures such as narrowing the targets for social protection benefits, reforms of pension and health-care systems, or increasing consumption taxes on basic products are implemented (ILO 2014a; ILO 2014b). The after-effects of these actions due in part to persistent unemployment, lower wages and higher taxes, include higher levels of poverty and social exclusion. It seems reasonable to expect that lower incomes will create lower demand and consumption and hence slow down the economy. The inverse should then also be true that social protection is a fundamental part of sound economic policy precisely because it contributes to the reduction of 'poverty, exclusion and inequality, while enhancing political stability and social cohesion' (ILO 2014b: 6).

The Australian context

A couple of these world trends mentioned earlier have impacted more specifically in the Australian context. The first is the devolution of services from central government providers to contracted community sector organisations. The process of entry of these providers into these fields has meant the instant creation of work teams in organisations that had not traditionally existed or been involved in this form of work.

Mission Australia (see case study) serves as a good example of these sorts of trends Iamamoto (2005) identified. The devolution of work to organisations like Mission Australia, has meant that they have grown exponentially as a result of this trend. However, it could also be read as regressive for workers and their employment conditions. In some instances this has meant the dismantling of parts of government, and government workers changing or losing their work. The idea and implementation of flexibility allows for the utilisation of high levels of technology and innovation into production. It can also lead to a similar expectation of flexibility in the employment conditions of the workforce itself as well. Potentially, social development is at risk as workers run the gauntlet of improving service and quality, as simultaneously their worker rights are put to the same sword of reducing costs and broadening profit rates. Crucially, in terms of the treatment of human beings we see again at work the wider neoliberal agenda of reducing coordinated rights like those won by worker's unions. The individual is expected to bear the expectation to be 'flexible' around their wages and their conditions and to bear these expectations individually. Unfortunately for social work, the same rationalisations occur in the workplaces social workers populate.

Iamamoto (2005, p. 144) makes the point that by streamlining work processes a number of strategies are employed: 'The work shift is intensified and increased, the number of work posts reduced and working conditions and labour rights become more precarious'. Ultimately, she argues, fissures and tremors occur in the types of values and ethics that construct workers' individual and group identities. This occurs in part because at the same time a wider project is at work in the company that requires workers to consent and adhere to company strategies and goals in the setting of an increasing lack of clarity of their own role. (Iamamoto 2005). The worker can experience a sense that their work holds little worth and indeed is more like process work bringing little meaning or reward for them. Iamamoto argues even further that workers become constructed as identities 'drained of history' (Iamamoto 2005, p. 144). This clearly operates in opposition to the goal of a civil society that critical social work advocates and strives for.

In the Australian context, we see the implementation of work conditions within these neoliberal parameters. Devolution of major social welfare work in the human services sector is being handed to 'flexibly' employed workers: flexible work hours, loads, qualifications and employee rights. It is true that social workers are assisted in the construction of their approach to work by their codes of ethics, practice culture, and the systematic production and dissemination of knowledge within the professional culture. They remain at the mercy, however, of the same flexible approaches which may sit contrary to their practices. They also sit with other workers who are employed in the very same work descriptions and sites but who may not have this background of knowledge and professional culture. Whilst the pay scales of each worker may be influenced by a worker's qualifications, little else differs in their shared neo-liberal constructed workplace.

Case Study: Mission Australia

At present Mission Australia run over 500 community services including community housing, employment and training, and programmes working with individuals who are homeless. While Mission Australia itself has existed as an organisation for over 150 years, in many respects their rise has been meteoric since they launched in their current form in early 2000 (Mission Australia 2010). Across Australia this organisation alone employs nearly 4000 workers. See Table 14.1 for a summary of the programs.

Table 14.1: Mission Australia Programs

Program area	Number of programs (2013)
Children and families	169
Youth	91
Homelessness	104
Work ready skills	41
Employment	167
Total	**572**

(Mission Australia 2013: 1)

Briskman, Pease and Allan state the: 'Dominance of economic paradigms reveals itself to social workers in a number of ways, including the increased corporatisation of the human services sector, including contractual arrangements which see services delivered less and less by government itself. Social workers are both perpetrators and victims in this process' (Briskman, et al. 2009: 8).

If this is true in the case of Mission Australia, how could Mission Australia be perpetrators and victims of economic paradigms and models? How could this affect how the service deals with their clients?

Aboriginal workers

One group of workers who are increasingly affected, perhaps as a result of this new era, are Aboriginal people. Since the 1960s or 1970s there has been a gradual increase of Aboriginals across the employment spectrum. Prior to now, the employment conditions for Aboriginal people in the workplace have been predominantly as para-professionals or workers without a formal qualification. The historical treatment of Aboriginal people left them at the margins of Australian society and resulted in little or no Aboriginal people graduating from higher education until the mid to late 1960s. Hence, it is not surprising that there are now small, but increasing, numbers of professionally trained Aboriginal and Torres Strait Island people. Graduates in education, social sciences, law and other areas through the 1970s, 1980s and 1990s, quickly found employment outside their formal area of training as many government bodies employed graduates into their graduate programs. The result has been that in areas such as teaching and health, there have not been as many who practised their profession, as there have been graduates. Early on, graduates could also get paid larger sums of money for being in government work and for impoverished families, this swayed their employment decisions.

As the availability of Aboriginal workers has increased, and flexibility and government programs including employment targets have made them desirable candidates to hire, it has now become the workplaces' challenge to incorporate and value Aboriginal employees in these workplaces. However, Iamamoto's (2005) argument suggests an interesting challenge for workplaces. On the one hand, workers are universally perceived as 'drained of history' but for an Aboriginal employee it is crucial that the workplace, and critical social workers, are aware of crucial historical markers in Australia's history. Dominant ideologies within the neoliberal project would argue that progress for Aboriginal people would be best created through the implementation of economic development strategies. Employment hence fits nicely into the neoliberal agenda. It is crucial though that the employment of Aboriginal people must consider historical, economical or experiential viewpoints, or those very workers could experience detrimental or harmful work environments (Briskman, Pease & Allan 2009).

Interestingly, the premise that the neoliberal approach to economic matters leads to social inequalities plays out in the campaign 'Stop. Think. Respect' by positive mental health organisation, BeyondBlue. This campaign launched in 2014 and it recognises that discrimination and racism are a common experience in the day-to-day life of individual Aboriginal and Torres Strait Islander Australians, and more than half of Australians surveyed had witnessed specific discriminatory behaviours. In fact, one in five (21 per cent) of the participants surveyed believed it was hard to treat Aboriginal people the same way as everyone else (BeyondBlue 2014). This might be misconstrued as emanating from within a 'positive discrimination' framework except for the complementary result that 70 per cent of the sample group argue that 'almost everyone is racist at some point in their lives' (BeyondBlue 2014: 6).

The survey goes on to examine two other related issues important to the discussion here. The first is that what actually constitutes discriminatory behaviour is not understood. For instance, 40 per cent of respondents did not consider telling jokes about Aboriginal people as an act of discrimination. Almost half of the respondents did not consider moving away when an Aboriginal person sits near them as discrimination. The second was that respondents (30 per cent) thought that while their acts of discrimination had occurred unconsciously, they appeared relatively unmotivated to change their behaviour (BeyondBlue 2014). This potentially holds serious implications for the workplace and the reflective practice of critical social workers in that workplace. The acts of discrimination discussed in the survey may occur regularly in the workplace, but it appears that individuals might not understand their acts to be racist and the neoliberal construct of the workplace which emphasises competition and the illusion of fairness does not encourage people to recognise that this may be occurring in a systematic way against a group of people. It would seem unreasonable that Aboriginal people, having fought numbers of campaigns for equal treatment in Australian society, are exposed to a greater number of racist acts because of the nature of the workplace itself.

There are another two findings in the research that are crucial to a critical social worker's reflective practice and practice standards. The first is that 75 per cent of respondents recognised that experiencing discrimination would have a negative personal impact on Aboriginal people, but that one in three respondents thought that those subjected to discrimination would not care that it had happened. However, there was a great awareness (81 per cent) that there may be a mental health impact on Aboriginal people resulting from the discrimination. Most importantly, 57 per cent said they would say something or intervene if they witnessed intolerance of discrimination against Aboriginal people but that percentage went up to 67 per cent if they had had more personal experiences of Aboriginal people (BeyondBlue 2014: 5).

Aboriginality as a skill

Critical social work practice means examining yourself and committing to personal and social transformation. Looking at the beliefs that we as individual social workers hold, and how we grapple with the questions raised by the contexts we work with, is core critical social work. Some of our reflections must involve considering how we operate with Aboriginal people as our colleagues, as fellow social workers or how we look within and reflect on our own Aboriginality. Briskman, Pease and Allan (2009) report that many organisations are reticent to engage or support engagement with critical and emancipatory concepts and actions. The question then is how does a social worker, whether Aboriginal or not, take up the challenge presented by self-reflection and emancipatory concepts when the organisational context is opposed to such considerations? Some workers choose to organise informal support groups with other like-minded individuals in their organisations. Some organise support outside their organisation; for instance, with their professional organisations, like the Australian Association of Social Workers. Some Aboriginal workers will also support each other in groups with agencies as well. It is essential that both social workers and organisations ensure unfair or inequitable employment conditions do not exist. This may, however, stand in the face of what the neoliberal agenda would prioritise.

The self-reflection of social workers also means addressing the predominant expectation that usually Aboriginal people in welfare organisations are the clients and not the fellow workers. When Aboriginal people have been employed at workplaces they have often been employed as liaison officers or consultants on cultural issues or as a conduit to engaging with other Aboriginal people. This has constructed assumptions of what an Aboriginal person brings to a workplace. Part of this is considering whether we are working on the assumption that the Aboriginal person has embedded 'Aboriginal cultural knowledge'. This leads us to examine whether we assume people have cultural knowledge and what happens when they do not hold such knowledge. It is important that Aboriginal people are employed for the expertise and skills they hold in the same way others are employed.

In some instances, the employment of Aboriginal people, in a conscious effort to respond to the needs identified in communities, is very important. The employment of Aboriginal people is right and just and in communities where they are a larger percentage of the population, they should be understood as one valuable resource to assist organisations to do their work. Due to past experiences and inequality, it is also true that Aboriginal people will make up part of the client group of community service agencies. Current statistics indicate that Aboriginal people tend to remain predominantly at the lower end of socioeconomic and health status measures.

The actual advertisement for Aboriginal people holding Aboriginality as one of their qualifications is another part of this interesting discussion. That is, if Aboriginality is a qualification, what is it that employers expect in this employee? One would imagine there is a conception of what Aboriginality is. So, is this recognition:

- of particular Aboriginal informed communication skills?
- of connections or family relationships in an Aboriginal community?
- of professional and private connections that the person can use to make their job easier?
- that the individual will be able to work to Aboriginal community norms?
- that the individual will be able to translate the employer's needs and norms for their Aboriginal clients?
- that workers identified as Aboriginal people will want to work with the organisation's Aboriginal clients?
- that the worker will want to be identified as an Aboriginal person within the organisation?
- that the worker may not be as qualified as a non-Aboriginal employee in their qualifications (for instance they may not necessarily be required to hold a degree)?
- to mean that their cases will be based on Aboriginal clients, if they are employed as a 'case-manager–Aboriginal'?
- that supervision will include both workload and the implementation of Aboriginality?

It is an important question for all social workers and organisations to ask if the Aboriginal worker is asked to utilise a large area of expertise. It is a good question to ask about how non-Aboriginal colleagues and employers support and supervise these workers and their work. It is also paramount that the workplace understands their expectations for that worker. The organisation also needs to reflect whether the worker is being paid for this expertise.

The current legal perspective according to the Australian Law Reform Commission of who is an Aboriginal person includes three parts:

> 'Aboriginal descent, self-identification and community recognition [when for] for determining eligibility for certain programs and benefits.'

On the other hand, when attempting to interpret the definitions utilised in Commonwealth legislaton, the courts tend to emphasise:

> 'the importance of descent in establishing Aboriginal identity, but have recognised that self-identification and community recognition may be relevant to establishing descent, and hence Aboriginal identity, for the purposes of specific legislation (ALRC 2014).

The *Anti-Discrimination Act 1977* (NSW) section 14 identifies that it is legally acceptable to target jobs or services to a particular group especially where, for instance, there is a perception of a 'special need' held by the group. Within these parameters, comes the ability to seek to employ Aboriginal people to Section 14 Exception-genuine occupational qualification '(d) providing persons of a particular race with services for the purpose of promoting their welfare where those services can most effectively be provided by a person of the same race' (AustLII 2014).

What aspects of Aboriginality then are translatable skills for the neoliberal constructed workplace and what does this mean for critical social work practice? Many positions are advertised, such as the two examples examined here, specifically for Aboriginal workers stating that being Aboriginal is a genuine occupational qualification as specified under Section 14 of the *Anti-Discrimination Act 1977* (NSW). Family and Community Services, the statutory body responsible for child protection in New South Wales, employs Aboriginal caseworkers whose major responsibilities include 'consulting and advising on Aboriginal children who are at risk, and the placement of Aboriginal children and young people who are in out-of-home care' (FCS 2014). This fits well within the perspective of employing the skills to suit the area of need, but it also reinforces a perspective of an almost interchangeable worker. In this case, the interchangeability is the signifier 'Aboriginal'; that one Aboriginal worker is the same or similar to other Aboriginal workers.

All caseworkers are expected to have skills in 'analysing and solving problems; planning and organising, building relationships, working with children and young adults' (FCS 2014). Coming into the job, you would be expected to have some experience via placements, volunteer work or previous paid work working with young people or families. Degrees in welfare, social science, social work and related disicplines are required for caseworkers.

So it may be assumed that the Aboriginal worker only requires their self-identification as Aboriginal to work with Aboriginal clients, whereas other caseworkers need a degree as a signifier of other required skills.

This illustration is perhaps made clearer in Wesley Mission's advertisement for an Indigenous Support Facilitator. In this advertisement, they state that the potential employee will hold relevant tertiary qualifications and substantial years of relevant experience or an 'equivalent level of expertise attained through previous appointments, service and study' (Wesley Mission 2014:1). What is crucial in this appointment is the identification and extrapolation of what Aboriginality might mean as a qualification in Wesley Mission's work. They identify essential criteria to include the following:

- Aboriginality and demonstrated ability to work with and understand the needs of Aboriginal communities
- ability to engage and work in a culturally appropriate way with culturally and linguistically diverse peoples
- comprehensive understanding of the local community and social determinants of health.
- experience in developing and maintaining effective networks and relationships, in particular with Aboriginal communities and health sector organisations.
- sound interpersonal and communication skills, including the ability to develop meaningful relationships whilst respecting traditional culture and values.
- demonstrated experience in building and maintaining partnerships across a broad range of sectors.
- a strong capacity to work with challenging issues, at both the client, service delivery and systems levels.
- ability to engage and work in a culturally appropriate way with Aboriginal and Torres Strait Islander people (Wesley Mission 2014: 1).

Increasingly, the outcomes of deliberate child removals and other destruction of Aboriginal communities and families, has led to people who claim Aboriginal heritage but are unfamiliar with their families, traditional country or community of origin and lack any insider knowledge of Aboriginal communication styles, lived cultures or norms. While this chapter is not challenging how these people's identities are formed or indeed their intentions, what it does illustrate is that an employing organisation may not gain the skills such as networking and an understanding of Aboriginal culture they thought they were getting by utilising the 3B Racial Discrimination Act exemption.

Organisations are concluding (or they must reach this conclusion) that there is the need to clearly articulate what skills are required. If the decision for legal or moral reasons exists to continue using the exemption, the skills audit must still be fulfilled. There will be some people who fulfil the skills audit who will not be Aboriginal. What does the personal experience of being Aboriginal bring to that organisation? Perhaps it is the other parts of the definition. For instance, are the skills required that they are known by the community and know the community, and that they know how the community works, who are the leaders and how to negotiate and operate within protocols and respect? Do they know those things because they are related to it and have an embedded place within it? Would it be enough that the person has the skills of communication but may be new to the community that they will be working with? Of course there are many non-Aboriginal people who live and love within Aboriginal communities.

There must be a very careful explanation of why an Aboriginal worker is required and how they will be supported once employed. The support provided must recognise the expertise that worker brings. They must also be prepared to work in the organisation as an advocate and activist against racism or bullying.

What does good practice look like?

How do critical theory-informed social workers work through these issues and what part then does critical social work have in this discussion? The International Federation of Social Workers (IFSW) advocates that organisations must ensure sufficient resources to meet needs and maintain standards of good practice. The organisations must uphold ethical practice standards and good-quality services through, for instance, good-quality ongoing training. The IFSW argue that the best services are those where employers work together with employees in a respectful and ethical manner understanding the work task together. Good practice is constructed within the framework of 'effective induction, supervision, workload management and continuing professional development' (IFSW 2012).

The IFSW also advocate that implementing and upholding principles of human rights and social justice are the basis of social work practice and thus any breach must be confronted. In the case of Aboriginal workers, those around them must be prepared to recognise the injustice of assuming Aboriginality is a qualification all Aboriginal people hold equally. History tells us this cannot be so, especially given the deliberate goal of assimilation policies to make Aboriginality disappear. It is also an injustice to assume Aboriginal people are not social workers or fellow professionals and are only ever the client.

The critical social worker must be able to access ongoing training and supervision, a reasonable workload, and an unthreatening, safe work for themselves and all employees of the organisation. A quality or a qualification, whether it is Aboriginality or a social work degree or both, are what helps gain initial employment but they are not what keep workers effective as workers. What is required is ongoing training, self-reflection, supervision and good organisation support. All organisations informed by a critical perspective will allow the strengthening and development of skills and knowledge, particularly as it allows organisations themselves to develop a better service model.

Part of building staff satisfaction and resilience includes understanding about each worker's career path. For Aboriginal people employed into liaison positions, this career path often has been non-existent. This means that little motivation will exist to develop advanced practice skills, particularly where the worker is understood to only be able to work with the Aboriginal client. This has a twofold disadvantage. One part is that the Aboriginal worker may be denied an opportunity for advancement. The other part is that other workers, in allocating Aboriginal clients to the Aboriginal worker, do not advance their own practice capabilities in this area. Unions and professional associations have always presented the opportunity to develop concepts of quality practice and what constitutes an appropriate working environment. Their continued involvement can assist the critical social worker gain understandings for their own practice and their own emancipation as well as broader social actions. Social work must continue to see the society wide implications of economic and social agendas.

Conclusion

This chapter has reinforced the impetus for social workers to understand their practice within the new world order of neoliberalism. While showing how neoliberalism has now constructed our nations and workplaces, it has also argued that we must continue to fight against it. The health and wellbeing of our nations and people within them is only benefited by the extension of social protectionism. At a micro level though, we as social workers, must remain aware of the inequities around us. We must look at our own practice and employment circumstances, and actively critique what is occurring to us and our fellow colleagues. We must continue to reflect within emancipatory ideals and understand peoples' lives as having history and value leading to their current stage of life. Structural inequality does exist and as the BeyondBlue organisation has shown, racism and discrimination have real physical and mental health effects on the people who experience them. Our actions, together with our colleagues and fellow citizens, must contribute to improving all people's lives. Part of this transformation must be opening our workplaces in diverse ways, including diverse ways of working and a diversity of the people who work in them. This requires workers to be acutely self-reflective but also externalise their anti-racist and anti-bullying stances. Critical social work is a life-long obligation but given that the challenges of our world will keep changing, so we must continue to re-articulate our commitment to social justice and fairness.

References

ALRC *see* Australian Law Reform Commission

AustLII 1977, 'Anti-Discrimination Act 1977—Sect 14', Australian Legal Information Institute (*AustLII),* <www.austlii.edu.au/au/legis/nsw/consol_act/aa1977204/s14.html>, accessed 16 June 2014

Australian Law Reform Commission (ALRC) 2014, 'The three-part definition', *ALRC,* <www.alrc.gov. au/publications/36-kinship-and-identity/legal-definitions-aboriginality>, accessed 16 June 2014

BeyondBlue 2014, 'Discrimination against Indigenous Australians: A snapshot of the views of non-Indigenous people aged 25–44', *BeyondBlue* <www.beyondblue.org.au/resources/for-me/ aboriginal-and-torres-strait-islander-people/stop-think-respect-campaign>, accessed 6 August 2014

Briskman, L., Pease, B. & Allan, J. 2009, 'Introducing critical theories for social work in a neo-liberal context' in J. Allan, L. Briskman and B. Pease (eds*), Critical Social Work: Theories and practices for a socially just world*, 2nd edn, *St Leonards:* Allen & Unwin, pp. 3–14

FCS *see* NSW Government, Family and Community Services

Iamamoto, M.V. 2005, 'Social work: Analytic contributions to professional practice'*, Revista Katálysis*, 8 (July-December), <www.redalyc.org/articulo.oa?id=179616343001>, accessed 4 August 2014

IFSW *see* International Federation of Social Workers

International Federation of Social Workers (IFSW) 2012, 'Effective and ethical environments for social work: The responsibilities of employers of social workers', *IFSW,* <http://ifsw.org/ policies/effective-and-ethical-working-environments-for-social-work-the-responsibilities-of-employers-of-social-workers-3>, accessed 6 August 2012

ILO 2014a, 'ILO: Invest more in social protection', *ILO,* <www.ilo.org/global/about-the-ilo/multimedia/ audio/WCMS_245388/lang—en/index.htm> , accessed 5 August 2014

—— 2014b, 'World Social Protection Report', *ILO,* <www.ilo.org/wcmsp5/groups/public/—dgre-ports/—dcomm/documents/publication/wcms_245201.pdf>, accessed 5 August 2014

—— 2014c, 'World Social Protection Report 2014/15: Building economic recovery, inclusive development and social justice', *ILO,* <www.ilo.org/wcmsp5/groups/public/—dgreports/—dcomm/ documents/publication/wcms_245131.pdf>, accessed 5 August 2014

International Labour Organisation *see* ILO

Mission Australia. 2010, 'Annual Report', *Mission Australia,* https://www.missionaustralia.com.au/ publications/annual-reports/annual-report-2010>, accessed 19 June 2014

—— 2013, 'Summary of the year 2012–2013', *Mission Australia*, < >,https://www.missionaustralia.com. au/publications/annual-reports/annual-report-2013 accessed 19 June 2014

NSW Government, Family and Community Services (FCS) 2014, 'Caseworker careers at Community Services', *FCS,* <www.community.nsw.gov.au/docs_menu/about_us/careers/caseworker_careers. html>, accessed 16 June 2014

Wesley Mission 2014, 'Partners in Recovery (PIR) Program—Indigenous Support Facilitator (Identified)'*, Wesley Mission,* <www.wesleymission.org.au/posvac/posvac/attachments/1262_-_ Application_Kit_-PIR_Support_Facilitator_-_Indigenous.pdf>, accessed 16 June 2014

15

Feminism under siege: critical reflections on the impact of neoliberalism and managerialism on feminist practice

Ann Carrington

Introduction

This chapter focuses on the 'doing' aspect of feminist practice in an Australian political and organisational environment, which I argue is steeped in the neoliberal agenda. The chapter discusses some key constraints and practical responses to feminist social work practice in terms of the sector that deals with domestic violence and sexual assault in the current climate of neoliberalism and managerialism. Through a critical reflective process, it is acknowledged that the culture, structure and policy frameworks articulated by neoliberal and managerialist positions have impacted on feminist practices. These impacts are often simply perceived as a negative; yet it is proposed here that tensions created in the current context may also provide an opportunity for subversive feminist practices with key organisations to further feminist agendas and social change. Although located in a specific sector, it is suggested that the experiences reflected upon here, and the practice responses discussed, are transferable. Through reflection on practice, five key areas impacted by the neo-liberal and managerialist agenda were identified: stifling of activism, collaboration and partnership, keeping gender on the agenda, management and education and training. Although these five key areas have been identified, these are all components of the larger threat of the current environment—that being attempts to dismantle feminist practices. This chapter speaks to the practical application of feminist social work in each of the identified areas with the overarching focus of practice being to maintain the feminist gains that have been made to 'hold the line' and to advance feminist practices in a hostile political environment.

Positioning the author and the reflective process

The personal is political, coined in Carol Hanisch's article first published in 1969 titled 'The personal is political', captures a core concept within feminism in that what occurs within the private spheres 'personal problems' (Hanisch 2006) are a result of the public or political sphere. As Phillips asserts, 'emphasizing that the personal is political, the women's movement forced private spheres of patriarchal domination in relation to sexuality, work and violence, onto the public policy agenda' (Phillips 2006: 203). In recognising that the personal is political, we see that individuals cannot be separated from the wider political context and that personal experience and what we do in the private sphere is also political (Hanisch 1969). As such, it is important to position myself and my engagement with feminism before addressing the focus of this chapter.

The reflections and practice responses presented in this chapter have been processed through my ideological positioning, world views and multiple identities informed by my personal life experience and professional life experience working in the sexual assault, domestic violence and women's sector. I cannot speak to the experiences of others' background and positioning and share the reflections in this chapter not as prescribed practices but as a point of reflection for readers to analyse and interpret through their own experiences, knowledge, positioning and world views. Critical reflection is an integral component of any critical and feminist social work approach and includes the practice of reflectivity and reflexivity (Morley 2009; Fook 2012). As mentioned, this chapter is based on my process of reflecting on practice in the specific context of women's services.

In line with critical and feminist methods that require the acknowledgement of one's own positioning or bias (Ackerly & True 2010), I provide some aspects of my identity that are relevant to the context of this chapter. I am a white, middle class, woman, able bodied, educated, social worker, mother of a son, sole parent, first-generation Australian of British descent, who is spiritual, and a feminist. Although each of these aspects of subjectivity could be further unpacked, the one that requires most attention is 'feminist'. Although I identify as a feminist, both personally and professionally, I do not label myself as a particular 'type' of feminist and I certainly do not feel I fit neatly into any one category of feminism. However, I do identify that major contributions to my practice and theoretical understandings are radical (Taylor 2007) and follow second-wave feminist principles (Dean 2009) with post-modern theory (Orme 2003) providing an additional complexity and dimension. The core and unwavering component that contributes to my feminist position and practice is my lived experience of being a woman in this colonised Australian society, within the global context, in this historical period.

The reflections presented in this chapter were further supported by a shared reflective process with the manager of a domestic violence service who has an Anglo-Celtic background from the UK and who identifies as feminist. We engaged in a process of shared reflection, which was audio recorded. The recording of our conversation has informed some aspects of this chapter and was a starting point for my further reflections, which continued through the exploration of literature and the writing process.

Contemporary understandings of feminism

While women's movements have been a constant presence throughout history, feminist theory within the social work context is somewhat newer and resulted from the women's movement of the 1960s and 1970s (Morley 2009). Feminist theory and practice is complex and includes a wide range of standpoints and influences. At the ideological level, the continuum ranges from conservative and liberal to radical and socialist (Taylor 2007). Liberal feminism focuses on achieving equality within existing social, economic and political structures (Taylor 2007). Radical and socialist feminism seeks change at a structural level in the form of dismantling the capitalist, racist, patriarchal system (Taylor 2007). Feeding into these different ideological positions are the different waves of feminism from the first wave, which focused on equal rights in areas such as property and voting, through to the emerging fourth wave which stills hold to the central tenet of equality but has less rigid parameters (Phillips & Cree 2014). Within the ideological spectrum and waves are a range of additional perspectives from black feminism to lesbian feminism. Each of these focuses on a specific concern or provides a further critique (Gray & Boddy 2010). Positioning within the modern or postmodern paradigms then adds a further layer of complexity. While the modern approach asserts collective social action by women from a universalist perspective, postmodernism emphasises the subjective experience, personal change and diversity among women (Morley 2009). These two positionings within the feminist context have created tensions that are still being resolved.

In spite of the diversity of feminist positionings and theories, there are some principles and methods that can be generally attributed to feminist practice. At a theoretical level, Weeks (2003) suggested there are four basic premises of feminist practice. First, that the personal is political as discussed above. Second, that structural change must occur to change the social, economic and political experience of women. Third, that personal pains or problems affecting women need to be recognised as a normal response to oppression and should be dealt with as such rather than blaming women. Fourth, that organisations are transformed to deliver appropriate services to respond to women's needs and issues.

To achieve these ends, a range of different practice methods have been developed and utilised by feminist practitioners. These include, but are not limited to, education or consciousness raising, empowerment and advocacy, group work, collective activism, normalisation, deconstruction of patriarchal norms, applying a gendered analysis, egalitarian relationships and reflexivity (Dominelli 2002; Weeks 2003; Payne 2014; Phillips 2015). Many of these methods are not exclusive to feminist practice and are common across critical approaches. In addition to these, Dominelli (2002) outlines a range of practices and principles that she claims are unique to feminist practice.

Having established the breadth of feminist parameters and practice approaches, it is important to note that although aspects of the principles and practices outlined above are discussed within this chapter, the focus is not on the specific details of these practices but rather on methods to resist attempts to dismantle feminist practice. It is also concerned with how to maintain and strengthen feminist approaches within the current context to achieve social change that benefits women. It is important to reiterate that as there is such diversity within a feminist approach that the reflections shared here are not universal and do not speak for the range of feminisms or all feminist practitioners. It is also relevant to note that the feminist application in practice and the organisation context is reflective of this diversity. Phillips' (2015) recent work further illustrates this in capturing that globally women's services are not only working from a range of feminist positions but also from positions not associated with feminism.

Stifling activism

Reflecting on the current constraints, there was a sense felt by my colleague and I that feminism and feminist practice was under siege. There was a fear, supported by Morley and MacFarlane (2008), that practice in public action and agitation may ultimately result in services losing funding or being engulfed by a larger, generic service, not specifically focused on violence against women where a feminist analysis may be diminished or lost. Ishkanian (2014) highlights similar fears within the sector in the UK and provides examples of instances where organisations lost funding contracts to generic agencies as a result of public agitation. Ishkanian (2014) argues that these incidences have worked to fuel fear and maintain compliance within the sector. This point was a major focus in the shared reflective process with the manager of the domestic violence service. She spoke at length regarding this fear and spoke of strategies to circumvent such outcomes. An example provided was the creation of new partnerships with larger agencies that did not necessarily align in terms of services but did align in terms of values. The idea being that if required, a joint application for funding would have a greater opportunity for success against a larger generic agency with no political voice or mandate in this area. If successful, this would stop the service from being engulfed by the generic organisation and allow for the continuation of feminist principles to inform the service.

This focus on survival has shifted the focus from public activism to resistance and subversive action within the current social structure (Thomas & Davies 2005). This approach is, as Wallace and Pease (2011) highlight, about finding the spaces to resist the neoliberal agenda and to maintain a feminist analysis. This resistance presents in practice as efforts to subvert (Carey & Foster 2011) the structures to actively promote feminist agendas, not from the 'outside-in' but from the 'inside-out' (Thomas & Davies 2005). Subversive action is not new to feminist practice, as both subversive and public actions have been used historically to great effect (Turiel 2003; Thomas & Davies 2005). Subversive action was particularly common for femocrats within the Australian (Chappell 2002; Pini, Panelli & Sawer 2008) and the international (Charles 2004) context. However, the need to increase the use of subversive practice and decrease public action may be due to fear of losing funding and other forms of reprisal within the neoliberal context.

Silencing the voices of feminism and the stifling of activism (McDonald 2005; Nichols 2011; 2013; Ishkanian 2014) emerge as the core impact of the neoliberal agenda. A further complexity to the silencing of feminist voices is the recognition that many of the constraints now being experienced are as a result of the successful activism of the past (Lehrner & Allen 2009). However, within the current context, activism was identified as the area most constrained and creates a filter-down effect substantially impacting the other key areas identified: collaboration and partnership, keeping gender on the agenda, education and training and management. In addition to the neoliberal agenda, the general backlash against feminism (Dominelli 2002) and the reduced support of feminist agendas by the public (Macy et al. 2010) further contribute to stifling feminist activism and add to the complexity when deciding between public activism and subversive action.

Collaboration and partnership

Collectivism and collaboration are foundational tenets of feminist practices (Payne 2014). The power and strength that came from the actions of collectives of women allowed agencies not only to give voice to issues affecting a diverse range of women, but to stand up and critique organisations and governmental policies that continued to oppress women (Macy et al. 2010). Within the current neoliberal context, these partnerships are being challenged and eroded to make room for forced collaborations and partnerships with the very agencies that feminists once spoke out against (Ishkanian 2014). This approach has the potential to silence the political voices of women's collectives and agencies and to jeopardise the continuation of small agencies, which are informed by feminist principles (McDonald 2005; Ishkanian 2014). As Charles (2004) asserts, to ensure women's issues are on the political agenda it may require that issues be framed in a way that resonates with liberal or dominant discourse which then changes how the problem is responded to. Although feminists often use this process to ensure services and funding, it ultimately moves away from radical ideas of changing underlying social structures (Charles 2004). In Australia, domestic violence is framed as a crime and places the response largely within the criminal and justice systems. This shifted the focus from changing patriarchal structures and power relations within society to focus on individuals within the context of the criminal and legal systems (Charles 2004). As a result, the old partnerships formed through a common goal of social change are being forcibly replaced by policy and funding body requirements. This replacement is achieved by establishing partnerships between domestic violence agencies and representatives from the legal and justice system.

This shift in partnerships or collaborations, although they're having a stifling effect, has also provided opportunities to have voices on the inside of key oppressive structures (Macy et al. 2010) and to guarantee issues such as domestic violence stay on the political agenda. The tension remains that while it is on the agenda, it is framed in a way that no longer defines the problem as an issue of men's violence against women (Charles 2004). The question then is how do we maintain feminist approaches within these partnerships that will address the underlying patriarchal structural causes of domestic violence? Strategic subversive approaches from within (Thomas & Davies 2005) these partnerships then become a must for feminist social workers.

The key to this approach being effective is in building strong and trusting relationships with significant partners. Through taking the time to build trusting relationships, one can advance feminist agendas through continuous consciousness-raising with key individuals inside organisations that perpetuate inequality. Reflecting on my practice, I found this allowed for change to occur at various levels through the education of key individuals with change then filtering throughout the partner organisations. This is done by building on the strength of the relationships of key people, then establishing trust with workers across organisations. An example of what can be achieved and some of the tensions that present within the context of a trusted relationship and subtle action from within partnerships are discussed in the following case study.

Case Study

This case study is an example from practice in which a partnership was tested after a local homicide. Members of the domestic violence service were to attend a public function and in recognition of the homicide being perceived as related to domestic violence had planned to wear the traditional red rose. An external partner with some power who would also be attending heard about this and promptly contacted the service directing them not to wear the red rose as it was not established that the homicide was a domestic violence incident. Following the conversation, members of the service and other supporting services wore the red rose that day with acceptance from the partner organisation.

What was achieved? Within this case study, the established relationship allowed this situation to be used as a 'teachable moment' to educate the partner organisation as to what wearing the red rose meant. With trust already established, the external partner's fears of public activism that would be disruptive and upstage the public event were appeased. The outcome was further building trust within the partner relationship as the action was no longer perceived as a threat, increased consciousness raising of the partner organisation as they now understood the meaning behind wearing the red rose, presence of a feminist analysis brought via the consciousness-raising process, maintenance of an intact partnership required by funding bodies as any room for miscommunication and aggression from either side was managed and a feminist activism achieved publically with acceptance, in the space of those who tried to oppose it.

In practical terms, such an approach to collaboration and partnerships over time assisted the organisation and workers within to use the knowledge and skills of the partners to the advantage of clients on a daily basis. This meant that advocacy for clients within these often hostile networks was more effective, ensuring not only basic health, wellbeing and safety outcomes but also more just and equitable treatment and outcomes for clients of the service.

Tensions that were present included the following one. There was the concern that an outside organisation could have such a powerful impact on the autonomy of the agency and stifle its political voice. Concern and fear of reprisal from the partner organisation and funding body needs to be considered in regard to providing services for clients. However, which is more important? Is it the continued partnership and ongoing funding to assist clients on a daily basis within the presence of such constraints? Or is it the public and political action that challenges the systems and structure for long-term social change? Noting that these are not exclusive, how does one balance these tensions when making decisions? In an act of resistance the red rose was worn and those who understood what it meant would have received the message. It was not explicitly explained, which meant that this moment of activism potentially did not reach the larger public audience. Although the partnership was intact and continued to support clients of the service, did it come at a cost? These are the tensions that must be navigated daily by feminist practitioners in the current context.

A further form of subversion and resistance in relation to partnerships and collaborations is the maintenance and nurturing of a traditional partnership. At a micro level, these networks allow for agencies to come together to achieve outcomes for individual clients that may not be possible in isolation, due to funding constraints. This is demonstrated by the following example from practice where four different organisations came together with a creative solution to help an extremely isolated and vulnerable woman escape a dangerous situation that did not neatly fit into any of the agencies' funding guidelines. However, together through the informal networks, they were able to rally and respond within a matter of hours. Working together they subverted the systems at the macro level and provided an immediate response at the micro level that would not be impossible within the normal constraints imposed by funding bodies. This approach is a strong remnant of the original beginnings of the feminist movement and a reminder that not all has changed or been lost.

Keeping gender on the agenda

The increased pressure to de-gender, pathologise and individualise many of the women's issues feminists have put on the public agenda places these issues and the services that respond to them at risk (Macy et al. 2010). Therefore, it is important that feminist social workers adopt practices that resist the move to gender neutral, individual and pathological explanations of social problems and apply a gender analysis and use gender language at all times (Morley & MacFarlane 2008). As authors such as Charles (2004), Morley and MacFarlane (2008) and Ishkanian (2014) argue, de-gendering women's issues changes how the cause of the problem is understood and how the problem is responded to. Using the language of domestic violence and framing it as family violence, not as men's violence against women, makes domestic violence the problem or pathology of the individual or family not a social problem that occurs due to the power imbalances within society (Lang 2000; Charles 2004). This framing changes the services and funding available and the experience of those service users (McDonald 2005; Nichols 2011; 2013). In regard to domestic violence, it often leads to victim-blaming processes and practice and continued re-victimisation of already vulnerable women (McDonald 2005; Nichols 2011; 2013). Women are now often prosecuted as using violence in relationships (Nichols 2011) with no consideration of the dynamics or who the predominant aggressor (Kernsmith 2005; Pence & Das Dasgupta 2006; Trujillo & Ross 2008) is or why the women may be using violence (Worcester 2002; Cavanagh 2003). In the broader context, this approach renders men and the patriarchal systems invisible and does not hold them to account.

The danger in this instance, as a feminist social worker, is that one may be convinced that adopting the gender-neutral language and forgoing a gendered analysis is acceptable if it means the continuation of services to women. However, in this instance I would argue that succumbing to the pressure of the current neoliberal context and reframing erodes the very foundations of feminist agendas, which is a cost too high.

The focus of practice in this area is on resisting the de-gendering wherever possible and to raise the consciousness of individuals, which in turn informs policies and practice at the agency and macro levels. Resistance to the gendering of social problems such as violence against women comes from all directions. For example, clients may find it challenging to see the gendered nature of domestic violence. The majority of women I have worked with over the years have been socialised into the dominant discourse believing not only that domestic violence is an individual problem as opposed to a social problem but that they as the victims are to blame. Critical social work process-orientations such as normalisation, consciousness raising and linking the personal with the political (see Chapter 4) are key when working with these women. These concepts allow them the opportunity to see their individual 'problem' from a different perspective (Payne 2014). Highlighting that they are not to blame and that there is a far larger social political dynamic at play that is impacting their private lives (Weeks 2003). Welfare work and social work students often ask 'What about the men?' or state 'Men are victims too'. In both my roles as an academic and a community educator, presenting a lecture or workshop and not having someone make such statements is the exception rather than the rule, even after providing a disclaimer addressing that men are victims too. Police, and those working in the legal system, maintain that domestic violence is equal and it was common to hear statements such as: 'They are as bad as each other' by lawyers, public prosecutors or police officers.

The continued use of gendered language and a gendered analysis in practice is integral in order to stop gendered issues becoming invisible or individualised and to keep the focus on the underlying structural issue that continues to perpetuate inequalities and the abuse of women. However, it is often the use of such language that will invite a negative response from others, at which point the feminist practitioner must be ready to respond with clarity and conviction as to the importance of maintaining a gendered position.

Management

Within the current neoliberal managerial context, the trend is to manage organisations and programs from a business model, often resulting in the employment of managers that have education and training in management but no background in welfare or social work (Macy et al. 2010). This leads to services being generically delivered with no consideration of the social issues addressed within the service and with limited understanding and professional knowledge of the social problems, the practicalities of working in a specific area or holding of feminist agendas. This works well from a managerial perspective but not so well for the clients or the workers on the frontline. It is a particular challenge for services that have historically been politically mobile or part of a political movement such as women's services.

The importance of the managers' ideological positioning in relation to how services were delivered is emphasised by Nichols (2013). In my reflections, it became apparent that although official organisational constitutions, missions, goals and values could be important in directing service delivery, the positioning of the manager often seemed to be more crucial. Reflections on two different organisations help to illustrate this point. The first organisation did not have feminism included in any of its official organisational documents but was run as a feminist organisation for women and children with men included in official mandate. The second organisation had feminist principles firmly embedded in the official organisational statements but was now being managed from a psychological and biomedical framework with no attention to gender analysis. The feminist manager within the 'non-feminist' organisation used the ambiguity of the official organisational statements to create the freedom to position the informal approach from a feminist perspective, while the non-feminist manager within the program that officially operated from a feminist position ignored the feminist principles and changed how services were delivered. This demonstrates the power in the position of the manager and management in directing the unofficial goals, values, culture, and service delivery based on personal and professional ideology. Phillips' (2015) recent works illustrate this pattern at a global scale where respondents to a survey of women's organisations globally recorded a wide range of responses as to whether they identified as feminist or not.

As a feminist social worker, this was an invaluable insight as it demonstrated the power of 'one' within the organisational context. With good management skills, one can expand a feminist position to an organisational approach rather than simply an individual approach. In the current environment of managerialism, core feminist social work skills need to include training and education in management to ensure such roles can be filled by feminist social workers. To enhance this training, it is essential for feminist management theory to be included. This training should pay particular attention to the lessons drawn from a femocrat approach in relation to the tensions and difficulties in changing the patriarchal nature of organisations (Chappell 2002).

Education and training

The effective use of education and training, in terms of power and influence, is important in a management role. This component of feminist practice is not just specific to the women's services field but also important within the academy. Nichols' (2013) work illustrated that non-feminist workers actively engage in feminist practice skills, not through personal identification with feminist ideals, but purely through training and education. This highlights that it is crucial to introduce feminist practices at a larger scale that not only resists the impact of neoliberalism through the training of staff in feminist principles, but also strengthens and maintains the use of feminist knowledge and practices. From a management position, one can direct what approaches are used within the organisation or program and provide the required training and education to staff to ensure these practices are maintained (Nichols 2013). Ensuring staff receive training informed by feminist analyses means that staff, feminist or not, will be practising in a way that is aligned with feminist ideals. The tension here is that although they may engage in the feminist practice, it is not ideologically informed, thus restricting the outcomes to micro practice and not social change (Lehrner & Allen 2009; Nichols 2013). This highlights the added importance of keeping gender on the agenda and providing education in feminist analysis.

Education and training within the practice setting also has a component of providing training to external agencies that is informed by a feminist analysis. This can be done both formally and informally. Many agencies still have provision within their funding to produce and deliver formal education and training to other agencies and the general community. This can be seen as an opportunity to not just resist the stifling of feminism, but as a consciousness-raising opportunity at the individual, agency and collective levels. Unfortunately, it is my experience the radical component of such training and education has somewhat been curtailed within the current political context and the public backlash towards feminism.

It is also important to recognise education within the universities in this context. However, it must be noted that the neoliberal and managerial agenda also influences the academy (Thomas & Davies 2002), with many of the risks associated with practice in the field also relevant in the context of the academy. Academics holding to a feminist agenda may experience pressure to let go of feminist content, with much of this pressure coming from students themselves. As a social work academic, this has been a point of concern for me given that social work is a predominantly women's profession (Weeks 2003) and that a majority of our practice and intervention are with and directly impact women and children (Orme 2003).

Although the neoliberal agenda has to some extent constrained how the feminist message may be delivered, it does not negate the importance of this role within a feminist approach. Education and training are still powerful methods, not only to resist, but to advance feminist agendas. Education and consciousness raising are cornerstone practices of feminism (Payne 2014) that require holding to in the current environment even if executed more strategically.

Conclusion

It is hoped that in sharing the reflections in this chapter, some aspects of feminist practice will be revitalised for students and practitioners. This chapter provides some possible practice responses to the constraints of neoliberalism and managerialism on feminist practice and it highlights further concerns in regard to the tensions present in this response. For those practising from a feminist framework within the current context, learning to negotiate the tensions created by the constraints, competing needs and outcomes is perhaps the most important practice skill to be developed. Deciding on a form of action, be it public or subversive, needs to be carefully considered in regard to the current constraints and the outcomes we wish to achieve; not just for clients now but in the future through continuing to inform social change.

References

Ackerly, B. & True, J. 2010, *Doing Feminist Research in Political and Social Science*, New York: Palgrave MacMillan

Carey, M. & Foster, V. 2011, 'Introducing "deviant" social work: Contextualising the limits of radical social work whilst understanding (fragmented) resistance within the social work labour process', *British Journal of Social Work*, vol. 41, no. 3, pp. 576–93

Cavanagh, K. 2003, 'Understanding women's responses to domestic violence', *Qualitative Social Work*, vol. 2, no. 3, pp. 229–49

Chappell, L. 2002, *Gendering Government: Feminist engagement with the state in Australia and Canada*, Vancouver: UBC Press

Charles, N. 2004, 'Feminist politics and devolution: A preliminary analysis', *Social Politics*, vol. 11, no. 2, pp. 297–311

Dean, J. 2009, 'Who's afraid of third wave feminism?', *International Feminist Journal of Politics*, vol. 11, pp. 334–52

Dominelli, L. 2002, *Feminist Social Work Theory and Practice*, New York: Palgrave MacMillan

Fook, J. 2012, *Social Work: A critical approach to practice*, Los Angeles: Sage

Gray, M. & Boddy, J. 2010, 'Making sense of the waves: Wipeout or still riding high?', *Affilia*, vol. 25, pp. 368–89

Hanisch, C. 1969/2006, *The personal is political*, <www.carolhanisch.org/CHwritings/PIP.html>, accessed August 2015

Ishkanian, A. 2014, 'Neoliberalism and violence: The big society and the changing politics of domestic violence in England', *Critical Social Policy*, vol. 34, no. 3, pp. 333–53

Kernsmith, P. 2005, 'Exerting power or striking back: A gendered comparison of motivations for Domestic violence perpetration', *Violence and Victims*, vol. 20, no. 2, pp. 173–85

Lang, L. 2000, 'Progress, trends and challenges in Australian responses to domestic violence', Issue Paper 1, Sydney: Australian Domestic and Family Violence Clearinghouse

Lehrner, A. & Allen, N. 2009, 'Still a movement after all these years?: Tensions in the domestic violence movement', *Violence Against Women*, vol. 15, no. 6, pp. 656–77

Macy, R., Giattina, M., Parish, L. & Crosby, C. 2010, 'Domestic violence and sexual assault services: Historical concerns and contemporary challenges', *Journal of Interpersonal Violence*, vol. 25, no. 1, pp. 3–32

McDonald, J. 2005, 'Neoliberalism and the pathologising of public issues: The displacement of feminist service models in domestic violence support services', *Australian Social Work*, vol. 58, no. 3, pp. 275–84

Morley, C. & MacFarlane, S. 2008, 'The continued importance of a feminist analysis: Making gendered inequalities visible through a critique of Howard Government policy on domestic violence', *Just Policy*, no. 47, pp. 31–8

Morley, C. 2009, 'Using critical reflection to improve feminist practice' in J. Allan, L. Briskman & B. Pease (eds), *Critical Social Work: Theories and practices for a socially just world*, 2nd edn, St Leonards: Allen & Unwin, pp. 145–59

Nichols, A.J. 2011, 'Gendered organisations: Challenges for domestic violence victim advocates and feminist advocacy', *Feminist Criminology*, vol. 6, no. 2, pp. 111–31

—— 2013, 'Meaning-making and domestic violence victim advocacy: An examination of feminist identities, ideologies, and practices', *Feminist Criminology*, vol. 8, no. 3, pp. 177–201

Orme, J. 2003, '"It's feminist because I say so!" Feminism, social work and critical practice in the UK', *Qualitative Social Work*, vol. 2, no. 2, pp. 131–53

Payne. M. 2014, *Modern social work theory*, 4th edn, New York: Palgrave MacMillan

Pence, E. & Das Dasgupta, S. 2006, 'Re-examining 'battering': Are all acts of violence against intimate partners the same?', *Praxis International*, Minnesota: Duluth

Phillips, R. 2006, 'Undoing an activist response: Feminism and the Australian government's domestic violence policy, *Critical Social Policy*, vol. 26, no. 1, pp. 129–219

Phillips, R. 2015, 'How "empowerment" may miss its mark: Gender equality policies and how they are understood in women's NGOs', *International Society for Third Sector Research*, Voluntas, DOI 10.1007/s11266-015-9586-y

—— & Cree, V., E. 2014, 'What does the "fourth wave" mean for teaching feminism in twenty-first century social work?', Social Work Education: *The International Journal*, vol. 33, no. 7, pp. 930–943

Pini, B., Panelli, R. & Sawer, M. 2008, 'Managing the Woman Issue', *International Feminist Journal of Politics*, vol. 10, no. 2, pp. 173–97

Taylor, G. 2007 *Welfare and ideology*, New York: Palgrave Macmillan

Thomas, R. & Davies, A. 2002, 'Gender and new public management: Reconstituting academic subjectivities', *Gender, Work and Organisation*, vol. 9, no. 4, pp. 372–97

—— 2005, 'What have the feminists done for us? Feminist theory and organizational resistance', *Organization*, vol. 12, no. 5, pp. 711–40

Trujillo, M.P. & Ross, S. 2008, 'Police responses to domestic violence: Making decisions about risk and risk management', *Journal of Interpersonal Violence*, vol. 23, no. 4, pp. 454–73

Turiel, E. 2003, 'Resistance and subversion in everyday life', *Journal of Moral Education*, vol. 32, no. 2, pp. 115–30

Wallace, J. & Pease, B. 2011, 'Neoliberalism and Australian social work: Accommodation or resistance?', *Journal of Social Work*, vol. 11, no. 2, pp. 132–42

Weeks, W. 2003, 'Women: Developing feminist practice in women's services' in J. Allan, B. Pease & L. Briskman (eds), *Critical social work: An introduction to theories and practices*, St Leonards: Allen & Unwin

Worcester, N. 2002, 'Women's use of force: Complexities and challenges of taking the issue seriously', *Violence Against Women*, vol. 8, no. 11, pp. 1390–415

16

Developing anti-ageist practice in social work

Tina Kostecki

Introduction

A critical approach to social work aims to achieve social justice, and redress inequality, marginalisation and disadvantage (Fook 2002; Briskman et al. 2009). Ostensibly then, critical social work should be the vanguard in its contribution to anti-ageist practice. A critically reflective position on ageing interrogates hegemonic cultural norms which produce systemic ageism, and challenges assumptions regarding what is considered as worthy, ageing lives. Theoretical frames which inform anti-ageist practice must be accessible and draw upon critical theories that fit professional settings (Rexhepi & Torres 2011), and aimed at addressing issues of power, values, authority and internalised privilege (Chambers 2004; Netting 2011). This chapter proposes the integration of perspectives from critical gerontology as a useful and abiding framework for social work in the development of anti-ageist practice and provides an example from research practice.

Ageing is an axiomatic experience for each one of us, and now it is more likely that we will live longer. It is estimated that 22 per cent of Australians will be over 65 years of age by 2061 and that the median age will rise from 37.3 years in 2012 to 44.5 years in 2061 (ABS 2013) due to greater life expectancy and lower levels of fertility in Western societies. Given that our experience of ageing is linked to our social, cultural and political contexts, the implications of growing older in greater numbers will increasingly transform how older people see their identities, and generate the need to reconsider our expectations and understandings of how ageing is conceptualised in society and the potential material circumstances of our later lives. Social work as a profession is yet to engage in a compelling way with theoretical perspectives, research and practice frameworks that adopt a critical approach to working with older adults, although there is some notable progress (for example, Chambers 2004; Crampton 2011; Duncan & Mason 2011; Hokenstad & Roberts 2011; Netting 2011; Ferguson & Schriver 2012). Mostly, deliberation regarding the cultural and social constructs of ageing, ageism, age narratives and social policy emerge from the fields of sociology and gerontology (for example, Phillipson 1998; Minkler & Estes 1999; Wilson 2000; Calasanti & Slevin 2006; Calasanti & King 2011; Aberdeen & Bye 2013).

Theorising age

In all categories of identity such as gender, class, sexuality and race, age is the least theorised (Krekula 2007). Age markers determine life experiences due to the effects of social, employment, housing and health policy as well as personal experiences with respect to how others will respond to us and make summations about competency and character (Sontag 1997; Westerhof & Tulle 2007). A critical theory approach to ageing explores how cultural norms construct age identities. This theoretical approach shows how the nature of individual experience is shaped by social structures, creating inequitable access to wealth and incomes, safety, healthy communities and quality health care (Holstein & Minkler 2003). Generally, practice and research in gerontology has privileged perspectives from functional health paradigms rather than query the 'existential and social challenges of adult ageing' (Biggs 2008: 116). In turn, this has influenced the nature of service provision and professional identity, not only in the health sciences but also in social work, at the expense of the critical recognition of ageism and how it constructs realities.

Additionally, anti-ageist practice in institutional care settings for older people is a significant area for consideration given that older people will constitute the largest group requiring assistance from health care professionals, and because the attitudes of health care providers is associated with quality of care (Eymard & Douglas 2012). Negative attitudes and stereotyping in aged care settings have been linked to psychological abuse, decreased involvement by residents in decisions regarding care, and use of restraints and inappropriate prescription practices (Eymard & Douglas 2012). Specifically in Australia, the devaluing of older people is structurally evident in a medical system that fiscally 'rations' health care for the elderly (Hitchcock 2015). From this perspective, anti-ageist practice frameworks and perspectives are not only relevant for frontline health care providers in terms of training but, in order to provide truly respectful places of care for older people, it is necessary to confront ageism at the cultural level, as well as at the program or policy level (Hitchcock 2015). Alongside this, the devaluing of formal and informal caregiving for older people, is at once, at the level of the structural (that is, the political and economic) and interpersonal, representative of ageism and gender inequity, since mostly, women comprise the majority of caregivers and older persons (Hooyman 2015).

Critical gerontology is an important perspective that, 'attempts a radical approach to adult ageing drawing on both the personal experience of older adults and their relationship to social and structural inequality' (Biggs 2008: 115), and, if embedded in social work, is a significant addition to practice and research. Critical gerontology has been developed by social gerontologists over some time (for example, Phillipson 1982; 1998; Minkler & Estes 1999; Cole et al. 1993) and furthermore, some theorists have fused aspects of feminism with critical gerontology (for example, Browne 1998; Calasanti 2004; Ray 2004; 1999; Calasanti & Slevin 2006; Estes 2006; Calasanti & King 2011; Freixas et al. 2012; Cruikshank 2013). Having been influenced by neo-Marxist theory and from civil rights movements (Biggs 2008), there are various complementary theoretical streams in critical gerontology (Phillipson 1998), including a focus on the political economy (Minkler & Estes 1999), ethical and historical considerations (Cole et al. 1993) and biographical or narrative perspectives that emphasise the meaning of ageing from the perspectives of older people themselves (Biggs 2001, 2004; Kenyan et al. 2008; Zeilig 2011). Theories associated with critical gerontology seek to interrogate the status quo (Ray 2008) and focus on exploring the dominance of biomedical models in research, the intersection of race, gender and class, normative constructions of age, (that is, how older people are usually represented in popular culture) the inclusion of the perspectives and narratives of older people in research, the nature and impact of ageism in society, and self-reflection in the academy (Ray 2008).

Thus, critical gerontology understands age as a fragmented, culturally derived concept: 'It signals the paradigm shift away from the dominant understanding of age, as represented in the positivism of the biomedical model, to the alternative view, a critical stance which exposes the underlying power structures and socially constructed "age conceptualizations" on both micro and macro levels' (Anderson 2011: 49).

Laws (1995) importantly highlights the connection between critical gerontology, feminism and postmodern theory in order to theorise age identity as being multiple and variable rather than an arrested or stable construct. For instance, the experience of ageing is experienced differently according to historical and social contexts, and the complex intersections of gender, class, race, ability and sexualities.

Similarly to the social work profession, critical gerontologists are concerned with critical reflection to explore how values are enacted, particularly in terms of how professionals may exert social control over older people (Ray 2003; Anderson 2011). There is recognition of how critical gerontologists are themselves ageing, and hence subject to and captured by normative cultural discourses. Thus, the emphasis is on the importance of self-reflection in terms of our own subjectivities as researchers and theorists (Ray 2003; Anderson 2011). In theorising age, it is important for social work to embrace critical gerontology since social responsibility, critical thinking and reflection, and a desire to develop theory approaches aimed at emancipation, are common to both disciplines (Anderson 2011).

The need for anti-ageist practice frameworks in social work

Socially constructed notions of ageing adults are mostly negative and can be attributable to ageism, a cultural construct which represents systemic patterns of discrimination, social exclusion and negative stereotypes that are deeply embedded in Western culture. In the main, these notions present older citizens as frail, unintelligent, weak, dependent, in need of care, and as objects of fear, derision and pity (Lee & Gupta 2007), such that ageism is, 'one of the most socially condoned, institutionalised forms of prejudice in the world' (Nelson 2004: iv).

Age stereotypes are developed in early childhood and continue during adolescence and adulthood. They are often reinforced and reproduced by social and cultural processes, notably through institutions such as the media (Bevan & Jeeawody 1998). Once established, ageist attitudes are difficult to change. Perhaps unsurprisingly then, in a profession such as social work, ageist values, assumptions and stereotypes are often deeply internalised among social work students (Gellis et al. 2003; Kane 2006; Allen et al. 2009) as well as social work academic staff (Papadaki et al. 2012), constituting one of the barriers to developing social workers who are appropriately skilled to work with older people (Wang & Chonody 2013). In Australia, as in the US and UK, there is concern that social workers are ill prepared to work with ageing populations, both in terms of the number of practitioners that will be required and due to a lack of preparedness regarding the development of knowledge, theory and skills in gerontology and critical perspectives (for example, Scharlach et al. 2000; Rosen et al. 2003; McCormack 2008; Ray et al. 2009; Hokenstad & Roberts 2011). The need for social workers to be knowledgeable about ageing extends to all areas of social work practice given the nature of changing social relations where older people occupy an increasingly diverse array of roles including, for example, the provision of primary care for grandchildren or great-grandchildren (Scharlach et al. 2000) and increasing participation in the workforce (Chou 2012).

New models of service delivery, theoretical perspectives, educational and research approaches as well as responses to policy arrangements will be required for the development of a critical social work approach to gerontology in light of changing demographics. For instance, Ferguson and Schriver (2012) discuss the need for social policy leadership at national levels in order to advocate and develop contemporary models of care. They suggest a more complex consideration of intergenerational diversity, differently ageing cohorts and the devolution of the notion of 'retirement' thus creating other possibilities for the nature of our later lives. Another example is discussed by Chou (2012) in regard to the need for a greater recognition of how ageism in the workforce impacts older workers and the resulting potential roles for social workers at the micro and macro levels. This includes counselling older workers and their families, providing employment services and advocating to achieve employment equity for older workers. Additionally, the nature of social work geron-tology in the future must include an invigorated advocacy role due to contemporary and emerging family or informal care networks. This is especially in terms of multi-cultural contexts. More advocacy is also required in policy reform that addresses health and wellbeing across the life span beginning in childhood (Crampton 2011), and the need for specialists in the provision of social and community services. An emphasis on community development perspectives that highlight the importance of social work in building, empowering and supporting coalitions of older citizens, and engagement with care-giving responsibilities of older people (Hokenstad & Roberts 2011) are also important future directions.

Critical reflection as a part of social work practice, on the 'stories' and narra-tives of ageing, whether in terms of identity or the social territory of policy, has the potential to create an opportunity to include alternative and diverse perspectives and to contest culturally normative expectations of what it means to grow old (Biggs 2001). Clearly, a critical perspective in social work on ageing has scope to develop a progressive approach to gerontology across a range of areas. These include lead-ership in policy advocacy and reform, the maturation of critical knowledge and practice approaches, and knowledge gained via the critical engagement with the cultural meanings of ageing.

A case study: hearing the stories of older women who experienced childhood sexual abuse

One of the ways that we may challenge ageism and begin to develop anti-ageist practices in social work is to hear and include the perspectives of older people in the development of services and examine our own ageist assumptions as practitioners. My research project explores the experiences and perspectives of older women who have experienced childhood sexual abuse, where I use critical gerontology as a theoretical basis. A methodological aim of the research was to privilege the views of the women and to position their experiences as a valid source of knowledge, particularly taking into account the diversity in perspectives among them. Gilfus (1999: 1252) uses a powerful and instructive metaphor for researchers of 'leaving home' in order to adopt a survivor-centred epistemology which begins with the survivor's ways of knowing and being in the world.

One of the themes in my research concerned the issue of how the women (aged between 57 and 82 years) perceived counselling as a strategy to manage the long-term impact of childhood sexual abuse. I was interested in how the women, given their historical and social contexts, supported the idea of counselling as a therapeutic framework, assuming that many may not have been exposed to or been offered this type of service during the course of their lives, particularly as children. Certainly, in professional practice, I had observed how very few older women accessed these services. In many cases, their views provided a contest to established or normative constructs of counselling and recovery. For example: 'I don't think it should even be called counselling. There should be a different terminology attached to it because counselling as I say has become a Mickey Mouse venture' (Bess, 65 years old).

Bess's point was based mainly on the lack of trust that she felt could be expected systemically from engaging in counselling when file notes are written from the perspective of the writer, as she explains:

> It doesn't have the value of absolute trust attached to it. It can be seconded into a court room . . . It's up for sale . . . up

for grabs . . . There's no defence against it . . . the pen is mightier than the sword in so many ways . . . The record keeping serves a bureaucratic and career purpose and it doesn't serve the purpose of truth . . . and truth is the first casualty of all these things.

Importantly, Bess told me about her own view that counselling was part of an industry which serves a function other than for its therapeutic value and hence her deep mistrust of the therapeutic process. Throughout our conversation, I also understood her response to be linked to her 'voice' being excluded and the lack of control she experienced.

Related to the question of counselling, I also asked about the notion of recovery. Rose (66 years old) provided a nuanced and challenging perspective that acknowledges how her view may differ from cultural expectations:

I'm not sure that you recover. I don't think you recover . . . How can you recover? You know if somebody knifes you and leaves a big scar in your side, you get over it but you don't recover from it . . . You get through it. I think it's more you get through it . . . I appreciate that not everybody's got the strength to do this. Maybe I was fortunate in some ways, coming from a tough background. I don't mean rough, I mean tough. This is what you did. If you didn't have anything to eat at the end of the week, nothing you can do about it. If we had a hole in your shoe, we used to mend them with leather from the mill. You had one pair of shoes . . . That's how it was and you didn't know any different.

Jane (76 years old) also expressed a distinctive view regarding the notion of recovery, which for her, means the pain of her experience is enduring:

Those words, 'moving on' and 'getting over it' especially say to me . . . oh forget about it, you know, it's all over. Done. Never done, not till the day you draw your last breath . . . It doesn't work that way. So moving on and getting over it has connotations for me anyway. You don't really. 'Dealing with it' is much better and 'living with' is better than 'moving on' . . . Telling it once is not going to cure it. I look at it this way . . . if I'm a tree. The tree was bent and it grew that way . . . It'll never grow up straight like as if nothing had ever happened . . . but like with the wind you know, by the sea . . . all the trees are bent. You need a strong stake . . . That means somebody who knows what they're doing . . . much pruning, getting rid of all the excess stuff . . . fertiliser, the encouragement . . . water, our tears . . . You cry a lot! And pain . . . until you can live with it and be the person you were meant to be . . . your tree . . . life . . . was bent . . . and grew that way . . . And then see the good things that came out of it. Not easy to do.

June (75 years old) also expressed strong scepticism of counselling but also a sense of her capacity to manage over her lifetime (as did Rose) as her following comments reveal: 'I've been a couple of times when I've got depressed . . . I went there but I didn't feel, "oh terrific I feel marvellous now!" Maybe I read too much! Maybe it's because I've done some psychology too . . . I'm thinking well I could have told myself that'.

These views are a small illustration of the perceptions of some older women in relation to particular issues for them in managing the impact of the abuse. In conversation with the women, I found that they challenged many normative narratives of counselling, and indeed, ageing. In order to develop an anti-ageist practice, social workers must centralise the perspectives and lived experiences of older people, since doing so reveals not only the resources and strengths that older people possess and use to resist oppressive social conditions that are linked to ageism and sexism, but also insights regarding how older people construct social problems. This includes attention to the personal biographies of older people that can uncover reasons why many older people do not access existing services. For instance, Harbison (2008) argues that domestic violence responses that are considered appropriate for younger women fail to address different needs and social conditions for older women and that services are rarely constructed according to the 'expressed needs of older people' (Harbison et al. 2012: 99).

Additionally, a reflexive approach to ageism can unearth assumptions that stereotype older people and particularly women as passive, helpless or inept. Older people are not a homogenous group and incorporating perspectives that explore the intersections of age, gender, race, class and sexuality contributes to the development of an approach that recognises diversity and various historical contexts. In the case of my own research, the women spoke about past oppressive conditions and the strategies they used for resistance and reconstruction. Social work practice which positions older people as 'knowers' (that is, having valid or legitimate knowledge) has the potential to incorporate their perspectives into direct practice at the level of the individual regarding ownership of information and choice of service, and group work (Duncan & Mason 2011), but also at the policy level where social workers may be influential more broadly, so that it is relevant and transformative (Ray 1999).

Conclusion

Critical gerontology as a theory to inform practice seeks to represent the varied stories of ageing lives and avoids essentialism (Holstein & Minkler 2003), focuses on politicising the issues of knowledge production (Browne 1998), explores stories of ageing from the 'inside' of ageing (Katz 2000) and uncovers 'hidden' social issues through giving emphasis to otherwise invisible voices (Formosa 2005). This is particularly the case for older women who are markedly absent in research (Freixas et al. 2012). Critical practice approaches assist to reconstruct normative age identities. In other words, it helps to develop new ways to conceptualise the identities of older people in positive ways to become a new norm. These approaches develop ways to theorise age in complex ways that acknowledge the particular and nuanced paths in which we grow old. Stories of ageing from diverse perspectives assist to 'open up new debates and redefine the meaning of ageing, the desire to embrace rather than elide the complexities of later life' (Zeilig 2011: 8). In this chapter I have argued for the inclusion of perspectives from older people in critical social work practice in order to inform direct service and use my own research with older women by way of example. The narratives of the women tell us that sometimes counselling frameworks are removed from what constitutes a meaningful exchange for older people.

Anti-ageist practice in social work must also include reflective practice and reflexive thinking (Fook & Gardner 2007). Critical gerontology, likewise, maintains a commitment to reflexivity as fundamental for theorists and practitioners in, 'trying to age critically and consciously in a world that still fears and resists ageing' (Ray 2008: 98). There is a symbiotic relationship between the shaping of knowledge and being fashioned ourselves by the very same concepts (Ray 2008).

As practitioners ourselves growing older or working with older people, it is necessary to adopt reflective processes that interrogate internalised ageism (Biggs 2008) if we are to engage with a shared commitment to the values and ethics of social work. Reflexivity requires a consciousness between generations that seeks, 'a relationship of complementarity rather than dominance' (Biggs 2008: 118) in order to build equality between generations (Biggs 2008). Wilson is instructive regarding ageism and the social construction of age when she tells us that, 'there is no universal old person' (Wilson 2000: 4). I discovered from speaking with the women in my study that my own views about ageing and direct practice were constantly challenged. When provided an opportunity to speak freely, they confounded many aspects of what I had previously considered to be helpful in the counselling process such as its relevancy which, from their perspectives, was variable. This prompted me to deconstruct my own practice and to advance the importance of privileging the narratives of the women who understand ageing from the inside.

References

Aberdeen, L. & Bye, L.A. 2013, 'Challenges for Australian sociology: Critical ageing research—ageing well?', *Journal of Sociology*, vol. 49, no. 1, pp. 3–21

ABS *see* Australian Bureau of Statistics

Allen, P.D., Cherry, K.E. & Palmore, E. 2009, 'Self-reported ageism in social work practitioners and students', *Journal of Gerontological Social Work*, vol. 52, no. 2, pp. 124–34

Anderson, A. 2011, 'How Critical Gerontology Challenges Anti-Ageing Ideology and Leads the Individual to a Self-Defined Later Life', MA thesis, Marylhurst: Marylhurst University, Accessed 9 January 2014, from Marylhurst Digital Thesis Collection

Australian Bureau of Statistics (ABS) 2013, *Population Projections, Australia, 2012 (base) to 2101, ABS*, Canberra <www.abs.gov.au>

Bevan, C. & Jeeawody, B. 1998, *Successful Ageing Perspectives on Health and Social Construction*, Sydney: Mosby

Biggs, S. 2001, 'Toward critical narrativity: Stories of ageing in contemporary social policy', *Journal of Ageing Studies*, vol. 15, no. 4, pp. 303–16

—— 2008, 'Ageing in a critical world: The search for generational intelligence', *Journal of Ageing Studies*, vol. 22, no. 2, pp. 115–19

Briskman, L., Pease, B. & Allan, J. 2009, 'Introducing critical theories for social work in a neo-liberal context' in J. Allan, L. Briskman and B. Pease (eds), *Critical Social Work: Theories and practices for a socially just world*, 2nd edn, St Leonards: Allen & Unwin, pp. 3–14

Browne, C.V. 1998, *Women, Feminism and Ageing,* New York: Springer Publishing Company

Calasanti, T. 2004, 'New directions in feminist gerontology: An introduction', *Journal of Ageing Studies*, vol. 18, no. 1, pp. 1–8

—— & King, N. 2011, 'A feminist lens on the third age: Refining the framework' in D. Carr & K.S. Komp (eds), *Gerontology in the Era of the Third Age: Implications and next steps,* New York: Springer Publishing Company, pp. 67–85

—— & Slevin, K.F. 2006, *Age Matters Realigning Feminist Thinking*, New York: Routledge

Chambers, P. 2004, 'The case for critical social gerontology in social work education and older women', *Social Work Education*, vol. 23, no. 6, pp. 745–58, DOI: 10.1080/0261547042000294518a

Chou, Rita Jing-Ann, 2012, 'Discrimination against older workers: Current knowledge, future research directions and implication for social work'. *Indian Journal of Gerontology*, vol. 26, no. 1, pp. 25–49

Cole, T., Achenbaum, W.A., Jakobi, P. & Kastenbaum, R. (eds) 1993, *Voices and Visions of Ageing: Toward a critical gerontology*, New York: Springer

Crampton, A. 2011, 'Population ageing and social work practice with older adults: Demographic and policy challenges', *International Social Work*, vol. 54, pp. 313–29, DOI: 10.1177/0020872810396257

Cruikshank, M. 2013, *Learning to be Old: Gender, culture, and ageing*, Maryland: Rowman & Littlefield Publishers Inc.

Duncan, J. & Mason, R. 2011, 'Older women reconnecting after sexual violence through group work', *Women Against Violence: An Australian Feminist Journal,* No. 23, pp. 18–28

Estes, C. 2006, 'Critical feminist perspectives, ageing and social policy' in J. Baars, D. Dannefer, C. Phillipson & A. Walker (eds), *Ageing, Globalization and Inequality, The new critical gerontology,* New York: Baywood Publishing Company Inc., pp. 81–101

Eymard, A.S. & Douglas, D.H. 2012, 'Ageism among health care providers and interventions to improve their attitudes toward older adults: an integrative review', *Journal of Gerontological Nursing*, vol. 38, pp. 26–35, DOI: 10.3928/00989134-20120307-09

Ferguson, A.J. & Schriver, J. 2012, 'The future of gerontological social work: A case for structural lag', *Journal of Gerontological Social Work*, vol. 55, no. 4, pp. 304–20

Fook, J. 2002, *Social Work: Critical theory and practice,* London: Sage

—— & Gardner, F. 2007, *Practising Critical Reflection: A resource handbook*, Berkshire: Open University Press

Formosa, M. 2005, 'Feminism and critical educational gerontology: An agenda for good practice', *Ageing International*, vol. 30, no. 4, pp. 396–411

Freixas, A., Luque, B. & Reina, A. 2012, 'Critical feminist gerontology: In the back room of research', *Journal of Women & Ageing*, vol. 24, no. 1, pp. 44–58

Gellis, Z.D., Sherman, S. & Lawrance, F. 2003, 'First year graduate social work students' knowledge of and attitude toward older adults', *Educational Gerontology*, vol. 29, no. 1, pp. 1–16

Gilfus, M.E. 1999, 'The Price of the ticket: A survivor-centered appraisal of trauma theory', *Violence Against Women*, vol. 5, no. 11, pp. 1238–57

Harbison, J. 2008, 'Stoic heroines or collaborators: Ageism, feminism and the provision of assistance to abused old women', *Journal of Social Work Practice*, vol. 22, no. 2, pp. 221–34

—— Coughlan, S., Beaulieu, M., Karabanow, J., Vanderplaat, M., Wildeman, S. & Wexler, E. 2012, 'Understanding "elder abuse and neglect": A critique of assumptions underpinning responses to the mistreatment and neglect of older people', *Journal of Elder Abuse and Neglect,* vol. 24, pp. 88–103

Hitchcock, K. 2015, 'Dear life: On caring for the elderly', *Quarterly Essay*, vol. 57, pp. 1–77

Hokenstad, M.C. & Roberts, A.R. 2011, 'International policy on ageing and older persons: Implications for social work practice', *International Social Work*, vol. 54, no. 3, pp. 330–43, DOI:10.1177/0020872810396259

Holstein, M.B. & Minkler, M. 2003, 'Self, society, and the "new gerontology"', *The Gerontologist*, vol. 43, no. 6, pp. 787–96

Hooyman, N. 2015, 'Social and health disparities in ageing: Gender inequities in long term care', *Generations, Journal of the American Society on Ageing*, vol. 38, no. 4, pp. 25–32

Kane, M.N. 2006, 'Ageism and gender among social work and criminal justice students', *Educational Gerontology*, vol. 32, no. 10, pp. 859–80

Katz, S. 2000, 'Busy bodies: Activity, ageing, and the management of everyday life', *Journal of Ageing Studies*, vol. 14, no. 2, pp. 135–52

Kenyan, G.M., Ruth, J.E. & Mader, W. 2008, 'Elements of a narrative gerontology' in V. Bengtson and W. Schaie (eds), *Handbook of Theories of Ageing*, Springer, New York, pp. 40–58

Krekula, C. 2007, 'The intersection of age and gender: Reworking gender theory and social gerontology', *Current Sociology*, vol. 55, pp. 155–71, DOI: 10.1177/0011392107073299

Laws, G. 1995, 'Understanding ageism: Lessons from feminism and postmodernism', *The Gerontologist*, vol. 35, no. 1, pp. 112–18

Lee, Yeon-Shim & Gupta, R. 2007, 'Ageism and social exclusion in the United States: Implications for social policy and social work practice', *Indian Journal of Gerontology*, vol. 21, no. 2, pp. 128–51

McCormack, J. 2008, 'Educating social workers for the demographic imperative', *Australian Health Review*, Vol. 32, No. 3, pp. 400–4

Minkler, M. & Estes, C.L. 1999, (eds), *Critical Gerontology, Perspectives from Political and Moral Economy*, New York: Baywood Publishing Company

Nelson, T.D. (ed.) 2004, *Ageism: Stereotyping and prejudice against older person*, Cambridge: Massachusetts Institute of Technology

Netting, F.E. 2011, 'Bridging critical feminist gerontology and social work to interrogate the narrative on civic engagement, *Affilia: Journal of Women and Social Work*, vol. 26, no. 3, pp. 239–49

Papadaki, E., Plotnikof, K. & Papadaki, V. 2012, 'Self-reported ageism in students and academic staff— the case of the Social Work Department in Crete, Greece', *European Journal of Social Work*, vol. 15, no. 5, pp. 696–711

Phillipson, C. 1982, *Capitalism and the Construction of Old Age*, London: Macmillan

—— 1998, *Reconstructing Old Age: New agendas in social theory and practice*, London: Sage

Ray, M., Bernard, M. & Phillips, J. 2009, *Critical Issues in Social Work with Older People*, London: Palgrave Macmillan

Ray, R. 1999, 'Researching to transgress: The need for critical feminism in gerontology', in J.D. Garner (ed.), *Fundamentals of Feminist Gerontology*, New York: Haworth Press, pp. 171–84

—— 2004, 'Toward the croning of a feminist gerontology', *Journal of Ageing Studies*, vol. 18, no. 1, pp. 109–21

Ray, R.E. 2003, 'The perils and possibilities of theory' in S. Biggs, A. Lowenstein and J. Hendricks (eds), *The Need for Theory: Critical approaches to social gerontology*, New York: Baywood Publishing Co., pp. 33–44

—— 2008, 'Coming of age in critical gerontology', *Journal of Ageing Studies*, vol. 22, no. 2, pp. 97–100

Rexhepi, J. & Torres, C.A. 2011, 'Reimagining critical theory', *British Journal of Sociology of Education*, vol. 32, no. 5, pp. 679–98

Rosen, A.L., Levy Zlotnik, J. & Singer, T. 2003, 'Basic gerontological competence for all social workers', *Journal of Gerontological Social Work*, vol. 39, no. 1–2, pp. 25–36, DOI: 10.1300/J083v39n01_04

Scharlach, A., Damron-Rodriguez, J., Robinson, B. & Feldman, R. 2000, 'Educating social workers for an ageing society: A vision for the 21st century', *Journal of Social Work Education*, vol. 36, no. 3, pp. 521–38

Sontag, S. 1997, 'The double standard of ageing', in M. Pearsall (ed.), *The Other Within Us: Feminist explorations of women and ageing*, Colorado: Westview Press, pp. 19–35

Twigg, J. 2004, 'The body, gender, and age: Feminist insights in social gerontology', *Journal of Ageing Studies*, vol. 18, no. 1, pp. 59–73, DOI: 10.1016/j.jaging.2003.09.001

Wang, D. & Chonody, J. 2013, 'Social workers' attitudes toward older adults: A review of the literature', *Journal of Social Work Education*, vol. 49, no. 1, pp. 150–72

Westerhof, G.J. & Tulle, E. 2007, 'Meanings of ageing and old age: Discursive contexts, social attitudes and personal identities' in J. Bond, S. Peace & F. Dittmann-Kohli (eds), *Ageing in Society*, London: Sage, pp. 235–54

Wilson, G. 2000, *Understanding Old Age: Critical and global perspectives*, London: Sage

Zeilig, H. 2011, 'The critical use of narrative and literature in gerontology', *International Journal of Ageing and Later Life*, vol. 6, no. 2, pp. 7–37

17

Working for equality and difference: (de)constructing heteronormativity

Jude Irwin

Introduction

Social workers, heterosexual and LGBTIQ (lesbian, gay, bisexual, transgender, intersex, queer) people have contact with LGBTIQ populations in all areas of practice, including health care, services for families, children and young people, aged care, alcohol and other drug users, those in correction institutions, those involved in the juvenile justice system, those with a disability, and community-based organisations. LGBTIQ people throughout Australia, (and in other parts of the world) face widespread discrimination on the basis of their sexual or gender identity or both in many areas of their lives such as in workplaces, families, and in the community (Irwin 2009). Since the 1960s, rights groups have fought tenaciously for equal rights for people from LGBTIQ communities and, as a consequence, in Australia over the last decade there have been numerous changes in federal, state and territory laws covering many, but not all, aspects of the lives of LGBTIQ people (Irwin 2009). However, these changes have not always been accompanied by changes in attitudes, values and behaviour and many LGBTIQ people still experience homophobic or heterosexist discrimination, threats and behaviour. Identifying, acknowledging and challenging such injustice has been central in critical social work, especially for groups and communities who are 'different', marginalised, excluded or disenfranchised. There is, however, barely any available literature that explores critical social work practice with LGBTIQ people and communities, especially on the topic of the pervasiveness of heteronormativity. This means that heterosexuality is seen as the only natural form of a person's sexuality. This literature also needs to discuss how these prejudices influences the way people engage with LGBTIQ people and communities.

The term heteronormativity is often used in contemporary theory to refer to the many ways in which heterosexuality is produced as a natural, unproblematic, everyday occurrence (Kitzinger 2005). In this chapter, I explore how social work practice with LGBTIQ people and communities can be premised on beliefs and assumptions of heteronormativity and heterosexism, how these can shape, produce and limit understandings and responses, and thus reinforce invisibility and contribute towards inequality in the lives of LGBTIQ people.

It is important to acknowledge that LGBTIQ communities are diverse in most areas such as age, education, income, class, racial, ethnic and cultural backgrounds, experiences, sexualities, political affiliations and beliefs, values and attitudes. What they have in common is some form of oppression related to their sexual orientation or gender nonconformity, which can result in marginalisation, exclusion and other negative life experiences. Normative heterosexuality intersects with the power and influences of patriarchy, racism, exclusion, misogyny and colonisation, which all contribute to provide meaning in their lives.

I begin this chapter with a brief history of the emergence of the gay and lesbian rights movements and link this history to the development of critical social work. I follow this by drawing on concepts and ideas from postmodernism to explore how heteronormative discourses shape understandings, beliefs and assumptions of LGBTIQ people. I discuss how these assumptions flow over to practitioners' engagement with LGBTIQ people and communities. I then explore how heteronormativity can limit services for particular groups in LGBTIQ communities, elders and young homeless people. I argue that unless these heteronormative influences are interrogated and challenged, people from LGBTIQ communities will remain invisible and struggle to access inclusive and appropriate services.

Setting the context: the LGBTIQ rights movement and critical social work

Both critical social work and LGBTIQ rights campaigns emerged from social movements; that is, groups of people or organisations or both who came together to fight collectively for specific areas of political, social, economic or cultural change, or a combination of these.

The gay and lesbian rights movements emerged in the 1960s, as gay men and lesbians joined together to protest their perceived second-class citizenship and fight for equality with heterosexuals, in order to challenge commonly held beliefs that they were deviant, 'sick' or 'sinful'. Their fight for equality and fairness has since extended beyond lesbians and gay men to include those who identify as bisexual, transgender, intersex and queer. Being in a similar situation to many other oppressed groups in the 1960s, the gays' and lesbians' experiences of ongoing discrimination, harassment and unequal treatment was the motivation for seeking change. LGBT activist movements formed in many parts of the Western world in the 1960s and 1970s, including Australia (Bullough 2002; Walton 2011). At that time, many lesbians were active in the women's movement that was fighting for gender equality and, because of their commitment to challenge patriarchal beliefs and practices, they chose not to participate in organisations and political activist groups that included (gay) men. They formed their own activist groups instead (Phelan 1989). The first lesbian civil and political rights organisation in the US, the Daughters of Bilitis, formed in 1955. 'Its very establishment in the midst of the witch hunts and police action was an act of courage, since members always had to fear they were under attack not because of what they did but because of who they were' (Faderman 1991: 190–1). It was an arm of the Daughters of Bilitis that was the first organised LGBT activist group in Australia, forming in 1969. Later that year, the Homosexual Law Reform Society formed in the Australian Capital Territory. It was, however, the Campaign Against Moral Persecution (CAMP) founded in Sydney in 1970 that galvanised the Australian Lesbian and Gay Rights movement (Willett 2000). Similar organisations had formed in some universities and in every capital city across Australia (for example, Society Five in Melbourne) to campaign and fight for LGBTIQ equality. Over the next several years, a number of other rights organisations formed and were involved in demonstrations and rallies seeking reform in all areas of life for lesbians and gay men. In Sydney in 1978, as part of the international solidarity celebrations, which grew out of the Stonewall riots in the US, lesbians and gay men marched through the CBD and along Oxford Street, Paddington, where they were stopped by police and 53 people were arrested; many of whom were beaten up in the police cells (Willett 2000). This march was later known as the first NSW Gay and Lesbian Mardi Gras (Willett 2000). This violent involvement of the police prompted protests and demonstrations over the next several months. Arrests continued until the laws on demonstrations, which had allowed the arrests, were changed in April 1979. This was seen as a major civil rights milestone that went beyond the gay and lesbian communities. All Australian states and territories have now amended homosexuality laws, which legalise sexual conduct between consenting males. LGBTIQ activist groups continue to be vocal and have been successful in obtaining broader law reform in many, but not all areas, at state, territory and federal levels. However, while laws have changed, there is not always the associated change in attitudes, beliefs and values. LGBTIQ people still experience exclusion, harassment and negative treatment because of their sexuality (Irwin 2009).

Radical social work was a precursor to critical social work, having its roots in the movements for social reform as early as the 1890s in the US. This is when social work activists worked for systemic change and challenged the individualistic and often pathological explanations of social problems (Benjamin 2007). This transformative period of social work was replaced by a much more individualistic, scientific, philanthropic approach where the focus was on giving social work a professional status and the maintenance of the status quo (Benjamin 2007). As discussed by Pease and Nipperess (see Chapter 1), radical social work re-emerged in the wake of the anti-Vietnam war demonstrations and the growth of social protest and rights movements in the 1950s and 1960s.

The LGBT liberation movement had an important influence in early radical social work with Don Milligan's (1975) ground-breaking chapter in *Radical Social Work*. It argued that the privileging of heterosexuality permeates our culture, resulting in the prejudice and discrimination of LGBT people. Adopting a similar approach to other radical social work writers, Milligan argued that social workers should actively challenge the structural basis of prejudice and discrimination towards LGBT people (Charing et al. 1975; Hart 1980). However, while sexual identity and sexual orientation have continued to be recognised in social work as sources of oppression and discrimination, they are often dealt with by simply adding LGBTIQ to the existing heteronormative framework. That is, rather than addressing the sociopolitical aspects of sexuality LGBTIQ are accommodated to the normative structures of heterosexual dominance (Hicks & Watson 2003).

Since the 1980s, various social justice-oriented approaches to social work have developed. They build on ideas and concepts drawn from structuralist, feminist, social constructivist, postmodernist and post-structuralist theories. While these approaches have differing views about the inclusion of postmodernist and post-structural concepts, it could be argued that there is broad agreement that post-modern and post-structural theories have contributed to greater understanding of the complexity and fluidity of some people's everyday lives and more nuanced ways of understanding social context, difference, diversity and identity. Discourse, language, subjectivity and power are concepts from postmodernism that I now explore in relation to LGBTIQ people and communities.

Discourses, language, power and subjectivities

Critiquing structuralists and humanists, who argued that human consciousness spreads out from the individual, and creates meaning as the person confronts the social world, Foucault (1977) argued that the individual is a social construction who is produced through discourses (language, thought, symbolic representations) that position subjects within a field of power relations and particular sets of practices. In discussing discourses Weedon picks up on the importance of discourse, language, subjectivity and power. She sees discourse as: greater than just the production of meaning and ways of thinking. She argues that:

> ... the Neither the body nor the thoughts or feelings have meaning outside their discursive articulation, but the ways in which discourse constitutes the minds and bodies of individuals is always part of a wider network of power relations, often with institutional bases (Weedon 1987: 108).

Central to this quote is the notion that discourse is part of the practices of everyday living; that is, a discourse constitutes reality and lived experience. The idea that what individuals can imagine, think say or do is both enabled and limited by discourse. The possible ways of being, produced by discourses, are bound up in relations of power. While social, cultural and historical contexts influence the construction of 'truth' and 'reality', language plays a pivotal role in shaping realities (D'Amico 2007) so that the way people see themselves in the world, their subjectivities, are both linguistically and socially constructed (Best & Kellner 1991).

People who identify as LGBTIQ live in a world where heterosexuality is the 'norm', and is seen as universal and synonymous with the human experience (Richardson 1996). Yep argues that heteronormativity is 'deeply embedded in our individual and group psyches, social relations, identities, social institutions and cultural land-scapes'(Yep 2002: 168). Heteronormative discourses saturate our lives and influence our understandings of how society works, and thus create a form of 'compulsory heterosexuality' (Rich 1980). The sociopolitical system regulates this 'compulsory heterosexuality' through laws, cultural practices, gender roles and institutionalised practices. Heteronormative discourses inform understandings of non-heterosexual sexualities and the language used. This shapes how LGBTIQ people view themselves and how they are in the world. To demonstrate the pervasiveness of this and the influence it has, I use the example of intimate partner violence (IPV) in lesbian relationships. This shows how dominant heteronormative understandings of IPV work to produce lesbian's understandings and experiences of violence in their own relationships.

Heteronormative discourses: the shaping of subjectivities

Second-wave feminist theorising of intimate partner violence (IPV) has provided a powerful discourse (knowledge and social practice) that did more than just describe the effects of violence. It produced understandings of both the violence and the people involved. Given the scale of male violence against women and the challenge to eradicate it, the focus was almost entirely on heterosexual relationships and, over time, discourses of IPV, influenced by radical feminist theorising have become normative (Irwin 2008a). The dominance of heteronormative explanations has meant there is both a silence and invisibility around lesbians' experiences of violence in their intimate relationships. This is reinforced by other socially constructed experiences of lesbian life, which have also shaped how lesbians understand IPV in their relationships. Discourses of lesbian utopia emerged in 1960s and 1970s as radical and lesbian cultural feminists challenged the dominant views of patriarchy (Williams 1996). Ideals of egalitarianism, non-violence and non-hierarchical practices replaced dominant patriarchal values that had shaped and limited women's lives. Discourses of lesbians as peace-loving, nurturing and non-competitive, yet assertive and independent, gained credence. As lesbian separatist communities emerged, these values became the basis for the 'ideal' community. They were embraced by many lesbian feminists, some of whom were actively involved in fighting for, and developing, specialist services for women, which were often modelled on these non-patriarchal values. Despite schisms over the notion of a lesbian utopia, following bitter recriminations in the women's movement over pornography, sadomasochism and butch/femme roles, lesbian relationships are still viewed as non-violent (Irwin 2008b). This presentation of IPV as heterosexual and lesbian relationships as non-violent combines with dominant discourses of masculinity (men as violent and aggressive) and femininity (women as gentle, caring and passive) to limit knowledge of IPV in lesbian relationships. The result is that IPV in lesbian relationships remains invisible and these stereotypes influence how lesbians experience, talk about, make sense of, and respond to violence in their relationships. The invisibility is also influenced by fear that exposure of violence between lesbians (women's violence) will challenge the political gains that were fought for so so long which were made about the extent and nature of violence against women perpetrated by men. The silence and invisibility of violence in intimate lesbian relationships does not mean that violence does not exist, rather it means that the language to talk about it is limited. As IPV between lesbians is not recognised, practice knowledge is limited, and appropriate health, human and community services are not readily available. The transposing of knowledge, understandings and interpretations from heterosexual IPV to lesbian's experiences discounts contextual issues and can erase lesbian's particular experiences. This reduces options for more nuanced understandings of the complexities of the violence.

Think about a community group or organisation you are familiar with and consider the following questions:

- What heteronormative discourses or stories circulate in this group or organisation about families, relationships and communities?
- What assumptions underpin these discourses?
- What are the origins of these assumptions?
- Who do these discourses privilege or limit participating in this group or organisation?
- What could you do to challenge this in terms of your own views and in terms of other people's views, and the community group or organisation's views?

While heteronormative discourses influence how LGBTIQ people and communities are constituted and understood, it is also important to take into account the structural, political, social and personal circumstances and the material lives of LGBTIQ people. In an environment that largely dismisses and devalues non-heterosexual sexualities, heteronormativity fosters heterosexism (the belief that everyone is, or should be, heterosexual). Cultural and institutional heterosexism in the form of discrimination systematically disadvantages and disempowers individuals who are not heterosexual. Religion, media and public discourse play an influential role in upholding the existing sexual hierarchy and power relations, and shape responses to different sexual and gender identities. For example, the denial of public rights, such as the right to marry, an aspect of institutional heterosexism, influences the legitimacy of LGBTIQ people's intimate relationships. This shapes how members of

LGBTIQ communities see themselves, and how their friends and families, and the general community constitute, understand and make meaning of their relationships. It is in this context that those who identify as LGBTIQ can protect their intimate relationships and be reluctant to acknowledge difficulties as this can be used as further evidence of the aberrance of their relationships.

In everyday discourse, LGBTIQ people are represented and talked about differently. Invasive questions, which would not be asked of heterosexual people are asked of LGBTIQ people on a regular basis. Words, tones and gestures can be used in ways that pathologise and degrade people. For example, in a televised interview with British talk show host Michael Parkinson in July 2014, Australian Olympian and world-champion swimmer Ian Thorpe came out publicly as a gay man after years of denying his homosexuality (Magnay 2002; Crouse 2014). In much of the print and online media it was commented that he 'admitted' he was gay (Harris & Rothfield 2014; Smith & France-Presse 2014) as though he had admitted to a serious crime. When has a heterosexual person had to admit being heterosexual?

It is the existence of institutional and cultural heterosexism that creates the opportunity for individual heterosexism and homophobia. This can have powerful and ongoing consequences, including being physically abused, marginalised, dismissed, excluded, humiliated, not taken seriously and being made invisible.

Heterosexism, in its many levels, plays out in the lives of LGBTIQ people in subtle and not so subtle ways. For example, 'coming out' or being open about one's sexuality is generally not an issue for heterosexuals as heterosexuality is assumed. However, for LGBTIQ people deciding whether (or not) to come out is an active choice. They make decisions about whether they are to be out and whom to be out to, and they consider the consequences of coming out to everyone, being selectively out or being completely closeted. Managing this in families, relationships, workplaces, community networks and the general community can be a juggling act (Markowitz 1991). In situations where LGBTIQ people are either closeted or selectively out, concern about being 'outed' can cause great anxiety and fear.

For the LGBTIQ community, the cumulative influences of living in a hetero-normative world bring up additional and complex issues as cultural, institutional and individual heterosexism and homophobia can result in LGBTIQ people being marginalised, their experiences being trivialised or denied by friends, family and service providers, which often acts as a disincentive for seeking support and assistance.

Heteronormativity and the shaping of health, human and community services

Many LGBTIQ people make choices about whether to seek help and support from community and human services organisations. Over the last decade, inclusion has become a priority in public policy. There has been an increasing awareness of the importance to ensure health, human and community services are accessible to a diverse population including the LGBTIQ community. However, the heteronormative assumptions that frame understandings of how LGBTIQ people are in the world also shape how service providers respond.

Health, human and community services and practitioners face particular challenges in planning and delivering accessible and inclusive services for people from LGBTIQ communities. To show how heteronormativity has influenced the delivery of services and to explore possibilities for change, I draw on the experiences of two groups from the LGBTIQ community: young homeless people and elders.

As heteronormative approaches have dominated aged care services, there has been little acknowledgement of the existence of LGBTIQ elders in either policy or practice (Harrison 2006). As Australia's ageing population is growing rapidly (ABS 2013), it is likely that greater numbers of older LBGTIQ people will require aged care services. The invisibility of older LGBTIQ people has meant that their needs have not been recognised (Fenge 2010). The heteronormative assumptions underlying practice and policy in social services supports this invisibility and many LGBTIQ elders choose not to disclose their sexual or gender identity, life history or needs to service providers as they consider it irrelevant or they feel unsafe or fear recriminations, or a combination of these (Harrison 2006). For many, this is linked to experiences of being LGBTIQ in a very different and much more oppressive era when lesbian or gay or transgender people were openly stigmatised for being sinful, deviant or mentally ill or all of these. Many have lived in constant fear of being 'outed', losing their jobs, being exposed to homophobic assaults, behaviour and treatment, being 'disowned' by families, and losing custody and contact with their children because of their 'unacceptable' lifestyle. These homophobic attitudes, behaviours and practices have profoundly shaped their lives. They have contributed to ongoing fears of being treated discriminatorily by staff and clients of services if they were to disclose their sexual identity. However, as the 'baby boomers', many of whom were activists in the LGBTIQ rights movements, are getting older and beginning to access aged care services, they are challenging exclusion and invisibility and refusing to accept being treated in discriminatory ways (Tolley & Ranzin 2006). Over the last few years, these LGBTIQ activists and organisations have been very vocal in drawing attention to the issues confronting LGBTIQ elders who are users of aged care services. They have begun to work with mainstream organisations about ways to ensure that services become more inclusive of the needs of LGBTIQ elders (Harrison 2006). This opens possibilities for change.

Unlike older LGBTIQ community members who have been invisible in aged care services, young homeless LGBTIQ members are very visible in homeless services for young people. A high proportion of homeless young people who access youth homelessness services in the US (40 per cent) and Australia (25 per cent), identify as LGBTIQ (Toms et al. 2007; Durso & Gates 2012). The majority leave home because their sexual or gender identity has resulted in being rejected by their family (Toms et al. 2007; Durso & Gates, 2012). Homeless LGBTIQ young people are more likely to have poor mental health and experience poverty than their heterosexual counterparts (Toms et al. 2007; Durso & Gates 2012). Transgender or gender-questioning young people are at much greater risk of homelessness, physical abuse, self-harm, suicide and poor academic performance (Toms et al. 2007; Durso & Gates 2012). Homophobic violence (verbal and physical) is regularly experienced by LGBTIQ youth who use homelessness services. Much of this violence is from other service users and although most services have a 'no violence' policy, this is not routinely monitored or enforced (Toms et al. 2007), which leaves LGBTIQ clients unsupported and unsafe, and the organisation complicit in the violence. Despite the large numbers of LGBTIQ homeless young people who access services, many agencies do not address the specific needs of LGBTIQ young people. They expect them to use the programs available for all homeless young people despite the risks of homophobic violence (Toms et al. 2007).

Both LGBTIQ elders and young homeless people can experience a lack of safety as they come into contact with services. To challenge this, it is crucial for heterosexual and LGBTIQ practitioners, to begin to analyse how heteronormative practices contribute to LGBTIQ people feeling unsafe. This can be done at both an institutional (macro) and an individual (micro) level. At an individual level, especially for heterosexual practitioners, interrogating motivations and benefits for tacitly supporting injustices can be a starting point. Asking questions such as the following ones:

- What are the assumptions underlying this?
- What do I gain from this?
- What do I lose from this?
- Who has the power in this situation?
- How does the organisation sustain this belief, value or practice?
- What can I do to challenge or further understand this?

Analysing a critical incident can also provide insight into the assumptions that underlie and support a practice. It can help to identify ways in which injustices are produced and acted upon. For a practitioner, a critical incident raises questions relating to beliefs, values, attitudes or behaviour. Analysing a critical incident can have a significant impact on personal and professional learning, and practice.

For example: Lena was a domestic violence worker at a women's health service. One of her roles was to support survivors of domestic violence, especially in terms of safety for themselves and their families. Marjo was referred to the health service by her local medical practitioner for assistance in locating emergency accommodation. Marjo had been with her partner, Chris, for five years. Over the last two years Chris had been both physically and emotionally abusive towards her. This had escalated over the last three months to the extent that Marjo now feared for her safety and the safety of her eight-year-old daughter. Lena found Marjo a little reticent about what was happening for her and it was not until well into the interview that Marjo said that Chris was a woman. Lena had assumed that Chris had been a man and was shocked by this assumption. She later discussed her reaction with her supervisor who suggested she analyse the incident to help her understand it better. Her supervisor suggested she begin by describing the incident and the context in which it happened. What made the incident significant? What were her concerns at the time? What was she thinking and feeling at the time? What did she think and feel after the incident? Was there anything particularly challenging about the situation? What societal messages exist that contributed to viewing the situation in that way? What assumptions had she made about Marjo and Chris, and their situation? What other ways could she have understood the situation? What could she have done that might be more helpful? How can this experience influence how she responds to a similar situation in the future?

Critically analysing everyday practice and activities (words, gestures, actions) is another rich source of identifying possible change. This can be done by using narrative techniques such as journalling, keeping notes and developing a critical consciousness. It can also be useful to do these activities with likeminded peers who have a commitment to change.

At the policy level, having a more nuanced understanding of the context is critical, specifically at an organisational level. Ask a series of questions aimed to make visible what has previously been invisible. Questions could include these ones:

- In what ways does existing policy and practice reinforce normative heterosexuality?
- Who gains from this?

- Who loses?
- What changes need to be made to address this?
- Who should be involved in the process of change?
- What resources are needed to achieve this change?

If the purpose is to have the frame of mind that is inclusive and free from discrimination, a rich source of knowledge can come from those who have experienced this discrimination as well as those who have done the discriminating, albeit unintentionally.

Challenging/deconstructing heteronormativity

Heteronormativity leads to social, cultural, political and interpersonal oppression of LGBTIQ people. It operates in an insidious way, in its 'natural', 'normal', 'taken for granted' presence. As Butler (2004) argues, normative social practices remain invisible, implicit and difficult to grasp. They can, however, be grasped and challenged as Kitzinger (2005) shows in her explanation of 'the implicit' in research using conversation analysis to show how heterosexuals continually reproduce themselves and others as heterosexual in everyday life conversations where sexuality is not the focus. Uncovering the 'implicit' is critical for practitioners, policymakers, educators and researchers in the health, human and community services if they are to challenge the power of heteronormativity. Interrogation and critical analysis of heteronormativity can expose the dominance of normative heterosexuality and how its oppressive practice affects the daily lives of LGBTIQ people. The development of a critical consciousness can lead to a change in power relations by identifying points of resistance. Then dominant ideas can be queried and challenged, acted on and meaning reconstructed, at both individual (micro) and institutional (macro) levels. Questioning assumptions that influence practice and the taken-for-granted practices in organisations can begin this process. Critically reflecting on the meaning of concepts that are often not queried, such as family, caring relationships, intimate relationships, household structure and community, can begin to make heteronormative practices more visible. For both heterosexual and LGBTIQ practitioners, the interrogation of everyday practices, such as talk and behaviour, can make an important contribution to further exposing heteronormativity, leading to greater social justice and equality for LGBTIQ people.

References

ABS *see* Australian Bureau of Statistics

Australian Bureau of Statistics (ABS). 2013, 'Feature Article 1: Population by Age and Sex, Australia, States and Territories', ABS, <www.abs.gov.au/ausstats/abs@.nsf/featurearticlesbytitle/1CD-2B1952AFC5E7ACA257298000F2E76?OpenDocument>, accessed 1 July 2014

Benjamin, A. 2007, 'Doing anti-oppressive social work: The importance of resistance, history and strategy' in D. Baines (ed.), *Doing Anti-Oppressive Practice: Building transformative politicized work*, Manitoba: Fernwood Publishing, pp. 196–204

Best, S. & Kellner, D. 1991, *Postmodern Theory: Critical interrogations*, London: Macmillan

Butler, J. 2004, *Undoing Gender*, New York: Routledge

Bullough, V.L. 2002, *Before Stonewall: Activists for gay and lesbian rights in historical context*, New York: Routledge

Charing, G., Deswardt, P., Henry, M., Launder, M., McDermott, A. & Pollard, N. (eds) 1975, 'Gay Issue'; *Case Con*, no. 18

Crouse, K. 2014, 'Ian Thorpe, Swimming Star for Australia in Olympics, Says He Is Gay', *The New York Times*, <www.nytimes.com/2014/07/13/sports/ian-thorpe-star-for-australia-in-olympics-says-hes-gay.html>, accessed 30 July 2015

D'Amico, M. 2007, *Critical Postmodern Social Work and Spirituality*, Master's thesis, Melbourne: RMIT University

Durso, L.E. & Gates, G.J. 2012, *Serving Our Youth: Findings from a national survey of service providers working with lesbian, gay, bisexual, transgender youth who are homeless or at risk of becoming homeless*, Los Angeles: The Williams Institute with True Colors Fund and True Palette Fund

Faderman, L. 1991, *Odd Girls and Twilight Lovers: A history of lesbian life in twentieth century America*, New York: Penguin Books

Fenge, L.A. 2010, 'Striving towards inclusive research: An example of participatory action research with older lesbians and gay men', *British Journal of Social Work*, vol. 40, pp. 878–94

Foucault, M. 1977, *Discipline and Punish: The birth of the prison*, London: Penguin

Harris, A. & Rothfield, P. 2014, 'Former world champion swimmer Ian Thorpe admits he's gay in Parkinson interview tonight', *The Mercury*, <www.themercury.com.au/news/former-world-champion-swimmer-ian-thorpe-admits-hes-gay-in-parkinson-interview-tonight/story-fnj4f7kx-1226987020616>, accessed 2 August 2015

Harrison, J. 2006, 'Coming out ready or not! Gay, lesbian, bisexual, transgender and intersex ageing and aged care in Australia: Reflections, contemporary developments and the road ahead', *Gay and Lesbian Issues and Psychology Review*, vol. 2, no. 2, pp. 44–53

Hart, J. 1980, 'It's just a stage we are going through: The sexual politics of casework' in M. Brake & R. Bailey (eds), *Radical Social Work and Practice*, London: Edward Arnold, pp. 46–63

Hicks, S. & Watson, K. 2003, 'Desire lines "queering" health and social welfare' *Sociological Research Online*, vol. 8, no. 1, pp. 1–21

Irwin, J. 2008a, 'Challenging the second closet: Intimate partner violence between lesbians' in B. Fawcett & F. Waugh (eds), *Addressing Violence, Abuse and Oppression: Debates and challenges*, Oxford: Routledge, pp. 80–92

—— 2008b, 'Discounted stories: Lesbians and domestic violence' in *Qualitative Social Work*, vol. 7, pp. 199–215

—— 2009, 'Lesbians and gay men: (un) equal before the law?' in P. Swain & S. Rice (eds), *In the Shadow of the Law: The legal context of social work practice,* 3rd edn, Sydney: Federation Press, pp. 192–207

Kitzinger, C. 2005, 'Heteronormativity in action: Reproducing the heterosexual nuclear family in after-hours medical calls', *Social Problems,* vol. 52, no. 4, pp. 477–98

Magnay, J. 2002, 'Thorpe straight as the line on the bottom of the pool', *Sydney Morning Herald,* <www.smh.com.au/articles/2002/11/17/1037490052340.html>, accessed 30 July 2015

Markowitz, L. 1991, 'Homosexuality: Are we still in the dark?' *Networker,* vol. 15, pp. 26–35

Milligan, D. 1975, 'Homosexuality: Sexual needs and social problems' in R. Bailey & M. Brake (eds), *Radical Social Work,* London: Edward Arnold, pp. 96–111

Phelan, S. 1989, *Identity Politics: Lesbian feminism and the limits of community,* Philadelphia: Temple University Press

Rich, A. 1980, 'Compulsory heterosexuality', *Signs: Journal of Women in Culture and Society,* vol. 5, pp. 631–60

Richardson, D. 1996, *Theorising Heterosexuality: Telling it straight.* Buckingham, Philadelphia, PA: Open University Press

Smith, R. & France-Prence, A. 2014, 'Aussie swimming legend Thorpe admits he's gay', <www.rappler.com/sports/world/63234-aussie-swimming-legend-thorpe-gay>, accessed 2 August 2015

Tolley, C. & Ranzjin, R. 2006, 'Heteronormativity amongst staff in residential aged care facilities', *Gay and Lesbian Issues and Psychology Review,* vol. 2, no. 2, pp. 78–86

Toms, M., Redshaw, S. & Twenty-Ten Association Incorporated. 2007, *"It may not be fancy . . . " Exploring the service needs of homeless gay, lesbian, bisexual and transgender young people.* Canberra: Commonwealth Department of Families Community Services and Indigenous Affairs

Walton, T. 2011, *Out of the Shadows,* London: Bona Street Press

Weedon, C. 1987, *Feminist Practice and Poststructuralist Theory,* Oxford: Basil Blackwell

Willett, G. 2000, *Living Out Loud: A history of gay and lesbian activism in Australia,* St Leonards: Allen & Unwin

Williams, C.R. 1996. *'Identity, Difference and the "Other"',* PhD Thesis, Campbelltown: University of Western Sydney

Part V

Towards collectivist and transformative practices in social work

18

Environmental social work as critical, decolonising practice

Mel Gray and John Coates

Popular interest in the environment has steadily grown in recent decades such that the environmental movement has been called the 'largest, most densely organised political cause in human history' (Brown 1995: xiv). Aided by the globalisation of communication, people in all parts of the world are increasingly alarmed by growing concerns about environmental changes, and the actual and anticipated threats to human and global wellbeing. In response, millions of small, locally oriented community groups and large globally influential organisations, such as Greenpeace, Worldwatch Institute, and Kairos have emerged (Hawken 2007; Turner 2007). While the focus initially was most frequently local pollution and habitat destruction, concern spread internationally as 'development' strategies, risky technologies, and waste disposal were transferred to nations in the Global South. Greenpeace advocates labelled this as 'toxic colonialism' (Koné 2010) and works such as Hofrichter (1993) and Pulido (1996) brought attention to the role of international financial institutions in the social injustices created by environmental degradation. Bullard (1993) argued the environmental justice movement brought issues of social inequality and power imbalances into the larger environmental movement and underscored the importance of connecting environmental and social justice issues. International organisations, such as the World Council on Environment and Development (WCED) and the International Panel on Climate Change (IPCC), added credibility to the feared consequences of environmental destruction.

The wide disciplinary interest in environmental issues, such as climate change, habitat destruction and species extinction, has resulted in a multidisciplinary perspective among scholars regarding discussions of causes, consequences and restorative actions (see Ife 2013). Critiques of the lack of effective action point to the need to challenge our extractive economy that views the Earth as a source of raw materials. Detailed reviews across many disciplines have critiqued the socioeconomic system for relentlessly extracting resources and exhausting the rehabilitative capacities of Earth (for example, Capra 1982; Berry 1988; Korten 2009). Despite the many benefits modern society has provided, there has been a dark side to growth (Capra 1982). Modern life has produced exploitation and inequality, and women, the poor, and indigenous communities suffer disproportionately more from the negative impacts of climate change and natural disasters (Alston & Whittenbury 2013; Hetherington & Boddy 2013). It is the focus on the 'intrinsically destructive relationship to nature' (Christopher 1999: 361) of modern economic and social beliefs, and practices as the root contributor to environmental and social problems, which makes environmental social work inherently critical. The concept of environmental justice suggests the nature of the environmental paradigm, which, for social work, requires a complete change in how we think about our practice. As we shall show, it also requires that social work names the obstacles standing in the way of the kind of just society we envisage, the preoccupation with progress, profit and efficiency that permeates contemporary policy and leads to the welfare austerity that is further exacerbating poverty and inequality (Gray & Webb 2013). We draw on critical thinkers who have, over the years, given concentrated thought to the idea of a just society, where principles of equality and fairness underline everything we do, and we marry this to the ways in which social workers might take action at all levels of practice toward environmental justice. Environmental scholars have identified the need to break free of the preoccupation with progress, profit and efficiency that act like blinkers to the severity of social and environmental injustices (for example, Berry 1999; Coates 2003). They have exposed the values, beliefs and destructive practices that have contributed to the exploitation of indigenous communities and their traditional territories, and to the Global North's benefits of elitist economic priorities and methods. They point to the multidimensional impact of globalisation, the impact of international trade and finance, deforestation, pollution, industrial agriculture, mining and dam construction. All of these involve human interventions that have severe consequences for the natural environment and people's lives, especially the most socially and economically disadvantaged in society most affected by environmental catastrophes. The movement to 'Decolonize Wall Street' exposed the gross financial inequality in society by highlighting the pervasive economic rationality dominating global governance.

Historical overview

The beginning of the modern environmental movement has been attributed to Rachel Carson's *Silent Spring* (1962), an exposé of the consequences of the unquestioned use of pesticides. Thereafter, concern for the environment grew exponentially in the public consciousness, receiving media attention worldwide. Scholarly publications began to surface (for example, Capra 1982) and the first World Commission on Environment and Development (Brundtland Commission 1987) was followed by government conferences and accords, such as the Kyoto Protocol (United Nations Development Program 1998) and the Intergovernmental Panel on Climate Change (2007). However, critical social work was late to engage with the environmental movement. Attention was first drawn to the ill-effects of environmental conditions on low-income and minority communities in Canada by Shkilnyk (1985), while in the US Chavis and Lee (1987) reported on the United Church of Christ's Commission on Racial Justice noting 'environmental racism' was contributing to the overrepresentation of minorities among those suffering the ill-effects of living near heavily polluting industrial and waste sites (see also Bullard 1993). This movement, known as 'environmental justice', since those most affected were low-income groups and not just racial minorities, began as a response to the social injustices arising from pollution and it is this focus on injustice and inequality that continues to give environmental social work its critical edge (Gray et al. 2013).

From the late 1980s onwards, church groups, and community and social service workers became concerned about environmental issues. Within a relatively short period, several publications emerged, and drew attention to the negative impacts of industrial pollution and harmful agricultural practices that were resulting in human exposure to toxins in water, soil and air (for example, Bullard 1993; Hofrichter 1993; Rogge 1994; Pulido 1996):

> Communities where people of color and people of low income live get disproportionate amounts of the harmful carry-overs which come from affluence and technology; get fewer of the benefits and are disproportionately excluded from the decision-making processes determining how toxic waste is managed (Rogge 1994: 53).

The first wide-ranging review of environmental issues for social work, and still a work of considerable relevance, was Hoff and McNutt's (1994) *The Global Environmental Crisis: Implications for social welfare and social work,* in which several chapters addressed how social work practitioners could and should be engaged in environmental issues. This was the only social work text on environmental issues that was published until a small group of social work scholars began to draw attention to environmental issues and concerns. For example, in Canada, Coates published *Ecology and Social Work* (2003) with his eco-social approach that focused on the unsustainable capitalist economic system; in Europe Mathies, Narhi and Ward (2001) explored sustainability in their edited book the *Eco-Social Approach in Social Work* and in the US Besthorn (2001) developed the 'Global Alliance for Deep-Ecological Social Work', a website to promote a more ecocentric or environmentally-based social work that went beyond the anthropocentric or human focused person-in-(social) environment perspective.

Despite these efforts, however, therapeutic models continued to dominate the North American centre from which this early work was emerging. The shallow, exclusively *social* interpretation of social work's longstanding 'person-in-environment' focus led to many academics being ill-equipped to connect social work and environmental issues. By and large, the profession has been quite reluctant to fully accept the importance of environmental issues for social work. There are many reasons for this; among them are the interdisciplinary nature of the terrain that involves a wide array of knowledge. This includes the once-contested science of global warming; scientific studies on air, water and soil pollution and their impact on people; habitat destruction and extinction of species; agricultural practices and policies; and globalisation and international trade policies, to name a few. Given the complex dimensions of global warming and environmental destruction, environmental interventions not only require interdisciplinary knowledge but also call for collective rather than individualistic solutions (Besthorn 2013; Ife 2013).

The range of disciplines within the environmental movement has brought social workers into alliances with scholars, community educators and social activists from many fields (for example, Coates & Besthorn 2010) and the issues requiring attention are diverse. For example, the area of disaster management includes working with others to rebuild communities following drought, mudslides, floods and hurricanes as well as dealing with environmental refugees displaced by such catastrophic events. The excessive burning of fossil fuels is the major source of carbon in the atmosphere and aided by industrial agriculture, excessive use of chemicals and packaging, the transportation of food thousands of kilometres, and the release of methane as the permafrost warms in the wake of global warming are all serious considerations that make climate change arguably the most severe crisis facing humanity (IPCC 2007).

With growing awareness of global warming and environmental destruction, social work's early focus on industrial pollution and toxic exposure began to expand. Critiques of neoliberal globalisation, deregulation, privatisation, commodification, consumerism, income disparities, food security, and social inequalities began to have an environmental dimension. In recent years social work has responded by expanding its theoretical considerations, and practice interventions to the physical environment have become more central to its discourse (for example, Mathies et al. 2001; Coates 2003, 2005; McKinnon 2008; Zapf 2009; van Wormer, Besthorn, & Keefe 2010; Dominelli 2012; Gray et al. 2013). Environmental realities have played a significant role in pushing social work to re-evaluate its interventions to address personal stress and family reactions to environmentally related issues, and significant lifestyle, community and public policy issues. This is to shift away from the current 'extractive economy' (Berry 1988) that exploits nature and the majority of humanity toward building a sustainable society (Mary 2008; Dylan 2013).

Environmental social work: expanding social work theory

Western knowledge systems, ideologies and methods of social care and development have been shown repeatedly to be inappropriate and totally inadequate for addressing the major crises confronting our planet (ecological, spiritual, social and economic) (Coates 2003; Gray et al. 2007). Mainstream Western ways of thinking focus on the individual and independence, as well as on social progress and economic growth. This has contributed to a competitive process of exploitation of Earth and its peoples, and resulted in social injustice and poverty. There are several areas of social work discourse where this critical awareness is changing the way in which social workers view their practice; among them are development and sustainability, environmental impacts on indigenous communities, and indigenous social work and spirituality.

Social work and sustainability

The discourse on social development and the environment is closely aligned to social work and highlights the importance of sustainable development (WCED 1987). Sustainable development is a contested concept, however, and is heavily political for those who claim it is a euphemism for economic growth. They see sustainability as a particular approach to serve the needs of the poor that requires authoritative structural and grassroots interventions (Mary 2008, Dylan 2013). Within this movement, there is increasing advocacy for a major shift from economic and industrial growth to sustainability; that is, meeting the needs of the present without compromising the ability of future generations to meet their needs (Brundtland Commission 1987). However, most social workers are situated mainly within human social services, where they offer psychosocial interventions. When it comes to 'community development, social planning and social policy within the framework of sustainable development' (Hessle 2005: 16), social workers enter a highly politicised, multidisciplinary area where they are often in a minority and lack power. Sustainable development, like social work, essentially concerns forms of resource management to promote social justice and human wellbeing, as well as vibrant and healthy natural ecosystems, with an eye to future generations.

Environmental impacts on indigenous communities

A number of scholarly publications have drawn attention to the severe negative impacts of environmental destruction and industrial practices on indigenous communities. Examples include relocation, water pollution and ill health as a consequence of mining operations on the traditional territory of indigenous peoples (Ross 2013), deforestation (Pulido 1996), toxic dumping (Rogge 1994) and mercury poisoning (Shkilnyk 1985). Frequently, governments have colluded with large corporations to exploit natural resources without compensation to displaced indigenous peoples. The structural adjustment programs of the International Monetary Fund (IMF) and World Trade Organisation (WTO) that demanded opening natural resources to international markets frequently contributed to these injustices (Hofrichter 1993). In Canada, Australia and the US, struggles to secure resolution of violations are ongoing (for example, Behrendt 2003; Ross 2013). An outstanding issue in Canada is the struggle of the Lubicon Cree to secure compensation for the pollution and exploitation of gas and oil from the Alberta Tar Sands (Amnesty International 2010). What this scholarship reveals is the direct relationship of environmental degradation to social injustices experienced by indigenous peoples and others.

Indigenous social work and spirituality

The profession's interest in indigenous social work and spirituality has also created a welcoming opportunity to discuss environmental issues. Coates et al. referred to this as the 'eco-spiritual' perspective 'to distinguish it from the more narrowly conceptualized, anthropocentric ecological perspective' (Coates et al. 2006: 388). Similarly, Zapf (2005) cautioned that limiting understanding of spirituality to the individual person risked missing the profound connection to the environment. As Gray stated, 'we need an outward focused eco-spiritual social work in which spirituality is "other" rather than self-centred, and not anthropocentric since it embraces all life forms as well as sustainability for the planet' (Gray 2008: 192). Morrissette et al. argued the distinctiveness of Aboriginal world views and traditions included their historical development 'involving a symbiotic relationship to the earth and a belief in the delicate balance among all things' (Morrissette et al. 1993: 93). They suggested this intimate and respectful relationship had resulted in a spiritual consciousness based on survival needs and a belief in people as caretakers of Earth's resources. In Australia several recent Aboriginal authors have added to this literature on indigenous world views and how they suggest a new paradigm for social work to be more consistent with an environmental perspective (Bennett et al. 2013; Muller 2014 Fejo-King 2013. The First National People of Color Environmental Leadership Summit (1991: 1) affirmed the 'sacredness of Mother Earth, ecological unity . . . the interdependence of all species, and the right to be free from ecological destruction'. This fundamental view of Earth as a sacred living thing is important to many indigenous peoples, and to a number of authors on the forefront of 'conscious evolution' (Berry 1988, 1999). This is a significant impact of critical environmental thought as it highlights the destructive capacity of the Western paradigm of progress and materialism, while it advances a holistic and more environmentally centred alternative (see Ife 2013). This view is in conflict with capitalist agendas based on exploiting Earth and dominant science perspectives that imply human control over nature because it cultivates harmony between humans and all living things. Critical environmental thought sees the entire world as interrelated and alive. These considerations lead us to the realm of environmental ethics and the 'ethical issues raised by human action in the non-human natural world' (Palmer 2003: 15).

Environmental ethics

Curry distinguished between environmental and ecological ethics. The former tends toward anthropocentrism with the focus on human interests, while the latter argues that ethics are intrinsic and should 'embrace the entire natural world' (Curry 2006: 1). Though Curry's reasoning has merit, in social work the term ecology is already intrinsic to mainstream, generic social work practice that has been largely focused on the relationship between humans and their social environment. Therefore, the term 'environmental ethics' is preferable since it denotes a new area of moral concern and social work theorising that emphasises the physical environment that has been neglected in social work. Where the profession stands on environmental social work possibly hinges on how it understands the relationship of humans to the rest of nature, and whether or not the non-human world has intrinsic or instrumental value. The intrinsic environmentally-centred stance sees the natural world as good in and of itself, while the instrumental people-centred view sees its value as derivative from human interests. Clearly, the profession needs to walk a fine line between enlightened self-interest, which saves nature so humans can survive, and an environmentally centred approach, which values nature for the sake of nature. Though the actions are often similar, the underlying philosophy differs. Actions that are independent of considerations for human benefit go against the grain of the humanistic foundations of social work, where values are seen as something owed to humans because of their dignity, worth and ability to reason, and because they are socially constructed and culturally specific. Especially in indigenous cultures, collective or group rights might predominate over individual rights and interests (Gray et al. 2008). In Western societies, human rights heavily inform codes of ethics, community and social policies, and theoretical frameworks tend to focus on individual benefit. Environmental ethics lead us to consider collective and group rights, not only of people, but also of ecosystems. Social work might embrace this broader, more inclusive view of rights by paying more attention to the third generation of human rights.

Environmental ethics highlights the difficulty humans have conceptualising nature as having other than instrumental value. Environmental social work encourages the profession to remove its individualistic and anthropocentric lens to consider our interdependence with other people and the physical world, which nourishes all that is human. It raises some perplexing questions for social work. While several writers have sought to capture the value of the physical environment, it would be extremely difficult to argue for social work to have a necessary role in environmental issues and problems without having a reference to human values and interests.

Environmental social work practice

It is in the context of this renewed ethical awareness and critical lens that environmental social work is emerging as an essential area of social work practice. Though there is a growing awareness of environmental issues, the practice of environmental social work continues to be under-emphasised despite the increasing role environmental concerns play in all communities and for all people across the world. Coates and Gray (2012) identified several broad themes in this emerging area of social work practice:

1. crisis intervention following disasters and traumatic events, including practice with survivors of natural disasters, and disaster relief services
2. social work intervention in times of drought
3. social work activism in relation to climate change

4. social work responses to toxic waste exposure, including practice with low-income communities to reduce children's exposure to toxins
5. food security, including community gardens, and urban and community-supported agriculture
6. environmental justice where racism, gender and poverty combine with climate change and environmental destruction so certain groups, like women and racial minorities, endure multiple oppressions
7. economic development, sustainability, and social capital to create employment, sustainable livelihoods and food security
8. community education relating to the environment, ecology, spirituality, and related matters
9. fossil fuels and housing adaptations with low-income communities
10. mining and industrial damage with those who have suffered at the hands of transnational corporations, especially mining companies.

These varied themes reflect the diversity of environmental issues with which social workers have been, and continue to be, engaged. However, this diversity raises questions about what position environmental social workers should take to engage in this issue. There is much work to be done in discerning the social work role and devising related practice models. Anecdotal evidence suggests many environmental social workers are practising on the margins; 'doing' environmental social work in their own time rather than as part of their daily jobs, but few are 'theorising' and 'writing' about their practice in these areas. While historically somewhat reluctant to embrace the environmental movement, social work, with its ecosystems, person-in-environment perspective is well placed to respond to the diverse challenges to environmental justice in contemporary life. However it needs a political dimension and critical perspective that sees human-made policies and structures as the cause of most environmental and social problems (Gray & Webb 2013).

Most social workers are mindful of the lack of resources available to meet the needs of service users. They see their role as strongly loaded towards those who bear the brunt of society's inequalities. As with efforts toward social justice, environmental social work broadens these arguments by highlighting the extent to which the poorest and most marginalised populations are hardest hit by the fallout of environmental destruction. Poverty remains one of the primary drivers of environmental degradation as impoverished people have the fewest options in industrially developed societies. The struggle for survival of the very poor in the Global South leads to habitat destruction, soil erosion and aridity, for example. At the other extreme, the excessive consumption of the wealthy is a significant driver of environmental decline.

Environmental social work sees a role for social workers in critically challenging local and national governments, and international organisations to enact policies that preserve habitat and species, and eliminate polluting and destructive practices carried out most frequently by, or on behalf of, large national and transnational corporations.

The causes and consequences of, and solutions to, environmental decline are complex. Many environmental problems impact large numbers of people and challenge social work's individualistic therapeutic and psychosocial focus. Similarly, international trade policies, industrial agriculture and forestry, and corporate economic practices contribute to the environmental problems that impact the basic elements of our lives, which are the air we breathe and the food we eat. To understand correctly how individuals, families and communities can be affected, it is important to understand the personal/economic/political interdependence at the root of the social injustice that accompanyies environmental destruction. It is becoming increasingly clear that global warming, habitat destruction, overharvesting, soil erosion and pollution are affecting human health and wellbeing, with consequent social injustices falling disproportionately on the most disadvantaged. These realities have raised serious challenges for social work and given rise to new ethical issues.

Ecological and spiritual social work as critical, decolonising practice

The discourses of environmental justice, spirituality and indigenous perspectives within social work have all highlighted the devastating consequences of modern economic and political practices. They have also critiqued the severe shortcomings of the colonising world view of modernity that dominates the world economy, popular culture and international politics. They have challenged the assumptions and values of the hegemony of modernity; that is, endless progress, the economic growth imperative, consumerism and faith in technology that leads to the exploitation of people and the planet for profit, and questioned the most fundamental assumptions of social institutions. These discourses of environmental justice see environmental and social problems to be the 'logical and unavoidable consequences of modern (that is, instrumental) rationality as expressed in the current structure of the most basic social and cultural institutions of modernity (that is, modern capitalism, industrial technology, individualistic morality, and mechanistic science)' (Christopher 1999: 361).

Scholars in many fields have proposed an alternative set of foundational values and beliefs with the potential to free humans 'from the straightjacket of modernity and markets' (Elshof 2010: 75). This framework shares foundational assumptions that recognise the interdependence between humans, and the relationship between humans and the non-human world; responsibility for self, others and the environment; connectedness of all things; and boundaries or limits to natural resources. These assumptions inform ecological and spiritual approaches that seek to provide a purpose to human life, a vision of the 'good' life, and a proper role for humans in relationship to one another and the planet. At heart, this reflects a relational world view. Such a relational world view finds expression in the principles of indigenous helping articulated by Hart (2009) including respect, sharing, balance, harmony, relationship and responsibility. The responsibility is both personal and collective in view of the impact of human behaviour on other people and Earth.

Ecological and spiritual approaches maintain that efforts to build a just and sustainable future must be founded 'on the awareness of the connections that bind us to each other, to all life and to all life to come' (Orr 2009: 125). Orr argues that every individual is 'stitched to a common fabric of life, kin to all other life forms ... Each ... is part of a common story that began three billion years ago' (Orr 2009: ix). Humanity can be seen to be at the threshold of a new age, where individual identity and wellbeing are connected to the wellbeing of Earth and future generations (Teasdale 1999). Ecological and spiritual approaches develop and build on interdependence, diversity and an inclusive framework that incorporates psychological, social, environmental and spiritual elements. This framework enables social workers to build on the assets of modernity (such as scientific knowledge and communication) yet also see through its constraints (such as exploitation and greed). They seek ways to challenge gross socioeconomic disparities and thus rectify persistent inequalities. They point to the need for a holistic world view that retains core modern ideas of human rights and social justice. Such integration expands the purview of mainstream social work, enabling it to more effectively engage issues of social marginalisation and economic exploitation that impact on all people, and Earth more generally.

Conclusion

Effective environmental social work is built upon a deep review of assumptions, values and actions, and as a result, to do environmental social work is to be political. Environmental social work draws critical attention to:

- the place of politics and ideology that informs and systemically supports social and ecological exploitation and degradation

- the connection between environmental degradation and poverty, sickness, exploitation, and numerous social injustices
- the individualistic, consumerist, and acquisitive values that dominate our world's economic and social planning
- the need for a critical exploration of constraints placed on the profession by its place in Western society.

Environmental social work provides an alternative framework that enables the profession to examine its roots (such as individualism, progress, consumerism, and materialism) and challenges social work to review and redefine its foundational assumptions. When social work challenges itself in this manner, the opportunity is created for the profession to consider an alternative foundation that enables significant social and political change.

References

Alston, M. & Whittenbury, K.L. (eds) 2013, *Research, Action and Policy: Addressing the gendered impacts of climate change*, New York: Springer

Amnesty International 2010, 'From Homeland to Oil Sands: The impact of oil and gas development on the Lubicon Cree of Canada', *Amnesty International*, <http://www.amnesty.ca/research/reports/from-homelands-to-oil-sands-the-impact-of-oil-and-gas-development-on-the-lubicon-cr, accessed 25 September 2014

Behrendt, L. 2003, *Achieving Social Justice: Indigenous rights and Australia's future*, Sydney: Federation Press

Bennett, B., Green, S., Gilbert, S. & Besarab, D. (eds) 2013, *Our Voices: Australian and Torres Strait Islander social work*, Melbourne: Palgrave Macmillan

Berry, T. 1988, *The Dream of the Earth*, San Francisco: Sierra Club Books

—— 1999, *The Great Work: Our way into the future*, New York: Bell Tower

Besthorn, F.H. 2001, 'Transpersonal psychology and deep ecological philosophy: Exploring linkages and applications for social work', *Social Thought: Journal of Religion in the Social Services*, vol. 22, no. 1/2, pp. 23–44

—— 2013, 'Radical equalitarian ecological justice: A social work call to action' in M. Gray, J. Coates & T. Hetherington (eds), *Environmental Social Work*, Routledge, Abingdon, pp. 31–45

Brown, L. 1995, 'Ecopsychology and the environmental revolution: An environmental forward' in T. Roszak, M. Gomes & A. Kanner (eds), *Ecopsychology: Restoring the earth, healing the mind*, San Francisco: Sierra Club Books, pp. xiii–xvi

Brundtland Commission 1987, *Report of the World Commission on Environment and Development: Our common future*, New York: Oxford University Press

Bullard, R. 1993, *Confronting Environmental Racism: Voices from the grassroots*, Cambridge: South End Press

Capra, F. 1982, *The Turning Point*, New York: Simon and Schuster

Carson, R. 1962, *Silent Spring*, Boston: Houston Mifflin

Chavis, B. & Lee, C. 1987, *Toxic Wastes and Race in the United States,* New York: Commission on Racial Justice United Church of Christ

Christopher, M. 1999, 'An exploration of the "reflex" in reflexive modernity: The rational and pre-rational social causes of the affinity for ecological consciousness', *Organizations and Environment,* vol. 12, no. 4, 357–400

Coates, J. 2003, *Ecology and Social Work: Toward a new paradigm,* Halifax: Fernwood Publishing

—— 2005, 'Environmental crisis: Implications for social work', *Journal of Progressive Human Services,* vol. 16, no. 1, pp. 25–49

—— & Besthorn, F.H. 2010, 'Introduction—Building bridges and crossing boundaries: Dialogues in professional helping', *Critical Social Work,* vol. 11, no. 3, pp. 1–7

—— & Gray, M. 2012, 'The environment and social work: An overview and introduction', *International Journal of Social Welfare,* vol. 21, no. 3, pp. 230–8

—— Gray, M. & Hetherington, T. 2006, 'An "ecospiritual" perspective: Finally, a place for Indigenous approaches', *British Journal of Social Work,* vol. 36, no. 3, pp. 381–99

Curry, P. 2006, *Ecological Ethics: An introduction,* Cambridge: Polity Press

Dominelli, L. 2012, *Green Social Work,* Cambridge: Polity Press

Dylan, A. 2013, 'Environmental sustainability, sustainable development, and social work' in M. Gray, J. Coates & T. Hetherington (eds), *Environmental Social Work,* Abingdon: Routledge, pp. 62–87

Elshof, L. 2010, 'Changing worldviews to cope with a changing climate' in R. Irwin (ed.), *Climate Change and Philosophy: Transformational possibilities,* New York: Continuum Press, pp. 75–108

Fejo-King, C. 2013, *Let's Talk Kinship: Innovating Australian social work education, theory, research and practice through Aboriginal knowledge. Insights from social work research conducted with the Larrakia and Warumungu Peoples of the Northern Territory,* Canberra: Christine Fejo-King Consulting

Gray, M. 2008, 'Viewing spirituality in social work through the lens of contemporary social theory', *British Journal of Social Work,* vol. 38, no. 1, pp. 175–96

—— & Webb, S.A. (eds) 2013, *The New Politics of Social Work,* Houndmills: Palgrave

—— Coates, J. & Hetherington, T. 2007 'Hearing Indigenous voices in mainstream social work', *Families in Society,* vol. 88, no. 1, pp. 53–64

—— (eds) 2013, *Environmental Social Work,* Abingdon: Routledge

Gray, M., Coates, J. & Yellow Bird, M. (eds) 2008, *Indigenous Social Work Around the World: Towards culturally relevant education and practice,* Aldershot: Ashgate

Hart, M.A. 2009, 'Anti-colonial Indigenous social work: Reflections on an Aboriginal approach' in R. Sinclair, M.A. Hart & G. Bruyere (eds), *Wicihitowin: Aboriginal Social Work in Canada,* Fernwood Publishing, Halifax, pp. 25–41

Hawken, P. 2007, *Blessed Unrest: How the largest movement in the world came into being and no one saw it coming,* New York: Viking Press

Hessle, S. 2005, 'Sustainable development and social work' in S. Hessle & D. Zavirsek (eds), *Sustainable Development in Social Work: The case of a regional network in the Balkans,* Studies in International Social Work, no. 5, Stockholm: Department of Social Work, Stockholm University, pp. 11–25

Hetherington, T. & Boddy, J. 2013, 'Ecosocial work with marginalized populations: Time for action on climate change' in M. Gray, J., Coates & T. Hetherington (eds), *Environmental Social Work,* Abingdon: Routledge, pp. 46–61

Hoff, M.D. & McNutt, J.G. (eds) 1994, *The Global Environmental Crisis: Implications for social welfare and social work,* Aldershot: Ashgate

Hofrichter, R. (ed.) 1993, *Toxic Struggles: The theory and practice of environmental justice,* Gabriola Island: New Society Publishers

Ife, J. 2013, *Community Development in an Uncertain world: Vision, analysis and practice,* Melbourne: Cambridge University Press

Intergovernmental Panel on Climate Change (IPCC). 2007, 'Climate Change 2007: Synthesis Report', IPCC, <www.ipcc.ch/publications_and_data/ar4/syr/en/contents.html>, accessed 25 September 2014

Koné, L. 2010, 'Toxic Colonialism: The human rights implications of illicit trade of toxic waste in Africa', *Consultancy Africa,* <http://www.consultancyafrica.com/index.php?option=com_contentandview=articleandid=473:toxic-colonialism-the-human-rights-implications-of-illicit-trade-of-toxic-waste-in-africaandcatid=91:rights-in-focusandItemid=296> [25 September 2014]

Korten, D. 2009, *Agenda for a New Economy: From phantom wealth to real wealth,* San Francisco: Berrett-Koehler

Mary, N. 2008, *Social Work in a Sustainable World,* Chicago: Lyceum Books

Mathies, A-L., Narhi, K. & Ward, D. (eds) 2001, *The Eco-social Approach in Social Work,* SoPhi, Jyvaskyla: University of Jyvaskyla

McKinnon, J. 2008, 'Exploring the nexus between social work and the environment', *Australian Social Work,* vol. 61, no. 3, pp. 256–68

Morrisette, V., McKenzie, B. & Morrissette, L. 1993, 'Towards an Aboriginal model of social work practice', *Canadian Social Work Review,* vol. 10, no. 1, pp. 91–108

Muller, L. 2014, *A Theory for Australian Indigenous Health and Human Service Work: Connecting Indigenous knowledge with practice,* St Leonards: Allen & Unwin

Orr, D. 2009, *Down to the Wire,* Toronto: Oxford University Press

Palmer, C. 2003, 'An overview of environmental ethics' in A. Light & H. Rolston III (eds), *Environmental ethics: An anthology,* Oxford: Blackwell, pp. 15–37

People of Color Environmental Leadership Summit 1991, 'Principles of Environmental Justice', *Environmental Justice Resource Centre,* <http://archive.is/No5x> [25 September 2014]

Pulido, L. 1996, *Environmentalism and Economic Justice,* Tucson: University of Arizona Press

Rogge, M. 1994, 'Environmental Injustice: Social welfare and toxic waste' in M. Hoff & J. McNutt (eds), *The Global Environmental Crisis: Implications for social welfare and social work,* Brookfield: Ashgate, pp. 53–74

Ross, D. 2013, 'Social work and the struggle for corporate social responsibility' in M. Gray, J., Coates & T. Hetherington (eds), *Environmental Social Work,* Abingdon: Routledge, pp. 193–210

Shkilnyk, A. 1985, *A Poison Stronger than Love: The destruction of an Ojibwa community,* New Haven: Yale University Press

Teasdale, W. 1999, 'The Interspiritual Age: Practical mysticism for the third millennium', *Council on Spiritual Practices,* <www.csp.org/experience/docs/teasdale-interspiritual.html>, accessed 25 September 2014

Turner, C. 2007, *The Geography of Hope: A tour of the world we need,* Toronto: Vintage Canada

United Nations Development Program (UNDP). 1998, '*Human Development Report*', UNDP, <http://hdr.undp.org/en/reports/global/hdr1998/>, accessed 25 September 2014

van Wormer, K., Besthorn, F. & Keefe, T. 2010, *Human Behavior and the Social Environment: Macro level: Groups, communities, and organizations,* 2nd edn, New York: Oxford University Press

World Commission on Environment and Development (WCED) 1987, *The Concept of Sustainable Development,* <http://www.un-documents.net/wced-ocf.htm> [25 September 2014]

Zapf, M.K. 2009, *Social Work and the Environment: Understanding people and place,* Toronto: Canadian Scholars Press

Zapf, MK. 2005, 'The spiritual dimension of person and environment: Perspectives from social work and traditional knowledge', *International Social Work,* vol. 48, no. 5, pp. 633–42

19

Taking it to the streets: critical social work's relationship with activism

Jessica Morrison

Introduction

This chapter explores ways that critical social workers can expand possibilities for social change. I examine some of the key foundations to social change-focused practice, and then explore ways that social workers can take up this challenge, both inside and outside workplaces. I also explore the link between the social work role and personal activism.

Context

There is a fundamental challenge for critical social workers. While the foundation of the approach is that the problem is structural oppression, and social justice is the core of social workers' professional identity (AASW 2010; IFSW 2004); it is very rare that 'overthrow the system' is part of our job description. The vast majority of the roles in most organisations steer workers towards the exhausting and gut-wrenching process of having to distribute a few crumbs to the starving masses, rather than ensure there is enough bread for us all. So what is the critical social worker to do? Accept that there are limited opportunities to change the system, and the best to hope for is to salve a few wounds and then have a good bath at the end of the day? I would hope not!

Social workers witness oppression and are therefore involved in the situations that make others suffer. As others have argued (Briskman 2008; Mmatli 2008; Allan 2009a), I suggest that it is social workers' responsibility to engage politically and participate in social change. One of the most fundamental contributions of post-modernism to critical social work is the notion that power is not static. The level of power a person or group holds depends on many factors, including individual decisions to fight for it (Bauman 1995; Fawcett & Featherstone 2000). One of the key limitations to practices of resistance is predominantly a reluctance to take up activism.

This is not a new idea; social work practice and activism have a long connection. One of social work's founding heroes in the US was Jane Addams who established settlement houses, was arrested many times for resisting war and protecting anarchists, and was a founder of Women's International League for Peace and Freedom (Linn 2000). There has been a constant stream of social workers since that time who have advocated for a strong engagement in politics and activism (Gray et al. 2002; Mendes 2008).

Foundations for activist practice

The first foundational building block for social change practice is to acknowledge that critical social work explicitly seeks to redress societal imbalances of power and resources (Mullaly 1997). This work will challenge those with power and wealth, something that is unlikely to be welcomed by those with disproportionate resources (Nzira & Williams 2008). Social change therefore involves direct conflict with people in power. This might come in many different forms, from official court hearings to confronting oppression within a group. Critical social workers therefore need to become comfortable with stirring up the hornets' nests of injustice and the tension that it creates.

The second foundational building block is that working from a critical perspective takes a significant level of commitment and a willingness to take risks; what some have called 'moral courage' (Briskman et al. 2009). Going along with a system is always easier than challenging it. Gandhi said that activism is 'experiments with truth' (Gandhi 1993) and we can never be sure of the results of experiments. In every situation, each person needs to assess what level of risk they are able to take. For example, to directly challenge an injustice in an organisation may affect promotion prospects or even job security. Similarly, to take up a campaign that is not part of your job description will require extra time as well as possible public exposure, which may be manageable, but it could also lead to some very grumpy partners, friends or kids if this is not negotiated.

The third foundational building block is a commitment to ongoing critical reflection. The first part of this is to always ask whether one's own life is replicating oppressive patterns in our society. This will be most pronounced for those who are more privileged: those who are closest to societally valued norms of race, class, gender, ability, sexual orientation and age. Good critical reflection allows us to honestly interrogate our own practice and life as well as provides an opportunity to develop new ideas and strategies. A period of reflection and fermentation of ideas with others preceded every single example of activist practice that I have been involved in.

A related aspect to critical reflection is being able to truly re-imagine relationships with equal power. I agree with Allan (2009b) that a foundational aspect of critical practice is about how we locate ourselves in relation to our 'client' or any oppressed 'other'. We can locate ourselves as the distant, expert other or as someone who is open to a relationship of mutuality. Activist practice must begin to 'be the change' in the way it operates, by seeking to build communities of resistance, which share power more equally. This can be particularly challenging for those of us who are privileged because we assume a place of power and a dominant role. For social change to happen, allies (such as social workers) must be open to dialogical relationships with people from oppressed groups and find ways to listen and learn together (see Friere 1970).

Ideas of how critical social workers can engage in activist practice can occur in three different settings: social change-focused organisations; mainstream organisations; and in our personal lives. These are of course artificial categories and the boundaries shift between them.

Basing ourselves in social change-focused organisations

There are organisations that wholly or largely aim towards social change. This is the easiest environment for a critical social worker as there is usually synergy between one's own values and that of the organisation. These organisations can be as diverse as peak bodies (for example, Australian Council for Social Services), advocacy groups (for example, Council for Single Mothers and their Children), and service-based organisations (for example, Flat Out Inc). Their similarity is that their key focus is social change. Critical social workers can be employed in a variety of roles and can support organisations in their vision.

I worked in one of these services, the Wellington People's Centre in New Zealand, which was established in the early 1990s due to major benefit cuts and a period of intense political action for the rights of people without paid work (Locke 2002; Locke & Stevens 2009). The organisation provided both services and advocacy, but its overall orientation was to change society. My role was to coordinate the advocacy services and I focused on boosting activist work in the organisation. We increased engagement in direct social policy advocacy, holding public debates with parliamentarians; meetings with Ministers; and worked with the media. We also focused on internal processes to better reflect the organisation's ideals. We had the difficult conversations about work quality and group dynamics that had previously been avoided (Morrison & Brannigan 2007). I was able to bring skills to this process, which included meeting facilitation and attention to processes such as critical reflection. In turn they challenged me about some class-based assumptions that I had, and assisted me to develop my own capacity to work in less hierarchical ways. The organisational structure, a self-help model with both advocacy services and professional health services, provided a difficult tension for us to negotiate.

Championing changes in organisational focus

In addition to organisations that are already focused on social change, social workers can also search for organisations that are open towards this focus. Perhaps the most famous example of this in Australia is the Family Centre Project organised by the Brotherhood of St Laurence in Melbourne in the 1970s. Previously a largely traditionalist welfare agency, this organisation's staff decided that clients needed power over resources, relationships, information and decision-making. They sacked their social workers and sought to give their service users more power and diverted money directly to the community members (Benn 1993). While the structure of the organisation is now very different, the orientation of the organisation towards social change has continued until today (BSL 2014).

One of my early roles as a social worker was in a small church-based agency, then called Sunshine Christian Community Services. The organisation had a very traditionalist orientation, and so did I. However, through the process of critical reflection and listening, as well as exposure to critical ideas, our organisation decided to reorientate towards social change. The first step in this was an internal cultural change, particularly focused on breaking down hierarchical structures in relationships. We opened up our physical space so people could meet. We held roundtable conversations and forums. Mentors were vital in this process and I spent a lot of time talking and brainstorming with social work staff and students at our local university, which was focused on critical social work. We began engaging in the social issues of our local community, from poker machines to access to housing, food security and the government's budget.

While working in social change-focused organisations is probably the easiest fit for critical workers, it requires commitment to all the foundational factors to work well. I worked many extra hours in Sunshine Christian Community Services and at the Wellington People's Centre because I wanted to achieve social change and support people who were being ground down by injustice. I also cringe about the ways that I operated from my middle-class privileges and assumptions. When we took up our first major campaign in Sunshine against a new poker machine venue in our community, I assumed the role of leader. It is only in hindsight that I look back with concern about my photograph being on the front page of the local paper on so many occasions. I suspect that my time would have been better spent in skill-share sessions with community members than being the poster girl for the campaign. It seems to take eternal vigilance to stop dominant power dynamics being replicated in organisations.

Strategic manoeuvring in mainstream organisations

It is a very small minority of organisations that are fundamentally oriented to social change, and very few critical social workers will be based in one of these organisations (Briskman 2008). Most social workers, however, will be employed by organisations that espouse a commitment to social justice. This is where critical social workers can use their influence.

I think strategic expansion of activist work within organisations can be some of the most important and exciting work as it opens up new possibilities. The following are some ways I have seen this happen in organisations:

- direct political challenge
- organisations and workers can lead or support activist campaigns. I supported a woman to organise a mini-campaign in her neighbourhood against her local bus company, which was threatening to reduce services. Events such as those that highlight social issues (Aids Awareness Day; NAIDOC week events) can be held in organisations. There are many discrete ways to engage in activist practices.
- challenge an aspect of organisational structure or culture.
- many organisational practices replicate oppression. In an organisation I worked for, there was a strict demarcation between toilets used by clients

and those used by staff, which were supported by false assumptions (for example, you can catch Hepatitis C from a toilet seat). Challenging these practices is significant and can lead to oppressive perspectives being changed.

- find ally organisations or groups to do the work that you cannot do.
- organisations do not feel able to lead campaigns and do not want their workers to be visibly involved. In these situations, social workers can link with organisations that can lead campaigns. There are many peak bodies, such as councils for social services, 'welfare rights' groups and others that we can engage with. In this way, we can provide direct examples of how particular policies are affecting people. Be very mindful when utilising people's stories in political advocacy. Do not 'own' someone's story, and continue to treat this story with the utmost respect and seek full consent in using it (see Goldsworthy 2001).

Many organisations have parent or sister organisations that can engage politically. In Sunshine Christian Community Services, our work was significantly multiplied by linking with the Uniting Church bodies in regards to advocacy and media attention. In one job I had, it was clear that methadone dispensing costs were a major stress for people. Later, when doing a short secondment with a peak body, I was able to use relationships in my home organisation, as well as form new ones, to write a report about this issue. Unions are also a clear way to engage with the political process. So are our formal associations such as the AASW (for example, Briskman & Goddard 2007).

While this work is often the most exciting, it also may require the most effort from workers. It is work that involves a strategic approach; that is, to identify the specific change that you seek, identify allies and reflect about how to implement this change. This is also the work that could involve the most conflict, as the change you seek is often in those who are very close to you. Often managers identify those who are agitating for change as 'problems'. I suggest only start to agitate for change when you are already seen as a strong asset to the organisation. It is also always a good idea to be very familiar with the context before you launch a direct challenge to it. In working in this way, social workers are able to support their clients to also realise their own capacity to exercise political power (Healy 1999).

Vignette: expanding activism in workplaces

I worked in a government-funded drug and alcohol service, where I was employed as a counsellor. A new senior counsellor was employed whose feminist practice had a profound effect on her work, particularly how she viewed power. She proposed we change our weekly group 'supervision' to 'co-visioning', to better reflect our mutual learning. Critical reflection processes assisted us to examine our own practice, the politics surrounding it and how we responded.

There were many small challenges to the system that we were able to work through at this time. When suddenly the funding formula changed to only cover six sessions per 'episode of care' we decided to periodically close an episode of care. Then we started a new episode of care a week later to ensure that we could give the service that was requested by clients without sending our organisation into financial crisis.

I also took on a personal responsibility to engage in social change in my own personal realm. As a Christian, I was exposed to some very judgemental views in churches about people who used drugs. Using my 'expert' position, I challenged these judgemental views whenever I saw them, such as by writing to denominational newspapers.

The counselling team also explored 'partnership accountability' (Hall 1994). We imagined and planned what it might look like to partner with our 'clients'. A discussion paper was written and circulated, redrafted and affirmed by the organisation's board members. The first meeting was wonderfully successful, including the attendance of many clients and former clients, various staff members and the chair of the board. The only difficult moment was when the chair of the board unilaterally announced that it was unlikely a client would sit on the board. This comment pre-empted any conversations that had not yet taken place and assumed clients were less competent. There were further meetings that embodied a sense of partnership and excitement about what was possible. A suggestion box idea was implemented, clients sat on an internal working group, and a 'Moreland Hall action group' was formed to be a voice in social policy reform regarding alcohol and drugs.

Then a major issue arose. One of the natural leaders among the 'client' group was interviewed as a spokesperson for the action group by the local paper. The result was a front-page article with the client's photograph calling for a trial of a safe-injecting facility in Victoria (a church agency in New South Wales had just established one in a direct challenge to state laws). The manager saw this as a major threat to the organisation and sought to censor both the client group and 'reign in' the client participation process. The counselling team staff were all chastised for not taking appropriate 'care' of our clients and they sought to classify the client participation process as a 'group program', which would be treated the same as any other therapeutic group (such as only two staff could participate). We were all horrified. Suddenly the expansive organisational processes and dynamics that we were seeking to establish were replaced in favour of a hierarchical model. The managers of the organisation were extremely directive towards staff and sought for us to show the same attitude towards clients. We resisted. Within six months, all of us had resigned under threats of disciplinary action (for more, see Beckwith 2000).

There are many things that I have learned from this process. The first is to never underestimate one's own power. In the midst of the conflict, I could perceive the way the management of the organisation abused their power. However, as time went on, I recognised that our counselling team had become a powerful group within the organisation. The clients, whose role had been previously very passive, had also quickly become a group of people whom the organisation could no longer control. If they had continued, I suspect they would have become a formidable voice for change in the drug and alcohol field.

The second key reflection is to realise that change is often slow and difficult. In this case, we had overestimated the support we had from other people in the organisation who had been deeply invested in hierarchical ways of operating. However, fifteen years later this organisation is playing a leading role in 'consumer participation' in the sector. So perhaps our experiment sowed the seeds of change.

Personal activism

The feminist axiom that the personal is political was powerfully demonstrated through my work as a social worker. My work provided a window into oppression that as a privileged person I had not previously had access to. It became clear that all my life decisions had political implications; where I live, who I hang out with, how I spend my time, how I talk about my role as a social worker and how I use my financial resources. I sought to make deliberate choices about all of these aspects of my life. Informed by my work and my critical thinking, social work led me to engage directly in social change work. It appears to me that this is an inevitable outcome of critical thinking. After becoming aware of how systems work to oppress people, it seems obvious we would seek to be both deliberate about how we engage in these systems and then seek to change them.

Research suggests that social workers are more likely to be engaged politically, whether this causes social workers to choose the career of social work or the effect of it is not clear. International studies have found that social workers are much more likely to vote for more progressive parties (Kriesi 1998), and that about one third of social workers engage in activism (Gray et al. 2002).

There are many ways to seek social change, including our engagement in political processes (lobbying, seeking election, writing letters or submissions to government agencies), awareness building, solidarity activities, demonstrations, and civil disobedience (blockades/culture jamming). All these tactics have valid roles in achieving social change and at different times I have been personally involved in all of them. There is a wealth of wonderful material that has been written to support creative and strategic activism (Burgmann 2003; Maddison & Scalmer 2006; Reinsborough & Canning 2010; McIntyre 2013; The Change Agency 2014).

It is vital for social workers to engage in social movements. Social movements are any sustained effort towards social change by a group of people. Traditionally these have been led by people experiencing oppression (racism, class inequality, gender inequality), and unions have played a significant role. In recent decades, movements have become more fluid in their organising, have more diverse tactics, and often have significant involvement from people not specifically impacted by a social injustice (Burgmann 2003; Eggert & Giugni 2012).

A key reason that social workers need to be involved in social movements is solidarity. Engagement in social change cannot be bound by the scope of our professional lives. This is where the critical social worker becomes a critical actor in society. Social workers also can bring particular skills and resources to social movements, which is another key reason to become involved.

Research indicates that social movements are 'disproportionately, indeed overwhelmingly, drawn from amongst the highly educated members of the new middle class, with a particular concentration among those employed in social and cultural services' (Kriesi 1998: 170). This suggests that already many social workers are taking up roles in social movements. It also suggests that as 'middle class' people engage, then it is likely that their role is to be working 'in solidarity' with others. Workers will need to be aware about replicating middle-class presumption of privilege when supporting movements.

Vignette: Occupy Melbourne

Occupy Melbourne was a rather spontaneous gathering inspired by events overseas. The people who led it had limited experience in organising campaigns, group processes or consensus-based decision-making. It had all the hallmarks of a new social movement. Occupy Melbourne sought to challenge the concentration of both wealth and power in the hands of the 'one per cent' of the population, and live out an alternative by physically 'occupying' public spaces. These reflected the aims that I had for society and therefore I sought to support the movement even though the tactic was unfamiliar (not only to me but also to the organisers).

I do not wish to give a commentary of the movement as this has been done elsewhere (Carson et al. 2012). However, I do want to briefly touch on the attempts to equalise power within the movement, and also the role of social workers.

Occupy Melbourne sought to practise what it preached regarding the sharing of power. Group decisions were made by large group consensus, and particular attention was paid to getting this process right. Voices who were often diminished were given a prominence. An Aboriginal and Torres Strait Islander solidarity tent was established as a priority, and people deliberately included people who were homeless. Many people learned to use a communication board to ensure each participant's voice was heard. This led to a movement that was much more inclusive than others I have been involved with. There was almost a visible tension between those who were from more middle-class, privileged backgrounds and others, as the group sought to equalise the power among people of different social classes.

Critical social workers and others in health and human services professions played very significant roles in Occupy Melbourne. It was clear that they had both skills to offer the larger group and a passion for the movement's aims. Critical social workers were particularly visible in the facilitation working group and they supported the large group to make decisions in general assemblies. It appears that social workers were among a relatively small group who had experience in group facilitation and consensus-building. Critical social workers were also significant in the debriefing process and the provision of personal support. When Occupy Melbourne was brutally evicted from Melbourne's Treasury Gardens, it was critical social workers who both led a large group debriefing process, located trauma in its structural context, and supported individuals in the immediate period after the eviction.

The third way that social workers were significant in Occupy Melbourne was in the 'First Aid and Care' team. It was the team that provided specific and direct support to activists within the movement, and it seemed the most attentive to the ways that the group replicated patterns of oppression. One of the most significant moments for me was when the First Aid and Care team made a collective and creative presentation about the ways that Occupy Melbourne camps were replicating patterns of patriarchy, often in violent ways.

Conclusion

This chapter has argued that social workers who profess a critical approach look for ways to be 'politicising all aspects of everyday life and engaging in efforts to transform society on many levels' (Baines 2007: 192). There are many opportunities to engage in social change both within workplaces as well as in broader social movements. For social workers to engage in social change work, a commitment and willingness to take risks is required as well as an honest interrogation of our own practice in the places we work and live. We need to be strategic in our own engagement, which includes that we know the issues thoroughly, position ourselves, and build alliances within our organisations and communities. Critical reflection and strategic analysis about how change is to occur is key to this process, as is the ongoing challenging of hierarchical ways of organising. Social workers are either directly challenging the conditions of oppression or are complicit in our silence.

References

AASAW *see* Australian Association of Social Workers

Allan, J. 2009a, 'Doing critical social work' in J. Allan, L. Briskman & B. Pease (eds), *Critical Social Work: Theories and practices for a socially just world,* 2nd edn, St Leonards: Allen & Unwin, pp. 70–87

Allan, J. 2009b, 'Theorising new developments in critical social work' in J. Allan, L. Briskman & B. Pease (eds), *Critical Social Work: Theories and practices for a socially just world*, 2nd edn, St Leonards: Allen & Unwin, Sydney, pp. 30–44

Australian Association of Social Workers (AASW). 2010, *Code of Ethics,* Canberra: AASW

Baines, D. (ed) 1997, *Doing Anti-Oppressive Practice: Building transformative politicized social work,* Halifax: Fernwood Publishing

Bauman, Z. 1995, *Life in Fragments,* Cambridge: Polity Press

Beckwith, J. 2000, *From Counselling to Client Partnership in Service Delivery: Towards a feminist psychological practice*, Master's thesis, Melbourne: Latrobe University

Benn, C. 1993, 'How the Family Centre changed the image of poverty and its contribution to research and social action' in C. Magree (ed.), *Looking Forward Looking Back: The Brotherhood's role in changing views of poverty,* Fitzroy: Brotherhood of St Laurence

Briskman, L. 2008, *Recasting Social Work: Human rights and political activism,* Eileen Younghusband Lecture, Durban, www.info.humanrights.curtin.edu.au/local/docs/Recasting_Social_Work.pdf, accessed 15 June 2014

—— & Goddard, C. 2007, 'Not in my name: The people's inquiry into immigration detention in D. Lusher, and N. Haslam (eds), *Yearning to breathe free*, Sydney: Federation Press, pp. 90–9

—— Pease, B. & Allan, J. 2009, 'Introducing critical theories for social work in a neo-liberal context' in J. Allan, L. Briskman & B. Pease (eds), *Critical Social Work: Theories and practices for a socially just world,* 2nd edn, St Leonards: Allen & Unwin, Sydney, pp. 3–14

Brotherhood of St Laurence (BSL) 2014, 'About the Brotherhood', BSL, <http://www.bsl.org.au/knowledge/about-the-research-policy-centre/our-history/ [1 July, 2014]

BSL *see* Brotherhood of St Laurence

Burgmann, V. 2003, *Power, Profit and Protest: Australian social movements and globalisation,* St Leonards: Allen & Unwin

Carson, N., Morrison, J., Marshall, C. & Mendelson, T. 2012, *Why Occupy Melbourne*, presentation at Ted X University of Melbourne, <www.ted.com/tedx/events/5517>, accessed 15 June 2014

Eggert, N. & Giugni, M. 2012, 'The homogenization of "Old" and "New" social movements: A comparison of participants in May Day and climate change demonstrations', *Mobilization, An International Quarterly,* vol. 17, no. 3, pp. 335–48

Fawcett, B. & Featherstone, B. 2000 'Setting the scene: An appraisal of notions of postmodernism, post-modernity and postmodern feminism' in B. Fawcett, B. Featherstone, J. Fook, & A. Rossiter (eds), *Practice research in social work: postmodern feminist perspectives,* Routledge, London, pp. 5–19

Friere, P. 1970, *Pedagogy of the Oppressed,* New York: Seabury Press

Gandi, M. 1993, *Autobiography: The story of my experiments with truth,* Boston: Beacon University Press.

Goldsworthy, J. 2001, *Telling Stories: Using case studies in advocacy and social policy,* Melbourne: Financial and Consumer Rights Council

Gray, M., Collett van Rooyen, C., Rennie, G. & Gaha, J. 2002, 'The political participation of social workers: A comparative study', *International Journal of Social Welfare,* vol. 11, no. 2, pp. 99–110

Hall, R. 1994, 'Partnership Accountability', *Dulwich Centre Newsletter,* no.2/3, pp. 6–28

Healy, K. 1999, 'Power and activist social work' in B. Pease & J. Fook (eds), *Transforming social work practice: postmodern critical practices,* St Leonards: Allen & Unwin, pp. 115–34

IFSW *see* International Federation of Social Workers

International Federation of Social Workers (IFSW) and International Association of Schools of Social Work 2004, 'Ethics in Social Work: Statement of Principles', IFSW, http://ifsw.org/policies/statement-of-ethical-principles, accessed 15 June 2014

Kriesi, H. 1998, 'The transformation of cleavage politics: The 1997 Stein Rokkan lecture', *European Journal of Political Research,* no. 33, pp. 165–385

Linn, J. 2000, *Jane Addams: A biography,* Chicago: University of Illinois Press

Locke, C. 2002, *Wellington People's Centre: Commemorating the tenth anniversary of the establishment of the WPC: Te Rauhitanga o te Whanganui-a-tara,* Wellington

—— & Stevens, J. 2009, *Unemployed movements,* Ideas Programme, Radio New Zealand National, <www.radionz.co.nz/national/programmes/ideas/20090816>, accessed 1 July, 2014

Maddison, S. & Scalmer, S. 2006, *Activist Wisdom: Practical knowledge and creative tension in social movements,* Sydney: UNSW Press

McIntyre, I. 2013, *How to Make Trouble and Influence People: Pranks, hoaxes, graffiti & political mischief-making from across Australia,* Oakland: PM Press

Mendes, P. 2008, 'Social workers and social activism in Victoria, Australia', *Journal of Progressive Human Services,* vol. 18, no. 1, pp. 25–44

Mmatli, T. 2008, 'Political activism as a social work strategy in Africa', *International Social Work,* vol. 51, no. 3, pp. 297–310

Morrison, J. & Brannigan, L. 2007, 'Working collectively in competitive times: case studies from New Zealand and Australia', *Community Development Journal,* vol. 44, no. 1, pp. 68–79

Mullaly, B. 1997, *Structural Social Work: Ideology, theory and practice,* 2nd edn, Oxford: Oxford University Press

Nzira, V. & Williams, P. 2008, *Anti-Oppressive Practice in Health and Social Care,* London: Sage

Reinsborough, P. & Canning, D. 2010, *Re:imagining Change: How to use story-based strategy to win campaigns, build movements, and change the world,* California: PM Press

The Change Agency 2014, website resource at

20

Social work, disability and social change: a critical participatory approach

Russell Shuttleworth

Introduction

At a time of rapid and widespread social and economic change, social work practice with marginalised groups in their struggle for social justice and access to social participation is becoming more urgent. Disabled people are a highly marginalised group who often experience complex daily discrimination that can restrict their social participation and prevent them from exercising their rights as citizens. The term disabled people is used in this chapter in preference to people with disabilities as a way of highlighting the process of social disablement. In this social model view, disability refers to the social factors and relations that function as barriers to access and participation. In using this terminology, I am not denying that people can have a wide range of impairments which intersect with racial, gender, sexual and other identities and that represent a diversity of subject positions. Advocacy and social action by disabled people has resulted in their increased participation in many parts of the globe. However, social workers, including critical social workers, have limited involvement in mobilising this group and working alongside them as co-participants in their struggle for inclusion. Social workers are involved with disabled people in a range of roles from counsellor to case manager but may not see their role as working for legislative change and policy reform that truly reflect this marginalised group's diversity of needs and aspirations. This is a generalisation and there are exceptions such as mental health. It is somewhat ironic given critical social work's espousing of critical and anti-oppressive principles that disabled people can still often be left off the agenda.

In this chapter, I provide a critical perspective on social work's minimal engagement with the social justice issues of disabled people and the disability movement in the struggle for social change. I also highlight a critical, participatory approach to working with disabled people on changes to policy, legislation and practice in their struggle for social access and participation. Several aspects of a critical participatory approach are considered, including deconstructing one's own values and attitudes, interrogating one's motivations and avoiding the assumption of the role of ally when working with marginalised groups. These ideas as well as others drawn from the critical tradition in social work may assist other social workers who choose to work with disabled people in a critical participatory role. I briefly describe my recent critical participation with a disability and sexuality advocacy group in Melbourne, the Sexuality and Disability Alliance (SDA), in helping craft a policy and research agenda for the use of facilitated sex.

Critical social work and disability

A critical reflection towards one's own discipline and practice has become crucial to many social science disciplines including social work (for example, Brown 1994; Fook 2012). In shining this light on social work, it can be seen that disabled people's issues have not often been considered a priority. In the Australian context, one only has to point to the core curriculum content required by the Australian Association of Social Workers (AASW) in its accreditation standards for social work education, which exclude disability except when relating to mental health (AASW 2012). The historical reliance on a medical model to frame the *problem* of disability has made it difficult for sociopolitical approaches to gain a foothold within social work (Meekosha & Dowse 2007; Soldatic & Meekosha 2012). As Meekosha and Dowse argue, social workers have often been 'unintentionally agents in [disabled people's] exclusion, influenced as they are by the medical and rehabilitative discourse of disability which views disabled people as either in need of treatment, cure or regulation' (Meekosha & Dowse 2007: 170). Social workers' roles within institutions and in providing services to individuals can work toward managing the non-normative or restoring the normative in working with individuals. As Johnson maintains, 'For social workers to work effectively with disabled people, they need to turn a critical gaze on both the knowledge that they receive and on the ways in which they exercise it in practice' (Johnson 2009: 200). Within the ascendance of the neoliberal policy environment in which social work is increasingly enmeshed, Soldatic and Meekosha argue it is paramount that social work education incorporate 'a disability studies emancipatory paradigm as an essential part of the curriculum' (Soldatic & Meekosha 2012: 246).

Within critical social work specifically, the concept of critical practice with disabled people is barely developed. While critical approaches have been more inclusive of disability as a disadvantaged category (for example, Sisneros et al. 2008; Johnson 2009), there is still an assumption that disability is less important than the issues relating to class, gender and race. A case in point is Ife (2013) who, while acknowledging that disabled people can face oppression and disadvantage, maintains a hierarchical view by implying that gender, race and class are more structurally pervasive social divisions than disability or sexuality. Disadvantages and oppressions are both similar to each other and different from each other across a range of social divisions and categories. Is there really anything to be gained by distinguishing between more and less structurally pervasive disadvantages? In the case of disability, most people if they live long enough will experience impairment(s) and suffer associated social stigma, oppression and disadvantage.

Several critical social work perspectives on disability have employed a discursive framing of disability drawn from post-structural perspectives (for example, Fawcett 2000; Johnson 2009). Post perspectives, especially Foucauldian approaches, have also gained ground in critical disability studies (for example, Allan 1996; Tremain 2005; Shildrick 2012). Shildrick (2007, 2012) employs what she refers to as a 'post-conventional' approach that transcends the oppositional binaries of modernist disability studies (such as medical model/social model, impairment/disability). Post-perspectives can indeed be strategically useful for critical social workers working with disabled people. However, since these approaches inherently deny any trans-contextual value, one needs to look elsewhere for any normative principle that can orient critical thinking and critical practice. Ife apprehends this problem and argues that post-modernist critique should be incorporated within a larger vision of critical theory because the latter 'fully [legitimises] social work's traditional commitments to universalist ideals of human rights and social justice' (Ife 1999: 222). The recent problematisation of the concept of human rights in the case of disability may trouble the specifics of Ife's point (for example, Meekosha & Soldatic 2011), but not the search for grounding, critical thinking in a trans-contextual, orienting frame.

Some social workers, counsellors and researchers have put forth transformative models for working with disabled people that recognise the need for *enabling practice*, incorporating sociopolitical models into one's perspective and sensitive to the various discourses of disability (Raske 2005; Swain, Griffith & French 2006; Johnson 2009). These models recognise the disabling effects of macro-level processes and structures on disabled individuals and that working toward social justice for this marginalised group is important. However, the discourse of these kind of approaches can often prioritise working with individuals to procure adequate material and social supports in the face of disabling social structures, which implicitly limits more direct involvement with disability groups and the disability movement in their struggle for social access and participation. While an important counter to individualised treatment within a medical model of disability, the transformative potential of such efforts will nevertheless be limited.

This prioritisation may be due to an inherent conceptual limitation of traditional social work frameworks for practice. In terms of social casework models, Pease (2003) argues that the person-in-environment paradigm is cast in a conservative mode. Thus, while the social worker in case-work or counsellor mode may be able to effect change for the individual and the individual may become more *empowered* in negotiating an ableist world, changing the discriminatory or oppressive hegemonies and ideologies within a society requires moving beyond the individual level. As Thompson points out:

> not only in terms of *understanding* but also in terms of tackling [these hegemonies]. This involves individuals playing their part in collectively challenging the dominant discriminatory culture and ideology and, in so doing, playing at least a part in the undermining of the structures which support, and are supported by that culture (Thompson 2006: 30).

Thus, given 'the material and discursive constraints on critical practice' (Pease 2003: 188), critical social workers need to work with disabled communities and the disability movement in their struggle for social access and participation.

A critical participatory approach to practice with disabled people

For the critical social worker engaged with disability issues and who works with disabled people to effect positive social change, they need to interrogate current everyday assumptions about disabled people, which fuel their oppression. A central task is to also link the everyday instances of discrimination and isolation to exclusion from broader social and community participation. The incorporation of a *critical participatory approach* to practice is also key. In a critical participatory approach, the social worker engages with disabled people on a particular issue or problem that requires legislative, policy or professional practice changes (or all of these) or some form of social action that is important in the struggle for social justice and social participation. Referring to Paulo Freire's critical and participatory approach to practice, Ife maintains that:

> 'In this form of practice, the knowledge and wisdom of the worker are not privileged over the knowledge and wisdom of the "client", and the relationship between the two is one of mutual education . . . and as a result they can together engage in some form of action which may have been impossible for each in isolation' (1999: 121).

There is by now a long history of participatory research with disabled people (for example, Sample 1996; Garbutt 2010), but this research represents a small minority of the research on disability. However, the concept of participatory practice (Ledwith & Springett 2010) has been less employed in reference to social and community work with this marginalised group. Ledwith and Springett argue that:

> participation (in a participatory practice approach) has to be understood as a transformative not ameliorative concept. The political dimensions of participation need to be framed within participatory democracy, a worldview in which communities are in control of the decision-making processes that affect their lives, giving voice to the most marginalised, giving greater power to local governance to influence policy-making thereby making institutions accountable (Ledwith & Springett 2010: 15).

In a critical participatory approach to research and practice, critical social workers and disabled people work together as co-partners to transform the current politics of disability. In this model, depending on the particular issue, the critical social worker might assist in gathering information, challenging received ideas, networking, advocating, theorising, analysing, interpreting, evaluating, advising, strategising and implementing; yet decision-making lies with the consensus of those disabled people who one is working with. While applicable to the political concerns of persons with a range of impairments, a critical participatory approach as defined here would need to be further elucidated in terms of social workers who work with people with intellectual disability. The issue is too complex to take up within this chapter. Suffice to say that the problem would involve social worker acknowledgement and critically and reflexively working through the inherent power relations between co-participants with different intellectual capacities.

In many ways a critical participatory approach might resemble a role that social workers have often taken up in community development. To some extent this may be true. However, concepts and understanding often require updating and theoretical and practice frameworks reconfiguring due to ever changing cultural and sociopolitical dynamics. As Lane, arguing for a postmodern emphasis on resistance in community development, implies:

> Does this offer a new approach to community development, or is it a statement, in different language, of a way of practising which has been around for a long while? Perhaps it is the latter, but we still need to bring it into focus to argue its relevance for the present (Lane 1999: 146).

If one takes this critical participatory approach seriously, an issue that social workers who work with marginalised groups must address is their possible complicity with and reinforcement of disability oppression and the hegemony of ableist norms. One issue that qualifies as worthy of interrogation within this critical participatory frame for social workers who work with marginalised groups is complicity. Pease (see Chapter 6) notes how some social workers who claim the ally role, that is working in collaboration with a marginalised group nevertheless remain complicit with prejudicial and oppressive attitudes towards these same groups. Thus, social workers must reflexively deconstruct and interrogate their own values and attitudes, which may reinforce oppressive social structures and cultural meanings towards the particular group they are working with. Necessary to add to this value and attitudinal deconstruction is a process-oriented interrogation of the hierarchising and negotiation of motivations and intentions that occur as social workers practice with and within marginalised groups and communities.

Interestingly, my own experience of the ally concept as used within disability rights movement in the US complicates this notion's typical usage. Practising at various times as a social worker and a personal assistant (support worker) for disabled people, I was involved for many years with the disability rights movement and consider myself a critical disability studies scholar. In contrast to the disability movement in Australia, the disability rights movement in the US has established a much stronger foothold in public disability discourse. The result is a more critical perspective towards academics, practitioners and others in the 'helping' professions. In this context, being an ally was not a role that people without a disability, in whatever capacity they worked with disabled people, could claim. Instead it was disabled people who conferred the ally status. A person without a disability committed to the disability movement's social and political agenda could be deemed an ally by disabled people, if that person proved themselves in challenging the everyday prejudices and structural disadvantage that disabled people face.

Being an ally was not just about supporting the disability movement ideologically but about standing up for the ideals of this movement and developing the trust of disabled people. It was not a role one could uncritically assume and indeed as an attributed status attributed to non-disabled people must be earned each day anew.

The above discussion highlights that the ally notion is not a neutral term and reveals a shift in power relations depending on whether the disabled person or the non-disabled person has the locus of control. This difference in meaning raises the issue of multiple interpretations of the concept which would be fruitful to pursue in future work. Despite the need for conceptual review of the term's diversity of meanings, critical social workers in whatever locale would be wise not to assume the role of ally but to simply work with marginalised groups in participatory ways and towards social transformation. Macfarlane argues, 'critical practice involves a shift in position from expert to co-collaborator . . . sharing power does not imply a "loss" of power or devaluing of one's expertise' (Macfarlane 2009: 204). Yet, becoming an ally (Bishop 1994) may in the above sense of the term not be up to the practitioner to decide. If disabled people increase their visibility and power within public discourse around disability issues in Australia, the ally status as conferred by non-disabled practitioners will likely be increasingly wrested from their control.

Reflections on critical participation with the Sexuality and Disability Alliance

The following briefly illustrates several aspects of a critical participatory approach to practice. The Sexuality and Disability Alliance (SDA) is a group of physically disabled young adults who came together in 2011 to advocate for sexual rights of disabled people in Melbourne. Focusing particularly on the barriers to sexual expression and sexual wellbeing for disabled people, this group's aim is to raise public awareness of a range of sexuality and disability issues. The members of this group view it as imperative to demonstrate that sexuality is part of their everyday lives, even if some of them experience barriers to their sexual participation. Over the course of the first year and a half of their existence, SDA created several strategies to change public perceptions of disabled sexuality. Several of these employ current communication media to good effect such as developing a Facebook page on sexuality and disability issues or creating short issue-related sexuality and disability videos for posting on YouTube.

Since their inception, I have critically participated with the SDA in advocating for the recognition of disabled people as sexual beings, deconstructing the barriers to sexual participation that disabled people encounter and developing strategies to address the barriers to their sexual participation and wellbeing. Given the need to focus its energy, the SDA had several specific meetings to prioritise what sexuality and disability issues to address in policy and research. A consensus of members decided that facilitated sex should be the first issue to contend with because of its importance for the sexual participation of many disabled people. This was an issue that I had raised among others. I presented an informed rationale for each one. Other members presented other issues. My experience as a social worker and support worker with disabled people and involvement in disability rights in the US, as well as discussions with disability advocacy groups and disabled people in Sydney while working there had made me aware of the significance of this issue for many disabled people. In my work with SDA, I provided the relevant details of my work and discussions with other disabled people. Members of the SDA discussed their own thoughts and experience on this issue and concurred with its significance in their lives. Together, members of SDA including me devised an approach to address this issue that would impact policy, disability services and support worker practice. We outlined tentative policy guidelines and a research plan.

Throughout the several SDA meetings, where issues for policy change and research were prioritised, I interrogated my own motivations regarding the issue of facilitated sex and examined the assumptions for my reasoning and for presenting it as a potential topic for the group's focus. This examination included the emotional investment I had in recognising its significance for disabled people in the contexts of the US and Sydney; the former in which I had often been termed an ally. In Sydney, I had gathered stories of disabled people's barriers to sexual participation. In presenting the issue to the SDA and the discussion that followed, I was at pains not to exert the authority of expertise. However, I had to adequately convey the complexity of the issue (for example, physical, emotional, psychological, social, political dimensions of the problem). I would have critically participated with the SDA on any issue deemed necessary in the struggle for the sexual recognition of disabled people.

The need for some kind of physical assistance to facilitate sexual expression and sexual participation can present a formidable barrier for many persons with significant physical limitations. There are many disabled people, representing diverse genders and sexualities who, depending on the type and degree of their impairments and functional limitations, may require particular kinds of physical support to express themselves sexually or in their sexual relationships (Tepper 2000; Shuttleworth & Mona 2002; Selina 2003; Browne & Russell 2005; Shildrick 2007; Shuttleworth 2007, 2010; Bahner 2012, 2013). For example, assistance might be required with positioning in order for a disabled person to masturbate comfortably or participate in sexual activity with a disabled partner (Tepper 2000; Mona 2003). Contrary to the misperception that facilitated sex is primarily about masturbating disabled men and providing them with sex worker services espoused by some academics (Jeffries 2008; Costel and Kimmel 2013), facilitated sex is crucial to the sexual participation and well-being of significantly disabled people, no matter what the gender. Facilitated sex is about providing some kind of physical assistance, support or accommodation to enable a disabled person to sexually express themselves and to participate in sexual activities; it does not mean that the person doing the assisting is actually a participant in these activities. Facilitated sex is also often uncritically assumed to be associated with the employment of a sex worker but these two issues should be viewed as distinct; in facilitated sex a disabled client is not employing someone to specifically participate in a sexual encounter with them.

The issue of facilitated sex and disability has had a difficult time making it onto the health and social welfare, policy and practice agendas because it transgresses Western values on sexuality such as autonomy and privacy (Shildrick 2007; Shuttleworth 2007). Negotiating this service is most often left entirely up to the disabled people and their support worker with the consequence that their sexual facilitation requirements are often not met. Both parties may be ill-equipped to deal with this experience (Selina 2003; Shildrick 2007; Shuttleworth 2007, 2010; Bahner 2012; 2013). Physically assisting another person to express their sexuality, if not supported by an appropriate policy and practice framework, can have ethical and legal ramifications (Mona 2003; Shildrick 2007). In such unregulated contexts, support workers run the risk of being perceived as sexual participants and, because payment is involved, may be legally liable in many jurisdictions (Mona 2003; Shildrick 2007). Currently, Denmark has the most progressive policy and practice guidelines on facilitated sex with a pro-sexuality perspective written into their disability policy. In Denmark, assisting with sexual concerns is a regular part of the job for support workers (Kulick 2013). There are no such regulations in Australia; appropriate policy and practice framework and guidelines regarding facilitated sex are absent. This includes the state of Victoria where the SDA is located.

In working with the SDA on the issue of facilitated sex, I presented an analysis of the 'Personal relationships, sexuality and sexual health policy and guidelines' for Disability Services in Victoria (DHS Victoria 2006). While several members referred to this document as providing a set of guidelines for interactions between disability services, support workers and disabled people, I drew out the imprecise language of this document for the specifics of facilitated sex. I did this to convey what kind of detailed description might be necessary to make these policy guidelines address their concerns. One member was particularly concerned about describing the actual kinds of sexual activities in which one might need assistance, while others saw that the current policy lacked power due to its vagueness and that clarity and detail was essential to address the requirements of facilitated sexual support. It took several meetings to finalise what degree of explicitness was necessary to clarify policy but not to cause offence. Through this process, a consensus of members perceived that the vagueness of the current guidelines also reflected their own sense of not knowing what the boundaries of this assistance might be. Indeed, both disability services/ support workers and disabled clients are often uncertain as to whether facilitated sex can be negotiated and, if so, where does 'the line' get drawn (Sexuality and Disability Alliance 2012)?

Along with facilitated sex guidelines for disabled people and their support workers, a research agenda on this issue was also developed. The group members decided that to provide the policy guidelines which emphasised empirical evidence research should be conducted before approaching disability services with the policy guidelines. SDA's facilitator, George Taleporos, who is disabled, and I are currently conducting research with disabled persons who employ support workers in Victoria on their thoughts regarding facilitated sex, their requirements for facilitated sex and what they feel are the barriers to accessing this kind of support. This research will likely fuel more discussions within the SDA as policy guidelines need to be tightened and presented to disability services and policy makers in Victoria. In both my research assistance and in these further discussions, I will play a critical participatory role working with disabled people as co-partners to transform the current politics of sexuality and disability. For several specific examples of disability policy analysis in the U.S. context employing a disability discrimination model see May 2005.

References

AASW 2012, Australian Social Work Education and Accreditation Standards. (ASWEAS) 2012,. 1.4, (revised July 2014) Canberra, AASW

Allan, J. 1996, 'Foucault and special educational needs: A 'box of tools' for analysing children's experiences of mainstreaming', *Disability and Society*, vol. 11, pp. 219–33

Bahner, J. 2012, 'Legal rights or simply wishes? The struggle for sexual recognition of people with physical disabilities using personal assistance in Sweden', *Sexuality and Disability*, vol. 30, no. 3 pp. 337–56

Bahner, J. 2013, 'The power of discretion and the discretion of power: personal assistants and sexual facilitation in disability services', *Vulnerable Groups and Inclusion*, vol. 4, pp. 1–22

Bishop, A. 1994, *Becoming an Ally*, Halifax: Fernwood Publishing

Brown, C. 1994, 'Feminist postmodernism and the challenge of diversity' in A. Chambon & A. Irving (eds), *Essays on Postmodernism and Social Work*, Toronto: Canadian Scholars Press, pp. 35–48

Browne, J. & Russell, S. 2005, 'My home, your workplace: People with physical disability negotiate their sexual health without crossing professional boundaries', *Disability and Society*, vol. 20, no. 4, pp. 375–88

Costell, B. and Kimmel, M. (2012) 'Seeing privilege where it isn't: Marginalised masculinities and the intersectionality of privilege,' *Journal of Social Issues*, Vol. 68, No. 1 pp. 97–111

Disability Services. 2006, *Personal Relationships, Sexuality and Sexual Health Policy and Guidelines*, Melbourne: Department of Human Services

Earle, S. 1999, 'Facilitated sex and the concept of sexual need: Disabled students and their personal assistants', *Disability and Society*, vol. 14, no. 3, pp. 309–23

Fawcett, B. 2000, 'Researching disability: Meanings, interpretation and analysis' in B. Fawcett, B. Featherstone, J. Fook & A. Rossiter (eds), *Practice and Research in Social Work: Postmodern feminist perspectives*, Routledge, London, pp. 62–82

Fook, J. 2012, *Social Work: A critical approach to practice*, 2nd edn, London: Sage

Garbutt, R. 2010, 'Exploring the barriers tos sex for people with learning disabilities' in R. Shuttleworth & T. Sanders (eds) *Sex and Disability: Politics, identity and access*, Leeds, The Disability Press

Ife, J. 1999, 'Postmodernism, critical theory and social work' in B. Pease & J. Fook (eds), *Social Work Practice: Postmodern critical perspectives*, St Leonards: Allen & Unwin, pp. 211–23

—— 2013, *Community Development in an Uncertain World*, Melbourne: Cambridge University Press

Jeffreys, S. 2008, 'Disability and the male sex right', *Women's Studies International Forum*, vol. 31, pp. 327–35

Johnson. K. 2009, 'Disabling discourses and enabling practices in disability politics' in J. Allan, B. Pease & L. Briskman (eds), *Critical Social Work: Theories and practices for a socially just world*, 2nd edn, St Leonards: Allen & Unwin, pp. 188–200

Kulick, D. 2013, *Disability and Sexuality: Who cares?*, public lecture presented at Monash University, Nexus: Monash Social Science, Humanities and Medicine Network, 17 May

Lane, M. 1999, 'Community development and a postmodernism of resistance' in *Social Work Practice: Postmodern critical perspectives*, St Leonards: Allen & Unwin, pp. 135–49

Ledwith, M. & Springett, J. 2010, *Participatory Practice: Community-based action for transformative change*, 2nd edn, Bristol: Policy Press

Macfarlane, S. 2009, 'Opening spaces for alternative understandings in mental health practice' in J. Allan, B. Pease & L. Briskman (eds), *Critical Social Work: Theories and practices for a socially just world*, 2nd edn, St Leonards: Allen & Unwin, pp. 201–13

Meekosha, H. & Dowse, L. 2007, 'Integrating critical disability studies into social work education and practice: An Australian perspective', *Practice*, vol. 19, no. 3, pp. 169–83

—— & Soldatic, K. 2011, 'Human rights and the Global South: The case of disability', *Third World Quarterly*, vol. 32, no. 8, pp. 1383–98

Pease, B. 2003, 'Rethinking the relationship between the self and society' in J. Allan, B. Pease & L. Briskman (eds), *Critical Social Work: Theories and practices for a socially just world*, 2nd edn, St Leonards: Allen & Unwin, pp. 187–201

May, G. 2005, 'The disability discrimination model in social policy practice' in G. May & M. Raske (eds), *Ending Disability Discrimination: Strategies for social workers*, Boston: Pearson Education, pp. 113–26

Mona, L. 2003, 'Sexual options for people with disabilities', *Women and Therapy*, vol. 26, no. 3–4, pp. 211–222

Raske, M. 2005, 'The disability discrimination model in social work practice' in G. May & M. Raske (eds), *Ending Disability Discrimination: Strategies for social workers*, Boston: Pearson Education, pp. 99–112

Sample, P. 1996, 'Beginnings: Participatory action research and adults with developmental disabilities', *Disability and Society*, vol. 11, no. 3, pp. 317–32

Selina, B. 2003, *Facilitated Sexual Expression in the Independent Living Movement in Ireland,* Master's thesis, Leeds: University of Leeds

Sexuality and Disability Alliance, 2012, *Minutes from July Sexuality and Disability Alliance Meeting,* Melbourne

Shildrick, M. 2007, 'Contested pleasures: The socio-political economy of disability and sexuality', *Sexuality Research & Social Policy*, vol. 4, no. 1, pp. 53–66

—— 2012, 'Critical disability studies: Rethinking the conventions for the age of postmodernity' in N. Watson, A Roulstone & C. Thomas (eds), *Routledge Handbook of Disability Studies*, Oxnon: Routledge, pp. 30–41

Sisneros, J., Stakeman, C., Joyner, M. & Schmitz, C. 2008, *Critical Multicultural Social Work*, Chicago: Lyceum Books

Shuttleworth, R. 2007, 'Critical research and policy debates in disability and sexuality studies', *Sexuality Research and Social Policy*, vol. 4, no. 1, pp. 1–14

—— 2010, 'Toward an inclusive sexuality and disability research agenda' in R. Shuttleworth & T. Sanders (eds), *Sexuality and Disability: Politics, identity, access,* Leeds: Disability Press, pp. 1–20

—— & Mona, L. 2002, 'Introduction to the Symposium: Focus on Sexual Access for Disabled People', *Disability Studies Quarterly,* vol. 22, no. 3, pp. 2–8

Soldatic, K., & Meekosha, H. 2012, 'Moving the boundaries of feminist social work education with disabled people in the neoliberal era', *Social Work Education*, vol. 31, no. 2, pp. 246–52

Swain, J., Griffiths, C., & French, S. 2006, 'Counselling with the social model: Challenging therapy's pathologies' in D. Goodley & R. Lawthom (eds), *Disability and Psychology*, Hampshire Palgrave Macmillan, pp. 155–69

Tepper, M. 2000, 'Facilitated sex: The next frontier in sexuality', *New Mobility*, vol. 11, no. 8, pp. 21–4

Thompson, N. 2006, *Anti-discriminatory Practice*, 4th edn, Palgrave Macmillan: London

Tremain, S. 2005, *Foucault and the Government of Disability*, Ann Arbor: University of Michigan Press

21

The structural, the post-structural and the commons: new practices for creating change in a complex world

José M. Ramos

Introduction

This chapter articulates new forms of critical social work and community work thinking and practice. By that, I refer to practice that engages with both the need to provide conceptual leadership in transforming existing structures and institutions, while simultaneously providing openings for conceptual diversity, interpretive multiplicity and opportunities for agency (Briskman et al 2009). My work has focused on global problems that affect most countries today, namely: challenging neoliberalism and articulating alternatives to it; the co-optation of political power by moneyed interests and the need to strengthen democracy; the problem of social atomisation and consumerist driven individualism and the need to develop peer-to-peer and solidarity cultures; and, the ecological crisis and the need to create ways of living which are in genuine balance with our integral life support systems. As might be recognised from this range of issues, my work and research has been typified by conditions of high cultural and conceptual diversity (Ramos 2010). This work has simultaneously engaged with both the question of developing agency that can create and transform global structures and systems, within communities in which there are a wide variety of interpretations on what those structures are, and diverse visions for change. This chapter provides an overview of the work of challenging neo-liberalisms many forms, and meta-networked efforts to create political, economic and cultural alternatives to it. The inner (or epistemological) dimension, and outer (or ontological) dimensions of 'meta-networking' practice for systemic change is explicated and explored.

In this chapter I therefore argue for a social work practice which integrates the structural and post-structural nature of the challenges and issues people face in addressing many commonly held social problems. Rather than accepting that diverse social perspectives are mutually exclusive, meta-networking offers an approach that can lead to the capacity for diverse actors and agents to collaborate on solving common challenges. Reflecting Jim Ife's (2012) core argument that social and community work needs to be coupled with a strong ethos of shared humanity and more extensively cultural forms of human rights, I argue the integration of structural and post-structural strategies through the practice of meta-networking is a pathway toward developing a practice that can develop the social 'commons' and common good at many levels, an approach fundamental to social work in the 21st century. If critical social work is to address the origins of social problems through systemically intelligent change strategies, meta-networking should be a key approach in the critical social work tool kit.

What is meta-networking?

Meta-networking is a process by which people work to create networks which facilitate flows of information and allow coordination and cooperation between otherwise disparate groups of people, with shared interests but with differing perspectives.

Meta-networking involves the linking or associational formation of disparate actors into a network, with the aim of helping the constituency to develop and meet its goals. It can be located as both a social research practice (Chisholm 2001) and an approach to community development (Gilchrist 2004). Trist (1979), as well as Carley & Christie (1993), were early developers of the thinking and practice of inter-organisational network development. Gilchrist (2004) locates it as a core community development practice and role, while Chisholm (2001) argues it is a type of action research.

Carley and Cristie (1993) describe inter-organisational network development aimed at sustainable development through 'action centred networks'. These use network strategies to solve complex sustainability dilemmas (Carley 1993, p. 180). In their approach to 'human ecology' and 'socio-ecological systems', they argue that 'meta-problems' are at the heart of many of the modern problems we face: 'meta-problems both exist in, and are the result of, turbulent environments which compound uncertainty, the root of the word problematique' (Carley 1993, p. 165).

Our era's meta-problems overwhelm the capacity for single organisations to cope with the challenges they face. What is required, they argue, is the development of 'action centred networks' that develop 'connective capacity' and undertake 'collaborative problem solving' (Carley 1993, p. 171). These networks can offer a variety of solutions; regulation, problem/trend appreciation, problem solving, support, political/economic mobilisation, and development projects (Carley 1993, p. 172). They argue for 'linking pin' organisations—organisations that provide a structure or platform for communication and coordination across groups, and thus can become a network of networks (Carley 1993, pp. 172–173).

If potential conflicts within action-centred networks are properly managed, such networks can lead to the capacity for innovative responses to meta-problems collectively faced. This innovation requires linking 'anticipation' (drawing from Godet's (2007) 'La Prospective') with collaborative mobilisation and practical and strategic action. They specifically called for approaches that develop such action centred networks (Carley 1993, pp. 180–181). Trist (1979, p. 9) argued that 'referent organisations' were a critical aspect of meta-networks in providing leadership for a problem area:

> Once ... a referent organization appears, purposeful action can be undertaken in the name of the [problem] domain. To be acceptable the referent organization must not usurp the functions of the constituent organizations, yet to be effective it must provide appropriate leadership.

Meta-networking as pathway to the commons

My research area on the World Social Forum (WSF), spanned a decade from 2001 to 2011. Early on, from 2001–2004, I saw the gathering at Porto Alegre as an emerging 'counter hegemonic bloc', where various civil society organisations would unite in common solidarity. This idea (originated by Italian political theorist Antonio Gramsci) contained the proposition that revolutionary change is preceded by a form of cultural activism—that is, when the key cultural institutions, churches, social organisations, etc. come together in a coherent opposition to a dominant consensus or 'hegemony' (a normative order), change then follows (Hansen 1997). I therefore hoped that with time, the various actors, organisations, activists and people brought together in the World Social Forum, would ultimately work through their differences, and come together in a strategic and ideologically coherent relationship. At the time George W. Bush was in power and the United States (US) invasion of Iraq—initiated on the false pretext of weapons of mass destruction—was in full swing. The connection between those with great political power and corporate/big oil seemed to be converging to satisfy each other's primal interests. It seemed at the time that, with the veil of corporate imperialism lifted for all to see, the 100,000 plus people attending the forum would be united in opposition, if not in a shared project to create an effective alternative to the problem.

In Australia, Social Forums were held in the major cities, and I was part of the organisation of the Melbourne forums, five of which were held between 2004 and 2010. In the seven or so years studying social forums and communities, fundamental assumptions I held were challenged. The idea of a Gramscian counter-hegemonic bloc made less and less sense in the face of participant diversity, indeed radical diversity, and the very different images of the future (of alternative globalisations) that were held by participants. In my quest to understand the various images of the future that a variety of different activist organisations and non-government organisations (NGOs) held, or what Castells (1997) termed the 'telos' of a group, I found that the discourses and visions that mobilise various actors in such events were not so easy to combine.

In fact a variety of mindsets converged at the forums in a maelstrom of discontent and radical activism, all which could be considered to be counter hegemonic (in their opposition to the dominant neoliberal capitalist vision). To give an idea of this diversity, represented were a variety of campaigns and projects. Indigenous justice campaigns critiqued the Australian state's approach to the sovereignty of Aboriginal lands. Advocates for relocalisation argued for the need to re-establish local economic systems that build community resilience. Eco-feminist critiques highlighted the patriarchal nature of globalisation as 'capitalist, masculine, white, middle—class, heterosexual, urban, and highly mobile' (Hawthorne 2002, pp. 32–3). Anti-war and peace campaigns in the context of the wars in Iraq and Afghanistan linked global economic interests with military adventurism and Western led neo-colonialism. Advocates for global governance solutions addressed the limitations of the nation state in solving global problems that transcend national borders. Science-based projects addressed the need to reduce carbon emissions and address global warming. These indicate a mere fraction of the diversity of the campaigns, activity and perspectives represented through the forums (Ramos 2010, p. 153). As can be inferred, both the histories and strategic visions of the various groups at the forums were distinctive and often hard to reconcile. It was not as simple as looking for and finding the 'telos' of how each fit into the umbrella of an anti-capitalist or post neo-liberal project. Understanding what was in play would require distilling and clarifying differences as much as creating conceptual similarities.

In the process, Latour's (2005) version of Actor Network Theory would be of great assistance, as it would show me that the way that a discourse frames the world does not just describe reality (the positivist view), but indeed it provides a template for strategic action for those who hold, use and disseminate a particular discourse or ideology (the constructivist view). As an organiser in such an event there was an aspect of letting go of the certainty of my particular frame of reference. I would need to listen beyond discourse, not just to discourse, but as discourse's relationship to people and action. I would need to become a discourse mapper, practice 'cognitive mapping' (Bergmann 2006) as a way of coming to grips with deep conceptual and discursive differences, while at the same time keeping my eye on deeper connections and indeed the structural dimensions that brought us together as diverse actors. Thus, for an issue like climate change, there was no denying that a Greenhouse Mafia in Australia has systematically thwarted any significant political action for decades— collusion and the convergence of corporate and political interests, on a variety of issues, was well documented (Hamilton 2007). The structural nature of power, however, did not negate that critiques of power come from diverse perspectives and discourses, which frame both the present situation and the future differently. This is what Inayatullah (1998) terms as levels of reality, an acknowledgement that both the post-structural (language, metaphor and discourse) and structural (geography, culture, power, economy etc.) are all in play.

In this way I discovered that post-structuralism was a pathway to building deeper coherence and strategic action between a variety of groups that may not neces-sarily speak the same conceptual languages. This is where I slowly began to learn the notion and practice of meta-networking. The naïve belief that the world could be organised and neatly fit into a single ideological or conceptual frame of reference did not make for very good social and community development work. In the quest for social change I was required to engage with people with often very different pictures and narratives of our situation. However, as a group with common concerns, we still needed to be able to challenge and transform shared structures, but this was better done across the embodied experience of diverse people. The post-structural turn, to honour a variety of embodied ways of knowing, was a healthy and important step beyond a naïve structuralism.

Post-structuralism—an approach that could appreciate and leverage multiple discourses and world views—was important but not enough. What was needed was inquiry toward a shared diagnosis of a problem, developing common ground vision and enabling collaborative collective action. The question remained over the why, what and how that brings us together—even when our discourses and perspectives differ.

In the World Social Forum and satellite forums (for example, Melbourne Social Forum or MSF), various actors, despite coming from often radically different perspectives, would collaborate to create change. Social theorist De Sousa Santos (2006, p. 168) thus argues that the *modus operandi* for the alter-globalisation movement (via the World Social Forum) is through 'de-polarising pluralities'. A pragmatic approach to diversity held sway, not by ignoring perspectives, but by making the diversity of thinking, what Santos (2006, p. 20) termed the 'ecology of knowledges', a resource that could be leveraged for co-analysis and collaborative strategic opportunities.

What emerged from this was an increasing appreciation for what brings us together despite our deeper differences. I have come to understand this through the language of 'the commons', as a keystone concept that may hold, if we construct it so, multiplicity and difference, but in dynamic relationship and synergy (Bollier & Heilfrich 2012).

Over the past ten years, I have been involved in a variety of processes that have taught me what it means to work across and integrate these dimensions of social and community work. The following account provides a brief overview.

The Melbourne Social Forum

The *Melbourne Social Forum* (MSF) emerged as an expression of the rich networks of counter-hegemonic actors in Melbourne. This included groups supportive of the WSF initiative, as well as groups and people who advocate or articulate for post-neoliberal and post-capitalist visions. Initially, the MSF founding group was inspired by the shared experience of the Mumbai WSF in early 2004 that led to the first MSF in late 2004.

Social forums were co-constructs, in which forum organisers facilitated a process in which the 'forum community' came together. Without a community of counter-hegemonic actors, there could be no social forum; yet without social forum organisers, there could be no social forums under the banner 'Another World is Possible'. A collaborative field existed between different groups with similar attitudes and values, which generated 'inter-alternatives'. A key form of agency was therefore collaboration among actors with a broadened conception of what a normative field meant—the aims and visions that guide action.

The actors that participated in the MSF were diverse, with close to 200 organisations, networks and groups. Modes of agency were correspondingly diverse. However, the process of 'midwifery' was key, giving space for the community to 'birth'; bring forth its alternatives, agendas and concerns. In this sense agency was facilitating the collaborative agency of others in enacting change—the meaning of 'meta-formation'.

Modes of agency could also be distinguished into that which was *outer* focused (change initiatives enacted on the world), and those that were *inner* focused, (initiatives that aimed to develop and strengthen collaboration and work between the network of actors). Movement building linked the two modalities of *outer* and *inner* focus: building the internal strength, knowledge, and capacity for collaboration, and the diverse modes of action used by networks in the enactment of structural and worldly change. Inner and outer movement building is represented by figure 1.

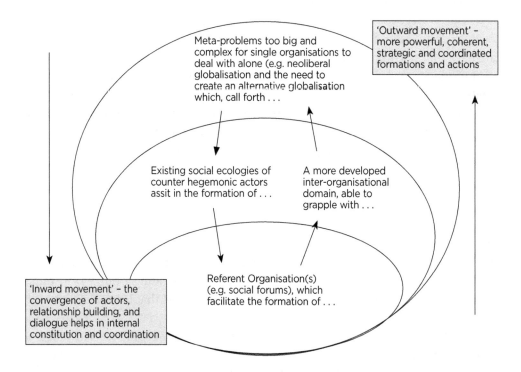

Figure 19.1 shows how the meta-problem represented by the pathologies of neo-liberal globalisation hastened the development of meta-networks of actors, which gave birth to the WSF and satellite forums (for example, MSF) as 'referent organisations'. In Trist's (1979, p. 9) view, the functions of a referent organisation includes, 'regulation . . . of present relationships and activities; establishing ground rules and

maintaining base values; appreciation . . . of emergent trends and issues [and] developing a shared image of a desirable future; and infrastructure support . . . resource, information sharing, special projects'.

'Referent organisations' fill the role of coordinating and holding the space for this new domain of inquiry and action. The diversity represented by the WSF process has confounded many, and yet the domain-related meta-problem(s) that actors addressed, however contested and debated, in Trist's (1979, p. 1) words:

> constitutes a domain of common concern for its members . . . The issues involved are too extensive and too many-sided to be coped with by any single organization, however large. The response capability required to clear up a mess is inter- and multi-organizational (Trist 1979, 1).

The forum had modest attendance between 2004 and 2010. Events were held in 2004, 2005, 2006, 2007, 2008, and 2009, bringing together an average of between 300 and 400 participants, and hosting 30–50 workshops per event. The initial forum in 2004 was a one-day event (which expanded to two days in 2005). In 2006 the MSF ran the G20 Alternative as part of the G20 Convergence (an aspect of the protest against the G20 meetings then). The year 2007 saw the largest MSF event attendance (with approximately 450 participants). This was followed by a mini forum in 2008, and a larger two-day forum in 2009. The last MSF events were held in 2010, and the remaining proceeds from the MSF organisation were given to the 'CounterAct: Training for Change' project. (See: http://counteract.org.au)

Meta-networking and social complexity

Meta-networking engages both epistemic and ontological complexity. Epistemic complexity refers to the diversity of viewpoints, standpoints and world views that converge within a process. Ontological complexity refers to the diverse array of organisations and groups and the issues they address that converge as part of a process. This epistemological and ontological complexity exists as part of what social change processes are (the composition of embodied participation), and as part of what social change processes aim to address (the composition of social issues). This can be seen as inner and outer dimensions of social complexity.

Table 21:1

	Internal composition of field (participants)	External composition of social issues to address
Epistemic complexity	The array of ideological positions, cultural standpoints and worldviews that exist in the actors and participants that take part in a process or convergence	The array of ideological positions, cultural standpoints and worldviews that are projected upon the various issues that actors and participants aim to address
Ontological complexity	The array of types of actors, such as social movements, NGOs, networks, ethnic groups, diasporic communities, and people as a convergence	The array of issues that actors and participants aim to address, and how they are systemically inter-locked and related

In the next section I will describe the inner (epistemological) and outer (ontological) dimensions of this emerging form of 'prismatic' work. The inner dimension refers to the thinking, emotioning and feeling that provide the foundations for this kind of practice. The outer dimension refers to the behaviours, structures and systems that these emerging practices employ.

Epistemic complexity and inner dimensions

In the early days of my PhD work I received some criticism from neo-Marxist colleagues. They saw my writing and, to them, it looked confused, without coherence, lacking a tradition. While I agreed with many of the propositions made by the scholars who have pioneered neo-Marxist analysis into contemporary globalisation (Robinson 2004; Sklair 2005), as an organiser working in projects that brought multiple perspectives together, holding a single discourse (as truth) for whatever we spoke about (globalisation, etc.) was unworkable from a practical point of view. Eventually I needed to engage in a dual movement with respect to well-established scholarship and perspectives on globalisation and its transformations. On the one hand, I needed to deepen my appreciation of such perspectives, by attending conferences, talking to proponents and through reading. I needed to appreciate where such perspectives made sense and what they explain well. Likewise, I also needed to allow myself to settle into a space and an identity that supported openness and curiosity with respect to various discourses and perspectives.

But it was not all about perspectives, and this was where Latour (2005) was crucial. For Latour, understanding the social was fundamentally about how elements associate. For him, the researcher-practitioner should try to not impose pre-existing theories or frameworks on an area of observation. What was needed was a way of seeing how ideas, institutions, machines and people all come together to form and reform the social. This kind of post-materialist empiricism was and is central. It transformed the role of discourse and ideas from that which explains reality (for example, post-positivist), into that which guides actors in their quest to understand and act—discourse/ideas are embodied and mediate people's strategic action. An idea's truth lay more in its utility and enabling effective and strategic action, rather than the presumption of universal or historical law.

The transformation of discourse from truth/false, in the positivist sense that theory can represent the world unproblematically, to the Latourian idea that theory (and discourse) guides the strategies of the actors that hold them, paralleled another shift. My inner perspective as a practitioner could see connections between various modes of analysis and action of the people that I networked with. There existed a field of thinking and activity which had deep relatedness, but which had not yet been connected. I could see the opportunities in this 'ecology of knowledges'. The idea of 'meta-networking' emerged to guide me (Gilchrist 2004). The meta-networker moves across multiple spaces, sometimes a chameleon, listening and looking for connections between various organisations, people, ideas, projects. Opportunistic and restless, to see the possibility of emergence from what currently exists.

Two metaphors also helped guide this. The first metaphor was of the 'bee and flower'. The bee and the flower both have unique characteristics (one coming from the insect family and the other from the plant family). Yet at some point a reciprocally beneficial relationship developed, as flowers relied on insects (like bees) to carry their creative genetic material, and bees relied on flowering plants for nutrients. While they do not communicate in the strict sense, they express signifiers that allow for a broader process of structural coupling (Maturana 1998). Their ontogenetic differences do not preclude either the codes needed for structural coupling nor a tacit shared interest. I found in my social work that this complex 'structural coupling' occurred across ontological diversities (organisations doing different types of work), epistemological diversities (organisations/groups with different world views) and thematic diversities (organisations working in thematically different areas), in creating 'ecologies of innovation' and the potential for 'meta-formation'.

A second metaphor also guided me—the bridge builder. The bridge builder works between and across diverse actors and their different ways of knowing, facilitating their processes of building coherent strategies for change. Whereas the bee and flower signifies that it was in-and-across the landscape of systems where creative synergy was to be found, the bridge-building metaphor was about the practitioner. It indicated that someone needed to provide the unique leadership to bring different elements/people together. The bridge builder created the spaces, platforms and language for people to relate across their diversities. The bridge builder's inner resources are key: cognitive mapping, to understand a broader spectrum of commonality that has the potential to connect disparate actors toward common goals and projects. In this regard, the practitioner's capacity to identify hegemonic and counter-hegemonic knowledges is critical.

The diverse field of alternative globalisation actors represented knowledges which have been marginalised or obscured by the dominant and official liberalist discourse on globalisation (as inevitable, necessary, progressive, developmental, etc.). Santos (2006, p. 13) argues it represents an 'Epistemology of the South', which expresses the legitimacy of the (multiple) knowledge systems of the world's marginalised and the social experiences which inform them. Whether they be Latin American indigenous groups struggling against the incursions of trans-national corporations, African peasants struggling against subsidised agricultural imports, Dalit (untouchables) struggling against an Indian caste system, Cuban or Australian permaculturalists, Buddhists teaching meditation for peace, or climate scientists arguing for the de-carbonisation of the global economy, together they represent knowledges coupled to diverse experiences, which challenge hegemonic expressions of neo-liberal globalisation and reality. In short, identifying counter-hegemonic discourse and knowledges was and is fundamental to the bridge-building efforts needed to create critically informed social change.

Ontological complexity and outer dimensions

An approach to the practice of meta-networking for social change cannot just rely on inner resources of practitioners, there are also the ontological dynamics and factors that accompany any effort that critically informs strategic action.

In my work I found that the recognition of the dynamics of power was central to informing my own reading of strategy. As the movements for another globalisation are fundamentally concerned with both politicising and transforming power structures (Teivainen 2007), we need ways to think about what structures of power mean in respect to globalisation. For example, in Sklair's (2002) analysis, the current global system is composed of three main spheres of power, the economic, political and cultural, and through this we witness the emergence of structural synergies of domination. This is carried forth economically through transnational corporations, politically through an emerging transnational capitalist class, and culturally through the ideology of consumerism (Sklair 2005, pp. 58–9). As Mills (1956) explored half a century earlier through his analysis of the circulation of power in the US between economic, military and political domains, Sklair also points out the emerging structural synergies in capitalist globalisation. Korten (2006), in a similar fashion, points out his vision of needed structural (cultural, political, economic) alternatives. In Table 2, I use both Sklair's and Korten's distinctions as examples of how alternatives presented within the alternative globalisation movement are structural in nature.

Table 21.2

	Capitalist globalisation (Sklair)	Alternative globalisation in AGM (Korten)
Economic	Trans-national corporations and their interests	Local living economies; Fair share taxation and trade; Democratising workplaces
Cultural	Culture-ideology of consumerism—worth based on possessions and accumulation	Post patriarchy feminine leadership; Narratives of an Earth community; Spiritual Inquiry
Political	Trans-national capitalist class—plutocratic systems of governance	Democratising structures of governance; Participatory and open media; Precautionary policy making

I discovered that social alternatives did not exist in the somewhat ambiguous territory of (global) civil society, but are directed at a variety of structures (Sklair 2002, p. 315) For counter-hegemonic alternatives to have the possibility of becoming social realities, this necessarily required that institutional anchors needed to be created across spheres of power (economic, political and cultural). My traditional role as a culture worker/academic/researcher was being challenged, I would need to engage across both the political and the economic. My reading of power also necessitated a reading of counter power. Counter-hegemonic alternatives form through new strategic couplings across these domains, such that a field of self-sustaining counter power may become resilient and influential in democratising core aspects of institutional life. My work became consciously about interlinking social ecologies and meta-networking which facilitated alternative formations of structural power. It needed to express a 'critical' methodology in building social capital, by opening up opportunities for interaction, informational exchange and collaboration as a counterpoint to elite forums of social capital development (for example, the Davos World Economic Forum) (Gilchrist 2004, pp. 4–7; Mayo 2005, p. 50). Importantly, the imperative to work across the domains of business, politics/policy, and culture (media/academia) further reinforced the need to integrate the three levels of structural, post-structural and the commons, as social change was identified more concretely with power structures, and yet the discourses across different power structures are diverse, and within this were potentials for identifying commonality and opportunities for collaboration.

Three 'Ps' are critical in the practice of meta-networking: processes, platforms and places. When bringing people together across diverse domains of social experience, there needs to be a place that can not only accommodate that diversity, but which can leverage or harness diversity toward mutual recognitions, common themes, strategic opportunities and collaborative action. People need places to meet that are safe and nurturing. Social spaces can be analogised with geographic spaces. Some are fertile ground to plant seeds, while others are deserts. In the early days of my organising, I was assisted by places in Melbourne which supported social and ecological justice causes and campaigns such as: Borderlands, Ceres, and Trades Hall which had a history of innovating social change and were themselves examples of counter-hegemonic alternatives. We also relied on the legacy systems of social democracy, public libraries and parks. Later, my projects had to have more systematic approaches to procuring spaces.

Platforms are structures that allow participants of a particular process to cohabitate for a time. Platforms are by design and can be created for a number of different purposes. They can be both live and/or online, and ideally both. In my work with the MSF, we took the lead from the global organisation and followed the open space method (Owen 1997). The open space method allows participants to design and develop their own thematic ideas and sub-processes. It is less programmatic and more diverse and divergent than traditional conference processes. Using open space we would host about 300–400 participants and approximately 30 workshops, mostly developed by participants. Participants would choose which workshops they wanted to attend. While open space helped to accommodate diversity and make critical connections, it did not necessarily facilitate collaborative or strategic action across the whole. Platforms are in a sense a convergence of a space and a method for people to come together in a particular way. Online platforms have developed substantially over the last 10 years, and there are now many options.

Process and methodology, which is entangled with both space and platform, is still an important distinctive element. Action researchers have developed a wide variety of approaches to large scale group intervention, such as search conferences, as a way of engaging in large-scale and systemic collaborative inquiry and action (Martin 2001). Recently methodologies include Collective Impact, developed in the United States (Kania 2013), and Living Labs, developed in Europe (Beamish et al 2012). These various approaches recognise that beneficial social change and innovation must connect across diverse sectors, harness and leverage diverse participants' perspectives, capabilities and resources, and build common ground for collective action and collaborative innovation.

When working with social complexity, I have learned that understanding the nature of the social complexity, the amount of time people have to come together, where they come together, and under what explicit or implicit motivations people come together, all matter. This requires preparation and a willingness to explore and research various participants and their backgrounds, and to begin to build the groundwork for a process that will genuinely serve the interests of people who engage, and which will create the possibility and opportunity for collaboration and innovation. These three 'Ps', processes, platforms and places, are all of fundamental concern in building meta-networks for positive social change in conditions of systemic complexity.

Conclusion

In my own work, an approach that posits the structural and post-structural as opposite binary positions is less useful than one which brings them together toward building common ground (the commons) toward critically informed social change. An approach that recognises the legitimacy of a diversity of viewpoints and discourses is an important aspect of social and community work in the 21st century. We live in a world in which more people from different backgrounds are coming together at various scales and geographies. Increasingly, we work across multiple cultural reference points. At the same time, the idea of 'wicked problem' has taken root, and we understand that the most intractable issues cannot be solved by solo stakeholders who are isolated from the vast majority of people and actors who inhabit those same 'wicked systems'. We need well-developed practices of meta-networking that can build common ground between diverse actors to solve complex social problems. We need a whole-of-system approach that brings people together from across the systems in need of change. While this is very different from traditional service delivery modes of engagement, deeper change requires systemic inquiry and action. Given the cultural and structural complexities we are increasingly engaged with, post-structuralist approaches and perspectives are needed to engaging with multiplicity, transforming diversity into a resource for systemic and collaborative innovation. At the same time, however, differing perspectives are not necessarily mutually exclusive. There is the relational in-between—our commonness, common humanity, participation in a commons and the active development of common ground through the practice of meta-networking.

References

Beamish, E., McDade, D., Mulvenna, M., Martin, S. & Soilemezi, D. 2012, *Better Together—The TRAIL User Participation Toolkit for Living Labs*, Ulster: University of Ulster

Bergmann, V. 2006, 'Archaeologies of anti-capitalist utopianism' in A. Milner, M. Ryan & R. Savage (eds), *Imagining the Future: Utopia and Dystopia*, Melbourne: Arena

Briskman, L., Pease, B. & Allan, J. 2009, 'Introducing critical theories for social work in a neo-liberal context' in J. Allan, L. Briskman & B. Pease (eds), *Critical Social Work: Theories for a socially just world*, 2nd edn, St Leonards: Allen & Unwin

Bollier, D. & Helfrich, S. ed. 2012, *The Wealth of the Commons: A World Beyond Market and State*, Amherst: Levellers Press

Carley, M. & Christie, I. 1993, *Managing Sustainable Development*, Minneapolis: University of Minnesota Press

Castells, M. 1997, *The Power of Identity*, Massachusetts: Blackwell

Chisholm, R. 2001, 'Action research to develop an inter-organizational network' in P. Reason & H. Bradbury (eds), *Handbook of Action Research: Participative Inquiry and Practice*, Thousand Oaks: Sage

Gilchrist, A. 2004, *The Well Connected Community*, Bristol: Policy Press

Godet, M. & Durance, P. 2007, *La prospectiva estratégica*, Paris: Instituto Europeo de Prospectiva Estratégica

Hamilton, C. 2007, *Scorcher: The dirty politics of climate change*, Melbourne: Black Inc.

Hansen, M. 1997, 'Antonio Gramsci: Hegemony and the Materialist Conception of History' in J. Galtung & S. Inayatullah (eds), *Macrohistory and Macrohistorians*, Westport: Praeger

Hawthorne, S. 2002, *Wild Politics*, Melbourne: Spinifex Press

Ife, J. 2012, *Human Rights and Social Work: Towards rights-based practice*, Massachusetts: Cambridge University Press

Inayatullah, S. 1998, 'Causal layered analysis: post-structuralism as method', *Futures*, vol. 30, pp. 815–29

Kania, J. & Kramer, M. 2013, 'Embracing emergence: how collective impact addresses complexity', Stanford: *Stanford Social Innovation Review*

Korten, D. 2006, *The Great Turning: From empire to earth community*, Bloomfield: Kumarian Press

Latour, B. 2005, *Reassembling the Social: An introduction to actor network theory*, Oxford: Oxford University Press

Martin, A. 2001, 'Large-group processes as action research' in P. Reason & H. Bradbury (eds), *Handbook of Action Research*, Thousand Oaks: Sage

Maturana, H. & Varela, F. 1998, *The Tree of Knowledge*, Boston: Shambhala

Mayo, M. 2005, *Global Citizens: Social movements and the challenge of globalization*, Toronto: Canadian Scholars Press

Mills, C.W. 1956, *The Power Elite*, London: Oxford University Press

Owen, H. 1997, *Open Space Technology: A users guide,* San Francisco: Berrett-Koehler

Ramos, J. 2010, *Alternative Futures of Globalisation: A socio-ecological study of the World Social Forum Process,* PhD thesis, Brisbane: Queensland University of Technology

Robinson, W. 2004, *A Theory of Global Capitalism,* London: John Hopkins University Press

Santos, B. 2006, *The Rise of the Global Left: The World Social Forum and beyond,* London: Zed Books

Sklair, L. 2002, *Globalisation: Capitalism and its Alternatives,* Oxford: Oxford University Press

—— 2005, 'Generic globalization, capitalist globalization and beyond: A framework for critical globalisation studies' *in* R. Appelbaum & W. Robinson (eds), *Critical Globalization Studies,* New York: Routledge

Teivanen, T. 2007, 'The political and its absence in the World Social Forum—Implications for Democracy', *Development Dialogue—Global Civil Society*, vol. 49, pp. 69–79

Trist, E. 1979, 'Referent Organizations and the Development of Inter-Organizational Domains', Academy of Management (Organization and Management Theory Division) 39th Annual Convention, Atlanta, Georgia

22

Education for critical social work: being true to a worthy project

Selma Macfarlane

Introduction

The aim of social work education is to prepare students for practice by introducing them to knowledge, skills and values required to engage in the profession. A sense of what social work is, and should be, shapes the path that social work education follows. Social work is both a reflection of and response to the social structures, discourses and systems in which it is placed. This chapter argues that neoliberal discourses, currently predominant in Western societies like Australia, have the potential to reduce social work education to acquiring competency-based skills rather than critically reflective, transformative learning. Such uncritical promotion of a form of practice aimed at maintaining the status quo, rather than critically analysing and challenging inequitable social structures and power relations, reshapes social work education towards conservative, market-led demands. This is aimed at producing technically proficient practitioners who conform to existing systems, who are unable to see the broader (moral and political) implications of their work. This chapter argues that if social work is to remain an ethical and emancipatory project, graduates need to critically respond to oppression disguised as progress, human suffering constructed as risk, and social control cloaked in the mantle of inclusion.

The challenges posed by neoliberalism may be a force that unites us as social workers in revisioning our practice.

While this entire book explores the meaning of 'critical social work,' a simple version that underpins this chapter pertains to a social work lens that acknowledges and addresses: structural inequalities and inequitable power dynamics; the impact of discourse on lived experience; the importance of diverse knowledge systems, social work values and ethics; and critical reflection for progressive practice. Such an approach most closely resembles the definition of our profession provided by our international body. This chapter explores how students' preparation to become critical social workers can be enhanced during the course of their qualifying degree. The question of what social work education is ultimately *for* is significant for educators, students, practitioners and the future of the profession.

Neoliberalism and higher education

Before discussing specific issues for social work education, I look briefly at some wider implications of neoliberal agendas for tertiary education. This includes university-wide shifts and emphases, expanding cohorts of university students, and industry demands. While much change is driven by economic imperatives of neoliberalism, it must also be recognised that neoliberalism is a political project aimed at generating particular subjectivities and norms of behaviour (Giroux 2010). Giroux paints a grim picture of neoliberalism as a 'powerful pedagogical force that shapes our lives, memories and daily experiences, while attempting to erase everything critical and emancipatory about history, justice, solidarity, freedom, and democracy itself' (Giroux 2010: 51). This view is echoed by Shahjahan who describes neoliberalism as a primary actor in the 'colonisation of our ways of being', undermining and replacing 'institutional practices and political subjectivities centered on social, intellectual and ethical rationalities' (Shahjahan 2014: 222) with technical and economic rationalities. Such a trend is antithetical to the notion of education as a public good: an important element of democracy in developing informed citizens (Johnstone 2014). Students, as well as educators, can easily comply with a view that higher education is a commodity to be purchased rather than a learning journey in critical thinking.

As higher education is remodelled to suit the needs of the market (Webhi & Turcotte 2007; Giroux 2010; McArthur 2010), education that will be 'occupationally useful' (MacKinnon 2009) is emphasised. However, the ideological underpinnings of such a term are often invisibilised and unquestioned. McArthur suggests the rightful role of all disciplines within universities is to resist the distorting influence of commercialisation and pursue the more emancipatory role of higher education

(McArthur 2010: 304) aligned with critical pedagogy and the alleviation of all forms of oppression, alienation and subordination (McLean 2006, cited in McArthur 2010: 313).

Alongside neoliberalism's emphasis on individualism and consumerism, is the insinuation that there is no alternative to these hegemonic norms (Deepak 2012), which may be the most 'dangerous and incorrect aspect of neoliberal dogma' (Stewart-Harawira 2007: 159). Neoliberalist higher education colludes with this discourse by training people to accept the status quo rather than developing critical social consciousness. However, education has historically been a place for social resistance and transformation based on the belief that other futures are possible (Stewart-Harawira 2007; Amsler 2011). Implementing critical programs may be particularly challenging in the neoliberalised context. Students may understandably find any form of social-justice education to be confrontational, uncomfortable and difficult to embrace (Preston & Aslett 2014).

Neoliberalism and social work education

The encroachment of neoliberal ideology on social work education is cause for concern. As critical social work becomes increasingly hard to do in current policy and service delivery contexts (Macdonald 2009: 243), what was meant 'as a challenge to the status quo' [i.e. social work] is in danger of being 'swallowed up by it' (Webhi & Turcotte 2007: 5). Education that emphasises competency-based approaches, narrowly defined forms of evidence and an over-emphasis on risk rather than more complex needs, takes away from the professional skills of social work and, while producing a set of skills the social worker can apply in a work setting, does not engender a capacity to think critically or reflectively (Mullaly 2007: 196). Mullaly (2007) cautions that such an educational emphasis does, however, create social workers who are easier to control, regulate and be quality assessed by their political masters. Social work, largely based in government-funded organisations, can be co-opted into uncritical acceptance of neoliberal discourses that support and entrench inequality in order to achieve 'quicker wins,' feeding the 'charity cycle ... [leading] us into a more palatable consumption of outrageous injustice' (Lorenzetti 2013: 2).

An important premise in this discussion is the belief that social work is always political, whether through action or inaction, resistance to or acceptance of the status quo: there is no neutral ground in social work (MacKinnon 2009; Lorenzetti 2013). Social work students and educators belong to a wider social work community committed to social justice, empowerment, liberation and community engagement; social work education has a responsibility to challenge the erosion of these basic values (Webhi & Turcotte 2007). An important element of social work education is to enable the development of students' critically reflexive voice, so they can deconstruct the discourses shaping the professional domain and see how they make sense of their place within it (MacArdle & Mansfield 2007). Otherwise, social work education may run the risk of creating 'competent technicians who can do the job they have been trained to do but are unable to see beyond the . . . work in hand to the wider society context and purpose of their work' (MacArdle & Mansfield 2007: 496). Education for critical social work aims to enable graduates to understand and challenge the unjust nature of society and oppressive elements in their own profession through their capacity to analyse power and social relationships as both personal and political (Campbell & Baikie 2012). The social-justice mandate of social work is inherently at odds with neoliberal paradigms. The question then, is how can education for critical social work thrive in increasingly challenging social and political contexts? I explore this question in the next three sections, finishing with a case study.

Education for critical social work: decolonising our minds, believing in possibilities

As mentioned earlier, one of the most dangerous aspects of neoliberalism is the implicit assumption that there is no alternative ideological or political positioning worthy of consideration or even possible in today's or tomorrow's world (Stewart-Harawira 2007). This adds to the challenge for social workers, faced with increasingly managerialist workplaces charged with implementing neoliberal policy, to believe in possibilities for social change. Unless a conscious effort is made, social work students, educators and practitioners may develop a sense that critical practice is not possible, and that activism is out of the question if one wishes to keep their job. Critical social workers can easily feel like failed activists (see Healy 2000; Rossiter 2001) or lone crusaders with few allies and many enemies (see Fook 2004; 2012).

Education for critical social work means moving beyond critiques of neoliberalism to create 'new ways of being, knowing and doing . . . through the injection of alternative . . . knowledge; in other words, a decolonising approach' (Shahjahan 2014: 219). This 'transformational resistance' involves first, recognising how easily we may become complicit with neoliberal and other oppressive discourses; second, our potential for agency within these discourses; and third, experimentation with alternative ways of knowing and being aligned with a vision for the future of human connection and interdependence (Shahjahan 2014). In social work, we do this, as students, lecturers and practitioners when we attempt to uncover our potential for agency and possibilities for more empowered practice through the practice of critical reflection, often based on specific practice incidents (see Fook 2012). The realisation that other alternatives are possible, not only in the visionary realm of social change, but in the day-to-day realities of working on-the-ground can be liberating for students, educators and practitioners. In this process, Taylor (2013) reminds us, it is important to focus on our own individual self-awareness and potential for changed practice and to interrogate the underlying meanings embedded in accepted helping practices and service delivery, which may be imbued with neoliberal or colonial premises or both.

'Educated' or 'critical' hope (Giroux 2004; MacKinnon 2009; Amsler 2011) can be a powerful subversive and mobilising force connecting critical education (which engages our thinking around social change), with political agency and concrete real-world translations of our vision into specific everyday-practice interactions (Giroux 2004). It is our broader vision of the mission of social work and a more socially just world, according to Fook (2012) that enables us to work in whatever context we find ourselves, expressing our critical social work values and ideals within the opportunities, small and large, that arise in our local and immediate practice settings. Sometimes, this may mean something as simple as changing the way our office or reception space is organised and the messages it conveys, or changing the way we write and talk about clients, or becoming more mindful of the cultural wisdom of others outside our profession. Education for critical social work involves developing awareness that we can work at both 'local and idealist levels simultaneously' because we do not see them as separate (Fook 2012).

Uncomfortable aspects of education for critical social work

As mentioned in the introduction, the penetration of neoliberal ideology into our expectations may make it particularly difficult for students, educators and practitioners to consider social and political alternatives (Preston & Aslett 2014). The commercialisation of higher education with its emphasis on producing satisfied customers (market-ready graduates who conform to existing social systems), has created what Amsler refers to as 'therapeutic education [that] prioritises feelings of wellbeing over either the acquisition of knowledge or the capacity for agency' (Amsler 2011: 50). As a critical educator, Amsler rues the accomplishment of the 'happy consciousness,' which, she says, is cause for alarm not celebration; it is discomfort rather than happiness that is the task of critical education (Amsler 2011: 55). Amsler proposes 'education must not only enable people to recognise and explain injustice through critical analysis, but also help them develop *critical affectivities* through which they are moved to change it' (emphasis added, Amsler 2011: 53). At a recent international social work conference, delegates were encouraged to bear witness and speak out about social injustice, to draw on an affective response of collective moral outrage to challenge the 'neoliberal tricksters' privileging of the rational over the emotional (Williams 2014).

In embracing critical social work we are constantly challenged to consider how we can accept the discomfort when wrestling with difficult issues such as opening our minds and hearts to notions of unearned privilege and oppression. A willingness to transform our own beliefs, assumptions and actions, whether we are students, educators or practitioners is not a singular event or accomplishment, but an ongoing element of critical practice (Taylor 2008: 13). Openly acknowledging and sharing with others the challenges we experience in trying to enact our espoused critical approaches can normalise the discomfort we feel when our emotional investment in maintaining existing world views comes under scrutiny.

Amsler (2011) suggests that the fundamental task of critical social work education is not so much to teach people how to feel about themselves or others, but to enable them to understand why they have certain feelings, desires and needs, and why they, or we, are not supposed to have others. This is particularly salient for graduating social workers whose abilities to critically question the often hidden norms of policy imperatives, service delivery and power dynamics are crucial (Nicotera & Kang 2009). In order to engage in these sorts of discussions, the development of a safe space in the classroom is necessary: a space where students and educators can engage in genuine examination of their own assumptions and social locations, as well as those deeply embedded and reflected in social work theory and practice. It is through the creation of safe spaces that discomforting experiences can be worked with. A pedagogy of discomfort is described by Leibowitz et al. as an invitation for students to 'critique deeply held assumptions and destabilise their view of themselves and their world' (Leibowitz et al. 2010: 84), acknowledging that learning about difference can be a painful experience, which may or may not lead to changed views or behaviours. Conversations, for example, about race and white privilege, require courage and the capacity to withstand and move through discomfort, to stay engaged in the presence of multiple perspectives. Rather than closing conversation down, Singleton and Hays (2013) observe that we need to engage *more deeply* when people speak their truth and provide opportunities to reconsider opinions; in this process of 'courageous conversations' we should expect and accept lack of closure and be guided by core social work skills of listening, inquiring and responding (Singleton & Hays 2013). The ideas of social workers such as Yuk-Lin Wong, who challenge our understanding of experiences such as discomfort, suggest that discomfort can be both a teacher and friend, and that leaving our comfort zones can lead to personal growth and social transformation (Wong 2004). Reframing discomfort in a more empowered way is strongly connected to the practice of critical reflection, which requires honest critique of and potential change to our own individual practice, as well as social work practices more generally.

Education for critical social work: curriculum content

As mentioned in the introduction, a critical social work lens acknowledges and addresses structural inequalities and inequitable power dynamics, the impact of discourse on lived experience, and the importance of diverse knowledge systems, social work values and ethics, and critical reflection for practice. Education for critical social work needs to clearly describe and discuss what is meant by 'critical social work' in the context of each specific unit. This is important as students are often grappling with contradictory messages around key terms.

Facilitating competency-based skills development and meeting the content requirements of the professional body is necessary. However, such requirements may mirror the power dynamics of the wider society (Bennett 2013) potentially minimising critical analysis of their ideological, political or theoretical underpinnings. A conscious and sustained effort is required to maintain a commitment to human rights and critical practice in educational and service-delivery climates saturated with neoliberal values and the view that all problems are private rather than social in nature (Giroux 2010). It is far beyond the scope of this chapter to detail what curricula content should include, except that it should reflect the core principles of critical social work.

The previous section outlined the importance of a critical approach to social work education if we are to deepen our understanding of oppression and privilege, and our own place within this dynamic. Critical social work education challenges conservative social work and neoliberal perceptions of clients as deviant, deficient, lazy or ignorant: that is, objects to be treated or controlled (Wright 2014). The construction of the stigmatised other is a powerful component of neoliberal and colonialist discourse that must be actively challenged by critical social workers. Speeches such as that given by Rosalie Kunoth-Monk (2014) 'I am not the problem' are potent reminders of how we may become complicit with the mind-numbing indoctrination of neoliberal and colonialist discourses that take us far away from the emancipatory intent of our profession.

Stewart-Harawira evocatively suggests that critical education aims at imparting 'an ontological vision that bespeaks humanity's wholeness and interrelatedness' (Stewart-Harawira 2005: 159). The process of decolonising our hearts and minds, and opening our eyes to the wisdom of 'marginalised' others requires more than a one-day workshop on cultural competence or a one-off presentation from a consumer or community group, although that may be a useful start. The normalised and entrenched nature of racism, colonialism and other forms of oppression means that we often do not recognise our complicity in oppressive practices (Kessaris 2006).

Despite our claim as a profession to value diverse knowledge systems, social work remains a heavily Westernised profession, with a knowledge base steeped in Western traditions and world views (Gray 2008). In a recent study canvassing the views and experiences of Aboriginal social workers in Australia, a consistent observation was that social workers without Aboriginal backgrounds often acted from an uncritical discourse of whiteness, ignorant of the real history of Aboriginal and Torres Strait Islander peoples and the role of colonisation and white privilege within themselves, social work and society (Bennett 2013). Resisting and transforming neoliberal and colonialist discourse means, in part, challenging limiting understandings of what constitutes 'real knowledge' for social work practice. Scheurich and Young describe how social groups, cultures and societies evolve different knowledge systems reflective of the social history of that group; however, 'all of the epistemologies currently legitimated in education arise exclusively out of the social history of the dominant White race' (Scheurich & Young 1997: 8), excluding the knowledge of other social groups. They refer to this as 'epistemological racism.' Indigenous scholars around the world, some of them social workers, contest this skewed construction of what constitutes valid knowledge (and how it is attained), articulating indigenous knowledge systems and Indigenist research practices reflecting Aboriginal world views, social mores and contexts, privileging the voices, experiences and lives of Aboriginal people and their lands, and identifying and redressing issues of importance *as defined by Aboriginal people* (Martin 2003). Far from being 'over the heads' of undergraduate students, these sorts of discussions and the new terms and concepts they introduce, can contribute to 'lightbulb' moments laden with possibilities.

Even with the best of critical intentions, Rossiter (2001) reminds us, the act of 'helping' is never entirely innocent; there is the potential for trespass whenever knowledge is employed, which is why critical reflection is a crucial component of education for critical social work. The principles of critical reflection have been extensively covered by Fook (2004, 2012), Taylor (2013) and others and will not be elaborated upon in this chapter. Essentially, it involves interrogating implicit values, beliefs and assumptions, identifying how these may be infused with ideas that support dominant power relations and structures through a two-stage process of deconstruction and reconstruction, leading to possibilities for changed practice (Morley & Macfarlane, in press). Through the process of critical reflection, study, and dialogue, students learn that no action is too small or insignificant, and that our heart and our imagination are as necessary as our rationality and logic.

Case study

This case study briefly describes some ways in which education for critical social work can take place in an Australian regional university setting, in the context of a four-year Bachelor of Social Work degree. It is by no means exhaustive and is open to ongoing improvement and change.

Developing and maintaining a focus on critical practice in a unit on mental health and illness: In response to the professional body's requirements for specific mental health content, a new unit was written to cover the required mental health content, also incorporating fields and methods of practice (Macfarlane 2009). In taking a critical approach, the meaning of 'critical social work' was clearly outlined in the first topic and remained a clear thread through each of the weekly topics, consistently encouraging students to consider 'what was critical about our approach to this week's concepts and issues?' When looking at mental health issues across fields of practice, consideration was given to how poverty, racism and sexism impact on individual experience and what social work has to offer in often highly medicalised settings. Demonstrating an understanding of a 'critical approach' to mental health issues was clearly built into both assessment pieces.

Reflecting a critical approach in assessment: To replace the mainstream psychology unit that Bachelor of Social Work students were required to complete, a new unit, with a more critical approach to psychological theories was introduced (Pease 2006) and developed (Furlong 2012). For example, in learning about theories of cognitive development, encouragement was provided to think critically about the social location and historical context of the theory's originator, the culturally bound nature of theories purporting to describe

---

universal 'human behaviour,' the lack of gender analysis that may be present, etc. Students, through keeping a weekly reflective journal, moved through four clearly articulated stages of critical reflection. First, they wrote about their initial response to the concepts they were studying and second where that initial response came from in terms of their own personal biography and social location. Third, they articulated their journey in further exploring the concept, and fourth, reflected on whether their view had changed through the process of moving 'from reaction to response' (Furlong 2012). Their second assignment involved an examination of their own life, in relation to an element of their structural location, drawing critically on concepts covered in the unit and concluding with a discussion of how privilege or oppression or both have shaped their experience and beliefs.

Drawing together a vision for social work practice: In one of the final units before graduation, fourth-year students are asked, in a major piece of writing, to describe their vision for practice and then illustrate how they would translate or enact their vision in a specific practice setting. Students describe, in their essays, possibilities for critical practice in changing and sometimes challenging contexts. Graduates from the program are invited to come in for conversations about how they attempt to practice critically across a range of settings. Alongside this unit, students undertake a core unit which takes them through in-depth shared deconstruction and reconstruction of practice scenarios, drawing on postmodern and critical theory to destabilise narratives of power and discourse that can lead to changed, more emancipatory practice (Fook 2004, 2012).

Students engage with reading material from a range of diverse cultures and knowledge systems; and, importantly students and educators share their ongoing journey in skill and knowledge development.

Conclusion

Critical social work education is not easy for educators or students. Sometimes it is 'too hard' or 'there's not enough time' or we don't really understand how to walk the talk. Students, educators and practitioners come to social work from diverse backgrounds, often combining study with work and caring responsibilities, motivated by a common desire to help people and make the world a better place; this will is tested by academic demands and the challenging nature of critical social work. However, as Ferguson (2008) puts it, critical social work is a profession worth fighting for: an ongoing moral and political project that attempts to reshape inequitable social structures, discourses and power relations. While the world is seldom changed in a day, and neoliberal agendas appear firmly entrenched, many small acts contribute to large changes and education for critical social work can and should be part of this endeavour.

References

Amsler, S. 2011, 'From "therapeutic" to political education: The centrality of affective sensibility in critical pedagogy', *Critical Studies in Education*, vol. 52, no. 1, pp. 47–63

Bennett, B. 2013, '"Stop deploying your white privilege on me!" Aboriginal and Torres Strait Islander engagement with the Australian Association of Social Workers', *Australian Social Work*, DOI: 10.1080/0312407X.2013.840325

Campbell, C. & Baikie, G. 2012, 'Beginning at the beginning: An exploration of critical social work', *Critical Social Work*, vol. 13, no. 1

Deepak, A. 2012, 'Globalization, power and resistance: Postcolonial and transnational feminist perspectives for social work practice', *International Social Work*, vol. 5, no. 6, pp. 779–93

Ferguson, I. 2008, *Reclaiming Social Work: Challenging neo-liberalism and promoting social justice*, London: Sage

Fook, J. 2004, 'The lone crusader: Constructing enemies and allies in the workplace' in L. Napier & J. Fook (eds), *Breakthroughs in Practice: Theorising critical moments in social work*, Whiting & Birch, London, pp. 186–200

—— 2012, *Social Work: A critical approach to practice*, 2nd edn, London: Sage

Furlong, M. 2012, *HSW219: Self and Society Study Guide*, Geelong: Deakin University

Giroux, P. 2004, 'When hope is subversive,' *Tikkun*, vol. 19, no. 6, pp. 38–9

—— 2010, 'Neoliberalism, pedagogy, and cultural politics: Beyond the theatre of cruelty' in Z. Leonardo (ed.), *Handbook of cultural politics and education*, Rotterdam: Sense Publishers, pp. 49–70

Gray, M. 2008, 'Editorial: Postcards from the West: Mapping the vicissitudes of Western social work', *Australian Social Work*, vol. 61, no. 1, pp. 1–6

Healy, K. 2000, *Social Work Practices: Contemporary perspectives on change*, London: Sage

Johnstone, M. 2014, 'Democracy's challenge: The tangled corporatization of citizenship and higher education in Canada', paper presented to Joint World Conference on Social Work, Education and Social Development, Melbourne, 11 July 2014

Kessaris, T.N. 2006, 'About being mununga (whitefulla): Making covert group racism visible', *Journal of Community & Applied Social Psychology,* vol. 6, pp. 347–62

Kunoth-Monk, R. 2014, 'I am not the problem', *Q & A program, Australian Broadcasting Corporation,* <_www.news.com.au/national/rosalie-kunoghmonks-inspires-with-her-qa-speech-i-am-not-the-problem/story-fncynjr2-1226949124486>, accessed 18 June 2014<_

Leibowitz, B., Bozalek, V., Rohlder, P., Crolissen, R. & Swartz, L. 2010, '"Ah, but the whiteys love to talk about themselves": Discomfort as a pedagogy for change', *Race Ethnicity and Education,* vol. 13, no. 1, pp. 83–100

Lorenzetti, L. 2013, 'Developing a cohesive emancipatory social work identity: Risking an act of love', *Critical Social Work,* vol. 14, no. 2

Macfarlane, S 2009, 'Opening spaces for alternative understandings in mental health practice,' in J. Allan, L. Briskman, & B. Pease (eds), *Critical socialwork: theories and pratices for a socially just world,* 2nd ed, Allen & Unwin, Crows Nest, NSW, pp. 201–213.

Martin, K.L. 2003, 'Ways of knowing, ways of being and ways of doing: A theoretical framework and methods for Indigenous re-search and Indigenist research', Voicing Dissent, New Talents 21C: Next Generation Australian Studies, *Journal of Australian Studies,* vol. 76, pp. 203–14

McArdle, K. & Mansfield, S. 2007, 'Voice, discourse and transformation: Enabling learning for the achieving of social change', *Discourse: Studies in the Cultural Politics of Education,* vol. 28, no. 4, pp. 485–98

McArthur, J. 2010, 'Time to look anew: Critical pedagogy and disciplines within higher education', *Studies in Higher Education,* vol. 35, no. 3, pp. 301–15

McDonald, C. 2009, 'Critical practice in a changing context' in J. Allan, L. Briskman, & B. Pease (eds), *Critical Social Work: Theories and practices for a socially just world,* 2nd edn, St Leonards: Allen & Unwin, pp. 243–54

MacKinnon, S. 2009, 'Social work intellectuals in the twenty-first century: critical social theory, critical social work and public engagement', *Social Work Education,* vol. 28, no. 5, pp. 512–27

Morley, C. & Macfarlane, S. (in press) 'Critical social work as ethical social work: Using critical reflection to research students' resistance to neoliberalism', *Critical and Radical Social Work*

Mullaly, B. 2007, *The New Structural Social Work,* 3rd edn, Ontario: Oxford University Press

Nicotera, N. & Kang, H. 2009, 'Beyond diversity courses: Strategies for integrating critical consciousness across social work curricula', *Journal of Teaching in Social Work,* vol. 29, no. 2, pp. 188–203

Preston, S. & Aslett, J. 2014, 'Resisting neoliberalism from within the academy: Subversion through an activist pedagogy', *Social Work Education: The International Journal,* vol. 33, no. 4, pp. 502–18

Rossiter, A. 2001, 'Innocence lost and suspicion found: do we educate for or against social work?', *Critical Social Work,* vol. 2, no. 1

Scheurich, J.J. & Young, M.D. 1997, 'Coloring epistemologies: Are our research epistemologies racially biased?', *Educational Researcher,* vol. 26, no. 4, pp. 4–16

Shahjahan, R.A. 2014, 'From 'no' to 'yes': Postcolonial perspectives on resistance to neoliberal higher education', *Discourse: Studies in the Cultural Politics of Education,* vol. 35, no. 2, pp. 219–32

Singleton, G. & Hays, C. 2013, 'Beginning courageous conversations about race' in M. Pollock (ed.), *Everyday Anti-racism: Getting real about race in school,* New York: The New Press

Stewart-Harawira, M. 2007, 'Cultural studies, Indigenous knowledge and pedagogies of hope', *Policy Futures in Education,* vol. 3, no. 2, pp. 153–63

Taylor, C. 2013, 'Critically reflective practice' in M. Gray & S. Webb (eds), *The New Politics of Social Work,* Palgrave Macmillan, Basingstoke, pp. 79–97

Taylor, E.W. 2008, 'Transformative learning theory', *New Directions for Adult and Continuing Education*, vol. 119, pp. 5–15

Webhi, S. & Turcotte, P. 2007, 'Social work education: Neoliberalism's willing victim?', *Critical Social Work*, vol. 8, no. 1

Williams, C. 2014, 'Reviving social work through moral outrage', paper presented to Joint World Conference on Social Work, Education and Social Development, Melbourne, 11 July 2014

Wong, Y. 2004, 'Knowing through discomfort: A mindfulness-based critical social work pedagogy', *Critical Social Work*, vol. 5, no. 1

Wright, K. 2014, 'The practical realities of implementing progressive social work: A case example in parenting education', *Journal of Progressive Human Services*, vol. 25, no. 2, pp. 133–53

Glossary

ableism is a term used for explaining an ideology in which able-bodiedness is privileged, often resulting in discrimination or prejudice against people with disabilities.

anti-discriminatory social work utilises the Personal-Cultural-Structural (PCS) model to address the disadvantage and oppression caused by different forms of discrimination including sexism, heterosexism, racism, ageism, ableism and religious discrimination.

anti-oppressive practice theorises and addresses the multiple, diverse and intersecting forms of oppression based on social divisions such as class, gender, race/ethnicity, sexuality, disability and so on.

anti-racist social work is an approach that draws on a range of critical race theories and seeks to address the discrimination and oppression caused by racism.

capital accumulation refers to profits that a company uses to increase its capital base. It involves acquiring more assets that can be used to create more wealth or that will appreciate in value.

classism refers to the entrenched oppression of those who must sell their waged labour (or be prepared to, as in people who are subject to unemployment) to survive, and those who care for them, by those who have control over the means of production.

classism – structural level is a component and practice of neoliberalism that normalises class-based structural violence against those individuals, families, groups and communities who are distanced by varying degrees from the mythical norm. This class-based structural violence includes unequal access by people to quality employment, education, housing, health, legal assistance, childcare, community infrastructure and welfare opportunities.

clear contracting means openly acknowledging the contradictions and conflicts between what social workers would like to be able to do, what the service user would ideally like and what the agency requires. This involves exposing the social worker's values, biases and limitations.

complicity means being an accomplice in, or having some involvement in, activities that are unlawful or morally wrong.

critical consciousness is the ability to perceive social, political, and economic oppression and to take action against the oppressive elements of society.

critical gerontology describes a broad spectrum of theoretical interests concerned with the construction and deconstruction of ageing and issues facing older people in the context of power and control in contemporary society.

critical questioning refers to using observation, thinking, listening, talking, learning with those involved, and analysis, to reveal and explore the impacts of the way institutions, organisations, relationships, socially accepted ideas and processes are organised that may produce oppressive and discriminatory outcomes.

critical postmodernism draws on poststructural thinking and modernist critical theories to inform critical social work practice.

critical social work is an umbrella term that describes a group of approaches in social work that are diverse but share a common commitment to both personal and structural change.

critical educationalist is an educator who uses critical pedagogy in their teaching, which is a philosophy of education and social movement, that combines education with critical theory.

critical incident analysis facilitates reflective practice and reflective learning in relation to critical incidents, which may cause someone to reflect on and rethink specific events.

critical theory–informed practice is practice informed by critical theory which is a school of thought that emphasises the reflective assessment and critique of society and culture by applying knowledge from the social sciences and humanities.

cultural humility involves a commitment to the ongoing processes of self-reflection and self-examination of our own social locations acknowledging the partiality of knowing how our own social locations impact how we understand and treat others.

culturally friendly attitude includes qualities of warmth, friendliness, curiosity and openness to learn from others that social workers can convey to signal to service users their genuine interest in them, and need to learn from them.

deprofessionalisation is a process which results in employers choosing non-qualified staff over qualified professionals in order to keep costs down, maintain competition and flexibility in service delivery and keep social service roles defined in narrow terms.

dialogical praxis is an acknowledgement of both the worker and those with whom they are working, as having expertise and opportunity to learn from each other. This collaboration involves the continuous cycle of critically assessing the value of practice and theories as they inform and are understood in the work with service users, communities, policies or organisations.

discourse analysis refers to a range of approaches that analyse texts (language both written and verbal). Critical discourse analysis is particularly concerned with how inequality, dominance and abuse of power are produced, reproduced and resisted by such texts.

essentialism is a view that categories of people (such as women and men, children and adults) have their own characteristics, which are intrinsic to all members of their category.

ethical listening aims to actively signal respect through demonstrating the listener's receptivity and interest to hear and learn from another's experience as contained in the values, cultural orientations, and feelings conveyed in the acts of being, speech, silence and listening. It is in listening that others can say what they want to say and the listener has the opportunity to learn.

feminist social work is an approach to social work that draws on feminist theories and seeks to address the discrimination and oppression caused by sexism.

gender analysis is a type of socio-economic analysis that uncovers how gender relations affect a problem.

gender role socialisation is the process of learning culturally dominant social expectations and behaviours associate with a person's apparent gender.

governmentality is a term coined by philosopher Michel Foucault, which refers to the way in which the state exercises control over, or governs, the people living under its jurisdiction.

grand narrative or meta-narrative, is a term introduced by Jean-Francois Lyotard in his writings, where he articulates a critique of the institutional and ideological forms of knowledge as constituting a totalising narrative that is authoritarian.

heteronormativity is the belief that people fall into distinct and complementary genders with natural roles in life. It assumes that heterosexuality is the only sexual orientation, or only norm, and maintains that heterosexual relations are the only acceptable form of sexual relations.

human rights-based social work is an approach that seeks to protect and promote human rights in social work practice.

indigenisation refers to adapting social work to non-Western settings; making it 'fit' rather than working from the local level to see what would be culturally relevant in that particular context.

individualisation literally means to make an individual distinctive and to discriminate them from the generic group to which they belong. However, it is also used to critique the idea of people's sense of identity being based on individual experience rather than from their relationships with others.

institutional ethnography is a feminist, critical, public sociological method of inquiry first developed by Dorothy E. Smith that aims to locate how and why the current actualities of social worlds are coordinated. This knowledge can then be used to inform action for social and political change.

intersectionality is a concept often used to describe the ways in which oppressive institutions (racism, sexism, homophobia, transphobia, ableism, xenophobia, classism, etc) are interconnected and cannot be examined separately from one another.

macro practice is professionally guided intervention designed to bring about change in organisational, community and policy arenas.

managerialism is a belief in the value of professional managers and the concepts and methods they use. It is associated with hierarchy, accountability and measurement, and a belief in the importance of tightly managed organisations.

meta-narrative see grand narrative.

micro practice focuses on the personal interaction between a social worker and client or consumer on an individual level or with a couple or family.

monocentrism is the political doctrine that human beings originated in a single region of the world and that all legitimate ideas flow from one legitimate source.

mythical norm is a socially constructed stereotype perpetuated by society, against which everyone else is measured forming a hierarchy under which others fall.

mutual consciousness-raising this term is used rather than consciousness-raising to acknowledge that social workers and service users have much to teach and learn from each other, as both are impacted in similar and different ways by social structures.

neo-conservatism refers to a return to a modified political ideology characterised by an emphasis on free-market capitalism and an interventionist foreign policy.

neoliberalism is an approach to economics and social sciences in which control of economic factors has shifted from the public sector to the private sector.

nihilism refers to the rejection of all religious and moral principles, often in the belief that life is meaningless.

normative morals are a code of behaviour that is accepted by the majority of people in a group, organisation, institution and / or society as the right, proper or only way to think and behave.

post structuralism is the name for a movement in philosophy that began in the 1960s. It rejects definitions that claim to have discovered absolute 'truths' or facts about the world.

poverty-aware and class cognisant (PACC) approach is an approach informed by the analysis of the class-based nature of the structural violence of poverty that informs and links social work practice in the day-to-day realities of working with people in organisations to the wider goals of transforming inequalities.

privilege refers to a special right, advantage, or immunity that is granted or available only to a particular person or group.

process orientations is a term used to identify that working from a critical social work perspective cannot be reduced to technical behaviours able to be understood or replicated without the critical theory and social justice value base.

radical social work is a form of social work that developed in the UK, North America and Australia in the 1970s that is centrally concerned with class oppression, capitalism, neoliberalism, austerity, inequality and social work practice.

relativism is the theory that value judgements, such as truth, beauty or morality, have no universal validity but are valid only for the persons or groups holding them.

social empathy is the capacity to increase understanding of, and response to, people, families, groups and communities through interacting with their life situations and as a result gain insight into the structural causes of their situations.

social location refers to one's social position in relation to both oppression and privilege as well as in relation to the various social dimensions of class, gender, race/ethnicity, age, ability, sexuality, religion and so on.

structural social work is an approach developed in Canada that is centrally concerned with the exploitative and oppressive structures or social divisions of society. It argued against the 'ranking' of social divisions (class, gender, race, age, ability/disability and sexuality) and emphasised the interweaving of these social divisions.

social-welfare feminism makes the link that the inequalities generated by the capitalist-market system underpins much social work practice.

subjugated knowledge is a term coined by French philosopher Michel Foucault to describe knowledge (and ways of knowing) that are left out, opposed or ignored by the mainstream dominant culture.

structural violence of poverty suggests that those individuals, families, groups and communities furthest from their society's 'mythical norm' are systematically subjected to the highest rates and impacts of the structural abuse of poverty. People and institutions can inflict harms such as discrimination and economic inequality on victims even when not in a direct relationship with them.

technicism refers to learning with a focus on compliance and achievement of set targets rather than engagement with deeper knowledge and experience.

truth claims are statements or propositions that are put forward as being true.

universalising focuses on the links between experiences that a person sees as unique and specific to them, and the experiences of others in similar situations. This involves use of social and personal empathy.

Index

critical social work
  common principles 5
  contradictions and 12
  criminal justice setting 164–6
  critical theory and 5–9
  definition 4, 5, 340
  emancipatory potential 25, 30
  Eurocentric bias 8
  good practice 223–4
  history of 4–5
  nature of 25–7
  neoliberalism and 11, 29, 177, 310
  new practices 310–23
  practice of 3
  process orientations 56–9, 113, 182, 343
  social justice and 26, 39
  state-based social work 3
  supervision 39–50
  theoretical approaches 5–9, 25–6, 42,
    52–68
critical theory 5–11, 42, 137
  critical social work practice and 5–9
  critical theory–informed practice 42,
    340
  mainstream social work and 9–11
  statutory context 137–8
  supervision informed by 42–7
cultural humility 57, 62, 340
culturally friendly attitude 57, 64, 66–7, 340
curriculum content 332–4
  disability excluded 299
  mental health and illness 334

deconstruction 28, 33, 54, 58, 64, 65, 67,
  114, 166, 303
determinism 29
'deviant social work' 14, 151
dialogical praxis 56, 61, 62, 114, 341
disability 18, 298–307
  able-bodied privilege 91
  alliance 303–4
  Centrelink services 152
  critical participatory approach 301–7
  critical reflection 299

critical social work 299–301
  discursive framing of 300
  diversity of needs and aspirations 299
  empowerment 301
  enabling practice 300–1
  facilitated sex 304–7
  marginalisation 298, 299
  oppression and disadvantage 300
  post-conventional approach 300
  post-structuralism 300
  rights movement 303
  Sexuality and Disability Alliance (SDA)
    299, 304–7
  terminology 298
  transformative models 300–1
discourse analysis 6, 341
discretion, use of 58, 64, 66, 67, 113, 159
discrimination
  Aboriginal people 217–18
  anti-discriminatory social work 5, 199,
    205
  LGBTIQ people 255, 256
  racism see racism
  religious 77–80
discriminatory practices 6, 63
  regulatory texts activating 182–3
  supervision to minimise 42
domestic violence
  Centrelink services 152
  child protection see child protection
  collaboration and partnership 231–4
  de-gendering problem 234–5
  engaging men emotionally in addressing
    95–7
  feminist social work 17, 226–38
  framing as crime 231
  gender power differences 61, 95
  intimate partner violence (IPV) 259–60
  lesbian relationships 259–60
  prisoners' backgrounds 164, 168
domination 27, 31, 42, 43

ecological approach 276, 277, 280–1
ecological ethics 277

meta-networking (*continued*)
  platforms 322
  post-structuralism 314–15
  processes 322
  referent organisations 312, 317
  Sklair's analysis 320–1
  social complexity and 317–18
  social forums 315
  'telos' of group 313, 314
  World Social Forum (WSF) 312, 313, 315
Mission Australia 214, 216
modernism 52–68
  critical modernism 52–68
  critical reflection and 27–35
  improving practices 33–5
  postmodernism and 52–68
  process orientations 56–9
  socialist-feminist social work 53–4, 59–64
moral courage 287
mutual consciousness raising 56, 61, 111,
  114, 182, 342
mythical norms 104, 109, 181, 342

neo-conservatism 39, 342
neoliberalism 11–12, 17, 19, 40, 104, 342
  activism, stifling 230–1
  capitalism 104, 106, 313
  Centrelink 151, 160
  challenging 11, 310, 333
  class-based hierarchy 105
  classism and 339
  'colonisation of our ways of being' 327
  critical reflection and 29
  definition 342
  de-gendering women's issues 234–5
  educators influenced by 17, 177, 180, 182,
    190, 237, 326–9
  feminist social work and 11, 17, 226–38
  globalisation 275, 316
  higher education and 327–8
  human rights and 76
  individualism 182, 328
  inequality 106
  Marxism and 7

mythical norms 104, 109, 181
neoliberal paternalism 108
practitioners in context of 211, 212, 215
responsibility 94–5
social work education and 17, 177, 180,
  182, 190, 237, 326–9
neo-Marxist theory 8, 243, 318
Network of Asylum Seeker Agencies of
  Victoria (NASAVic) 207
networking meeting 115
normative morals 52, 343

Occupy Melbourne 294–5
oppression 6, 9, 16, 25, 89–101, 199, 287, 293
  anti-oppressive social work *see* anti-
    oppressive social work
  asylum seekers 199, 205, 206
  awareness of 92
  class-based 7
  complicity in 89, 93–4
  critical modernist theories 27
  critical social work responding to 43, 326
  denial of 90
  disabled people 300
  education system 44
  hegemonic 33
  human rights-based social work 82
  Marxist view 7
  postmodern view 8
  power relations causing 17, 163–5
  prisoners and 164, 165
  privilege and 89–101, 293
  responsibility 94–5
  supervision to minimise 40, 42, 43
  systemic 89

partnership accountability 292
partnership and collaboration 10, 232–4
paternalism 108, 113, 153
patriarchy 94, 99, 313
pedagogy of discomfort 97–8, 331
pedagogy of privilege 91–3
peer supervision and critical reflection
  30–1

354

privilege 16, 48, 89–101, 343
  awareness of 91–2, 98
  complicity in oppression 89, 93–4
  contrapuntal deconstruction 100
  definition 343
  denial of 90
  engaging men emotionally regarding
    95–7
  epistemology of ignorance 90
  guilt about 98
  human rights-based social work 82
  McIntosh's work 91
  oppression and 89–101
  pedagogy of 91–3
  pedagogy of discomfort 97–8, 331
  politics of privileged identities 98
  racism and 97–9
  social work education and 331
  structural forms 90
  supervision to minimise 42, 43
  whiteness and 42, 45, 47, 82, 89, 91, 94,
    97, 333
process orientations 56–9, 113, 182, 343
professional practice standards 176–90
  AASW Code of Ethics 180, 183, 185
  ASWEAS Guidelines 180–4
  human rights and 183
  institutional ethnography 179
  regulatory texts 179–83
  shared understandings of theory 178
  social justice 179, 183
professional supervision *see* supervision
public confidence in social workers 40

quality-of-life goals 163, 173

race 8–9
  white privilege 42, 45, 47, 82, 89, 91, 94,
    97
racism 8–9
  Aboriginal people 217–18
  anti-racist abolitionists 99
  anti-racist social work 5, 83, 98, 339
  complicity in 93, 94

  empathy with sufferers 97
  human rights-based social work 82, 83
  privilege and 93, 94, 97–9
radical casework method 5
radical social work 5, 7, 8, 11, 12, 25, 137,
  257
  definition 343
  gay rights movement 256–8
  LGBTIQ people 257
reconstruction 28, 33, 35, 249
reflective practice 13, 27–8, 218
  critical reflection see critical reflection
  drawbacks and attributes 27–8
reflectivity 58, 64, 65, 67, 200
reflexivity 28, 58, 59, 65, 67, 200, 249
reframing 160, 182
refugees *see also* asylum seekers
  Australian immigration policy 197–8,
    201, 204, 205, 206
  Australian visas for 197, 206
  Convention on the Status of Refugees 80,
    196, 197, 198
  definition 196, 197
  human rights-based social work 77–85
  Humanitarian Program 197–8
  religious vilification 77–80
  statistics on 197
regulatory texts 179–86
  AASW Code of Ethics 180, 183, 185
  accreditation of university courses and
    185
  ASWEAS Guidelines 180–3
  discriminatory effects 182–3
  dominant discourses 179, 180
  examining 113, 179–83
  exerting control 179
  human service organisations and 185–6
  identifying 180
  individualism, enforcement of 182
  mythical norms, regulation of 181–2
  neoliberalism 180, 182
  organising normality 113, 179, 180
  technicism 185–6, 344
  'text-reader conversation' 179

relationship building
  mental health practice 128–9
  prison practice 170–4
relativism 56, 343
religion 79
  discrimination/vilification 77–80, 83
  human rights-based social work 77–85
  Islamophobia 79, 84
  right to freedom of 80, 84
research 59, 64, 66, 67
resistance 57, 58, 182, 249
  possibilities for 30
  small-scale acts of 13, 14
  transformational resistance 329
responsibility 30, 94–5
Richmond, Mary 4

Schon's reflective model 27
Scott, Dorothy 139
'self-help' method 4
Settlement House movement 4, 287
Sexuality and Disability Alliance (SDA)
  299, 304–7
social change-focused organisations
  288–9
social empathy 343
social inequality 26
  denial of oppression and privilege 90
  guilt about 98
  modern life producing 272
  poverty and class and 104
  privilege see privilege
  psychological disorder and 133
  redressing power imbalances 287
social justice 26, 39, 137, 179, 328
  critical social work and 39, 164, 223
  empowerment and 144
  environmental justice 271–5, 279, 280
  oppression while espousing 89
  practice principles 179, 183
  prison social work 164
social location 68, 79, 105, 170, 200, 331,
  334, 343
social movements 294

social protections
  advocating for 213–14
  ILO research 213–14
social welfare feminism 108–9, 343
social work education see education and
  training; field education
social work educators see educators
social work practitioners 211–24
  Aboriginal 212, 217–23, 333
  activism see activism
  advocating for social protections 213–14
  Australian context 214–15
  changed employment conditions 211
  critical theory 212
  flexible employment 215
  global perspective 212
  good practice 223–4
  Mission Australia 214, 216
  neoliberal agenda 212, 215
  ongoing training 223
  political engagement 287, 293–4
  staff satisfaction and resilience, building
    223–4
  streamlining work processes 215
  supervision see supervision
social work students see field education
social work supervision see supervision
socialist-feminist social work 53–4, 107–10
  child protection case study 59–64
  class-based inequalities 107
  institutional ethnography 109–10
  PACC practice 110
sociological imagination 12
solidarity 177, 182, 188–9, 294, 295, 312
solution-focused social work 9–10
spirituality 276–7, 280–1
state, role of 12
strength-based social work 9, 10
  child protection 137, 144
Strier's 'class-competent social work' model
  110
structural dominance 61
structural social work 5, 25, 311, 343
  child protection practice 137, 138